The GOLD COAST CURE'S

FITTER FIRMER *FASTER* PROGRAM

The GOLD COAST CURE'S

FITTER FIRMER *FASTER* PROGRAM

Get a Killer Body Without Killing Yourself

Ivy Ingram Larson

Andrew Larson, M.D.

Health Communications, Inc.
Deerfield Beach, Florida

www.hcibooks.com

Library of Congress Cataloging-in-Publication Data

Larson, Ivy Ingram, 1973-
    The gold coast cure's fitter, firmer, faster program : get a killer body without killing yourself / Ivy Larson, Andy Larson.
      p. cm.
    Includes bibliographical references.
    ISBN-13: 978-7573-0556-6 (trade paper)
    ISBN-10: 0-7573-0556-3 (trade paper)
    1. Reducing diets. 2. Health. 3. Exercise. I. Title.
    RM222.2.L344 2007
    613.2'5—dc22

2006028751

Publisher: Health Communications, Inc.
          3201 S.W. 15th Street
          Deerfield Beach, FL 33442–8190

Cover design by Larissa Hise Henoch
Inside book design and formatting by Dawn Von Strolley Grove

For our dear son, Blake.
You give our lives meaning.
We love you always.

Contents

Acknowledgments

It's hard to believe we've now completed our second book together. After all, working with your spouse to write about living healthfully can sometimes fall short of connubial bliss. However, we feel so fortunate to be able to say we genuinely love what we do, and we feel even more privileged knowing the two of us can do what we love together. We've been very lucky.

Anyone who has undertaken a project such as this knows it takes more than two lucky persons in love to write a book, it truly does require a team. So many people have worked so hard, for so long, to help us realize our dreams. We are, of course, indebted to our loyal readers, without you we wouldn't be writing books! Our deepest appreciation goes to our parents, Gail and Norman Ingram and Elaine and Ken Larson for their unrelenting support from day one. They have continued to encourage us through the ups, downs, twists and turns. They have continued to believe in us, even when we doubted ourselves. They inspire us to be the best we can be. They have remained our biggest fans; they proselytize our *Gold Coast Cure* lifestyle to anyone willing to listen. They have even changed the way they eat and the way they live to reflect the healthy habits we endorse! A most special and heartfelt thanks to Ivy's mom, Gail, for the tremendous effort she has put into helping bring our recipes to life. Gail's culinary skills and her passion for entertaining motivated Ivy to learn her way around the kitchen from an early age . . . lucky for Andy! Gail generously creates, donates and advises us on recipes and she supplies more inspiration than she realizes.

Our HCI family is outstanding! To our editor, and good friend, Allison Janse, you gave us the opportunity to make this dream come true. You believed in us first, and you had a vision for our book even we could not see. Your dedication, guidance, intellectual insight and friendship have been priceless. We will never forget what you have done for us. Kim Weiss, the stars must surely have been aligned when we were given the chance to work with you. So much of the success of our first book was contingent on your remarkable, highly effective public relations efforts. Peter Vegso, you took a chance on us and offered us the opportunity to reach for the stars before we had any idea how far away they lie. We will always continue reaching and always continue to be grateful for the opportunities you have provided. We wish we could thank everyone individually, from the sales team to the art department; all of you in our HCI family make the publication journey a joy.

We also want to express sincere gratitude to Erin Glynn and Regina Gausepohl who helped bring our *Gold Coast Cure* lifestyle to the public. You supported us before we even had a contract. To our trusted agent, Barbara Neighbors Deal, who always has our best interests at heart. To Jack Nicklaus, for reaching out to assist us when we needed it most. To Dr. Gloria Hakkarainen, Penny Linch and the entire staff at the Palm Beach Weight and Wellness Center, we offer our deepest thanks for the support you have given our *Gold Coast Cure* and for allowing us the opportunity to work with your patients to acquire testimonials for this book. To Natasha Graf for helping us "tighten" up!

Finally, AJ, we still remember why we started writing in the first place, and we will always remember you.

Introduction

Getting Real About Getting Fit

Let's face it: The market is glutted with diet books that promise to help people lose weight. Unfortunately, as we see working with our patients and clients every day—myself, as a general surgeon, and my wife, Ivy, as a fitness trainer—most programs are so restrictive and extreme that without amazing willpower or access to a personal chef, the average person falls off the wagon and puts the pounds back on—and then some. The *Fitter, Firmer, Faster* program, which grew from the success of our first book, *The Gold Coast Cure*, has helped thousands of people lose weight and gain health. This is a diet plan for *real* life, for people who *have* a life.

Think of this program as the Anti-Extreme Makeover: You can lose pounds and inches in five weeks, and prevent or reverse inflammatory conditions without starving yourself, without spending hours at the gym and without saying good-bye to most of the foods you love—foods you may have been told were bad for weight loss. You have the green light to enjoy pasta, potatoes, bread, chocolate and even a glass of wine or beer a day—every day. How do you lose weight on a "diet" like this? The answer is found in whole foods.

No Willpower? No Problem

It's a medical fact that the healthy foods you *don't* eat have just as much to do with why you can't lose weight as any bad foods you *do* eat. Whether your body burns food for energy or stores it as fat is determined by a number of chemical reactions that take place . . . or not. Since these reactions depend upon certain key nutrients, even a slight deficiency caused by eating a low-fat diet or a diet that eliminates certain food groups like carbs, can actually increase your risk of getting and staying fat. For example, being deficient in omega-3 essential fats or chromium or even vitamin C all contribute to stalled weight loss. All of these nutrients are best obtained by eating a balanced "whole foods" diet. In this book we'll show you how.

What's more, the nutrients found in natural whole foods are nature's flab-fighters: They curb your appetite, control food cravings and most important, improve your body's ability to burn fat instead of storing it. That's why our philosophy is to ditch the concept of "dieting" altogether, and instead embrace the concept of eating to get the *nutrients* your body needs for optimal health. In other words, don't count your food; make your food count! Our philosophy about choosing foods because they are nutrient rich (as opposed to low calorie, low carb or low fat) is one of the fundamental differences between our diet and all of the other diets out there—and it's the difference that will allow you to reach your weight-loss goals.

By changing your attitude toward food, making simple dietary swaps, doing a specific type of exercise thirty minutes three times a week, and supplementing your diet with a few nutrients, you can truly transform your body inside and out. You'll effortlessly achieve ideal health and the body that goes with it without going to extremes.

The One-Size-Fits-All Way to Reach Your Ideal Size

Fitter, Firmer, Faster is not a fad diet. It's a medically proven diet supported by studies in publications including the *New England Journal of Medicine, The Lancet* and the *Journal of the American Medical Association.* Unlike some other plans, it's healthy for almost anyone—from toddlers to teens, marathoners to moms-to-be, young families to senior citizens. It's a lifestyle plan that healthy women follow to shed a few pounds and tone up, while their husbands follow it to improve their cholesterol ratios and lower their blood pressure. New moms have used the plan to safely shed their pregnancy weight while keeping their energy up, while people with heart conditions and diabetes follow the program to stay healthy and control their symptoms. This is truly a healing diet . . . and we know this firsthand.

How We Found the "Cure" ... and Each Other

Before we were married, in 1998, Ivy was twenty-two years old when she received the devastating diagnosis of multiple sclerosis. Already experiencing numbness and weakness in her legs, as well as overwhelming fatigue and severe bladder problems, she worried what her future held. For a variety of personal reasons, Ivy didn't want to take prescription drugs to manage her symptoms if she didn't have to. At the suggestion of her neurologist, she decided to try lifestyle modification as her first course of action. Since Ivy and I were childhood friends who grew up on the Gold Coast of Florida, she called me at medical school and asked for help in researching any reputable studies that linked diet and MS. Together we started researching a way to put her symptoms into remission. Before her diagnosis, Ivy's diet was a disaster (even she admits this!). She rarely ate nutrient-rich "whole foods"; always on the run, she relied heavily on packaged, highly processed foods loaded with refined flour and sugar. We soon realized her diet was highly inflammatory, and since the symptoms of MS are brought on and made worse by inflammation, her diet needed a major overhaul. She began by following an MS diet developed by Dr. Roy Swank, outlined in the *Multiple Sclerosis Diet Book* (Doubleday, 1987). Unfortunately, Ivy quickly became bored with the limited and somewhat bland diet and began tinkering with the recipes. Over time, we expanded upon the diet, updating it to reflect new research and adding exercise and nutritional supplementation. Fairly quickly Ivy noticed a marked improvement in her symptoms: She got the strength back in her legs, her bladder problems improved ... and by the time we walked down the aisle two years later, we both knew we meant it when we vowed to be together "in sickness and in health." And she's been healthy ever since.

Although I didn't have a specific health or weight problem, after our wedding I began following Ivy's diet and exercising with her. I decreased my blood pressure, which was borderline high, and decreased my body fat percentage from 16 percent to 10 percent.

Ivy stuck to the diet throughout her pregnancy, gained a healthy twenty-five pounds, delivered a 7 pound, 15 ounce baby boy and then quickly regained her shape. After Ivy weaned our son, Blake, he too began eating our healthful "whole-foods" diet. Blake is now five years old, and (knock on wood!) he has rarely been sick; in fact, he's only required antibiotics once in his life even though he goes to preschool.

Excited by what the lifestyle had done for us, we took our program to several established medical and fitness facilities. The results have been consistently impressive: Our plan not only helped people with inflammation-mediated diseases such as MS, heart disease, arthritis and allergies, but as a "side benefit" it helped people lose weight, tone up and keep the weight off. For example, in one of our most recent 4-week Fitness Challenge where we partnered with Cuts Fitness for Men (*www.cutsfitness.com*), the forty-three men who participated in our program lost an average of 7½ pounds in four weeks, decreased their body fat percentage by an average of 7½ percent, and lost an average of 4½ inches from their waist and hips. The three men who lost the most weight on the 4-week program lost an average of 14 pounds, decreased their body fat percentage by 11 percent and lost 7 inches from their waist and hips. In another Fitness Challenge, we teamed up with board-certified bariatrician Dr. Gloria Hakkarainen at the Palm Beach Weight and Wellness Center in West Palm Beach, Florida. The women who participated lost an average of 7 pounds, decreased their body fat by 6 percent and lost a total of 4 inches from their waist and hips. Keep in mind, these results were seen without restricting calories or portion sizes, without counting carbs, without counting fat grams while exercising as little as thirty minutes at a time, three times a week!

Time and again we've helped folks from all walks of life lose weight, decrease their cholesterol levels, reduce their blood pressure, improve their health and look better, too! Unlike other diets, the *Fitter, Firmer, Faster* program doesn't just result in a loss of pounds; it reshapes your entire body, speeds up your metabolism, strengthens and tones your muscles, lowers your body fat percentage, and strips inches from your waist and hips.

How Does the Program Work?

By combining cutting-edge research, we've developed a three-pronged lifestyle plan consisting of a whole-foods diet, six nutritional supplements, and thirty minutes of resistance circuit training exercise three days per week. Fully functional, nutrient-rich whole foods keep your body optimally nourished to curb food cravings, support a healthy metabolism, help your body burn fat for energy and naturally control your appetite. Healing oils and healthful omega-3 fats fight inflammation and insulin resistance—two leading culprits in weight gain and degenerative disease. Six nutritional supplements work synergistically to enhance the health and weight-loss benefits. Finally, the custom-designed resistance circuit training workout burns fat *three times* faster than aerobic exercise alone by building metabolically active muscle and increasing excess post-exercise oxygen consumption, which, in turn burns fat fast.

Why This Program Works in the Real World

The whole-foods diet we recommend provides your body with the optimal nutrients it needs and craves. You will literally feel more satisfied eating fewer calories. You'll enjoy hunger-free weight loss. You'll be fueling your body with the nutrients it needs to support a healthy metabolism, improve your sensitivity to insulin and burn fat for fuel. Not only will you not be hungry, you're going to love the taste of whole foods. In fact, our clients report they actually enjoy eating the foods we recommend better than the foods they were eating before!

We include plenty of quick and easy recipes plus 30-minute family-friendly meals. What if you don't cook? We provide a complete "figure-friendly" convenience foods shopping guide specially designed for those of you who cannot or will not cook. We've built these convenience foods into our meal plans. How about Chocolate Blackberry Brownie Pudding or Cherry Upside-Down Cake? Yes, you can even enjoy a sweet treat every day! Even coffee and wine are allowed. Rest assured you won't go hungry, and you won't be deprived.

Most important, because our health plan is realistic enough and enjoyable enough to truly live up to the concept of being a "lifestyle plan," you'll not only lose weight, but you'll also have the chance to reach your ideal weight. How many times have you read weight-loss "success" stories in which someone successfully loses fifty pounds yet remains thirty pounds overweight? With our plan you'll shed the fifty pounds and the thirty pounds—it won't be overnight, but it will happen. You will eventually reach your ideal weight and maintain that weight. This is how we define success.

How This Books Differs from Others (Including Our Own)

In our first book, *The Gold Coast Cure*, we explained how diet can fight and even reverse the symptoms of up to ten chronic conditions. In this book, we focus solely on weight loss. For those of you already familiar with our *Gold Coast Cure*, this book provides a multitude of new tips to supercharge your already healthful lifestyle.

We provide more tools to help you follow our whole-foods diet, more delicious ethnic and gourmet recipes, an expanded "figure-friendly" convenience foods shopping list and an all-new chapter featuring "nearly homemade" meals that can be ready in less than thirty minutes. This time we bring your entire family to the table with our brand new "Family-Friendly Meals" section. We devote an entire chapter to kids, letting you in on our secrets for getting your children to eat and enjoy healthful whole foods. We teach you how to take your fitness routine to the next level with updated, shortcut training techniques and a complete, all-new, more-advanced workout routine that combines the best of yoga, calisthenics, core toning and high-repetition strength-training exercises that work synergistically to deliver a tight, firm and streamlined physique. Finally, we've included additional help in designing your vitamin supplementation regimen by offering many more brand-name product suggestions.

From what to eat and what brand-name products to buy, to how to prepare healthful meals quickly, to how to get fit and firm exercising less than two hours a week, we'll let you in on all of our secrets and solutions. We'll present you with a get-real plan for transforming your body *and* your life, and we'll open the door for you to reach your ideal weight and enjoy optimal health. We're going to show you how to lose weight and gain health. We're confident our *Fitter, Firmer, Faster* program is the get-real comprehensive lifestyle solution you've been looking for. Let's get to it!

—Andrew Larson, M.D.

www.goldcoastcure.com

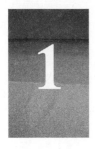

1

Ditch Dieting and Go for Whole Foods

We want you to forget everything you've been taught about dieting. Forget what you've been told about carbohydrates and fats. Forget about protein shakes and fat-burning meal-replacement bars. Forget about tallying up points and counting calories. Forget about trying to figure out how to muster up the psychological self-discipline necessary to avoid eating. The truth is that the diets most of us use don't work—they don't work for lasting weight loss, and they certainly don't work for improving health.

It turns out the best way to lose weight—and keep it off—is to approach weight loss from an entirely new perspective: Focus on health first, and the side benefit is lasting weight loss. Instead of obsessing over the number of calories in your food and the number of carbs, learn to think about getting more bang for your nutritional buck. Make your food count; don't count your food. The way to do that is to eat balanced meals consisting of carbohydrates, fats and proteins from healthy "whole" foods.

Whole foods are unrefined "real" foods, packaged the way nature intended. We're talking potatoes, not potato chips. We're advocating corn, not corn flakes. We'd rather you eat an apple instead of apple sauce. We'd rather you choose oatmeal instead of oat flakes. Go for grapes not grape juice. Go for eggs, not egg substitutes. The point is, the more unrefined "whole" foods you eat and the less refined, "packaged" foods you eat the healthier you will be and the easier it will be for you to manage your weight. We're not saying you can never have another bowl of cornflakes again, we're just saying you are much better off choosing corn on the cob instead.

Balanced whole-foods diets work for weight control and more. The human body has evolved over thousands of centuries to consume all-natural whole foods. Research now confirms that the same whole foods your body needs to prevent disease and maintain health can help you look your best and maintain your ideal weight. Whole foods are nature's flab fighters.

Whole Foods Fight the "Malnourished Munchies"

It is possible to be overweight *and* malnourished. How? Easy: Malnutrition refers to inadequate *nutrition,* not necessarily inadequate *calorie intake.* Even though it's possible to obtain plenty of calories, or more likely too many calories, on the typical American diet, it is rare to obtain adequate nutrition this way. It is entirely possible to be one hundred pounds or more overweight and still be malnourished. If you don't get the nutrients your body needs, your body signals hunger because it assumes more food is needed in order to obtain these crucial nutrients. You crave these nutrients, not necessarily the doughnut or the bagel in the break room.

While some hunger is psychological, most of it occurs in an attempt to motivate you to satisfy natural, appropriate cravings for the nutrients your diet lacks. Cravings, as most people know, hinder the success of most fad diets. Only a balanced whole-foods diet supplies your body with all the nutrients it needs to curb food cravings.

Unless you have supernatural willpower you'll ultimately surrender to these cravings and end up eating more calories than your body really needs in an effort to obtain adequate nutrition. It doesn't take too many of these extra calories to make a difference on the scale. Even as little as two hundred additional calories per day (the equivalent of one granola bar) results in a weight gain of forty pounds over the course of two years!

Whole Foods Keep Your Blood Sugar from Going Berserk

Diets rich in overly processed, quickly digested carbohydrates result in a surge of insulin followed by a sharp drop in your blood sugar level. Low blood sugar levels cause increased appetite. A balanced whole-foods diet includes healthful fats that keep you feeling satisfied for hours as well as plenty of filling, slowly digested, high-fiber carbohydrates. Your blood-sugar level remains stable, and your appetite remains naturally suppressed.

Whole Foods Turn Off Your Body's Fat-Storage System

Whole foods reduce your body's tendency to store energy as fat. Insulin is a hormone that promotes the absorption and storage of calories as energy. More insulin means more fat storage. Insulin is released in large quantities when you eat carbohydrate-rich foods—especially empty-calorie carbohydrate foods such as refined flour, white rice and sugar. Very little insulin is released when you eat a balanced whole-foods diet containing fiber-rich carbohydrates, healthy fats and lean protein.

Your body needs a certain amount of insulin for transporting nutrients and energy into your cells. If your body is accustomed to having only small amounts of insulin in its blood stream, its cells remain very sensitive to insulin, and only small amounts of insulin need to be secreted. If your body is accustomed to having large amounts of insulin in its blood stream, its cells adapt to the overload by becoming less sensitive, and more resistant, to insulin. Even more insulin is secreted in response to this problem. From a weight-loss standpoint these abnormally high insulin levels encourage abnormally high amounts of fat storage. A healthy whole-foods diet helps reverse this process.

Whole Foods Stoke Your Metabolism

Certain nutrients present only in whole foods actually speed the process of burning fat for energy. For example, vitamin C, various B vitamins, calcium and, especially, the good omega-3 fats found only in whole foods are all needed to maintain a healthful, rapid metabolism. Deficiencies in these nutrients slow your metabolism, making it harder to lose weight, break through plateaus and keep off the pounds.

The Types of Fat You Eat Can Either Help or Hinder Weight Loss

Our whole-foods diet contains the proper balance of omega-3 fats and omega-6 fats. Achieving this balance increases your cells' sensitivity to insulin, therefore decreasing the amount of insulin your body need to produce. As you now know, the less insulin your body needs to make, the easier it is for you to lose weight and keep it off.

Whole Foods Keep You Feeling Full on Fewer Calories

If you eat a balanced whole-foods diet containing plenty of fruits, vegetables, whole grains, beans, nuts and seeds, you'll be getting lots of fat-fighting fiber without very many calories. Even though you'll be eating fewer calories, you'll still feel full and satisfied because the fiber-rich whole foods take up a lot of space in your stomach and provide a large volume of food. Studies show the more fiber you eat and the greater volume of food you eat, the more satisfied you'll feel and the fewer number of calories you'll eat in a day. For example, you'll feel more satisfied and less hungry after eating a 130-gram serving of fiber-rich beans containing just 120 calories as opposed to the typical 52-gram fiber-less doughnut containing 200 calories. You will feel more satisfied after eating a voluminous, fiber-rich 150-calorie bowl of oatmeal compared to a condensed 200-calorie, sugary, low-fiber granola bar. When all is said and done, feeling full on fewer calories will help you lose weight.

Whole Foods Reduce Inflammation to Help You Gain Health *and* Lose Weight

The foods you eat can either increase systemic inflammation or decrease systemic inflammation. To feel and look your best you want to avoid pro-inflammatory processed foods and instead choose a healthy and balanced anti-inflammatory whole-foods diet. An anti-inflammatory diet will improve your health and help whittle your waistline. Researchers have discovered the common denominator linking many modern degenerative diseases is inflammation run amok. Seemingly unrelated conditions, such as heart disease, multiple sclerosis, asthma, allergies, arthritis, acne, Crohn's disease and fibromyalgia, all share one common link: inflammation. All of these conditions are made worse when systemic inflammation remains unchecked.

We can take this conversation one step further. We now know obesity and inflammation are also linked. Being obese in and of itself increases systemic inflammation because excess fat cells are active endocrine organs that directly and indirectly put your body into a constant pro-inflammatory state. Fat cells send inflammation signals throughout your body, affecting the health of your skin, your heart, your joints and even your brain. There is growing evidence that the inflammation-enhancing signals secreted by these fat cells actually promote obesity itself and even the development of type 2 diabetes. Whole foods fight obesity; less obesity means less inflammation. Whole foods also fight inflammation; less inflammation means less obesity. While doctors continue to prescribe medications to calm inflammation and improve their patients' disease symptoms, it is becoming more and more common for cutting-edge doctors to prescribe anti-inflammatory diets and lifestyles, too. This is because some foods, such as highly processed white flour and trans fat, dramatically worsen inflammation, while other whole foods, such as walnuts, fish and whole grains, can actively decrease inflammation. Our whole-foods diet has the power to reduce inflammation, helping you not only to lose weight but also to improve your health.

More Than Just Weight Loss

The *Fitter, Firmer, Faster* diet contains a wide spectrum of vitamins, minerals, antioxidants, phytonutrients, fiber and essential fats that work *synergistically* to protect you from many different diseases.

- **Type 2 Diabetes.** Unstable blood sugar levels, the resulting excess insulin production and obesity itself all play a major role in the development of prediabetes and the exacerbation of type 2 diabetes. Any lifestyle plan that combats insulin resistance by keeping your blood sugar level more stable is guaranteed to work toward reversing type 2 diabetes. The *Fitter, Firmer, Faster* exercise program also decreases your body fat percentage and increases your muscle mass, further decreasing your body's need to produce insulin. All in all, you have a multifaceted approach for reversing the insulin resistance that ultimately leads to type 2 diabetes.
- **Osteoporosis.** Whole foods rich in vitamin D, calcium, magnesium and essential fat decrease your risk of developing osteoporosis as does an increased intake of soy and flax.
- **Cancer.** Achieving and maintaining a healthful weight, increasing your dietary intake of fiber, soy, fruits, vegetables and natural phytonutrients, along with decreasing your intake of saturated fat–rich and trans fat–rich foods all contribute to a decreased risk of developing many types of cancer.
- **Heart Disease.** Recent studies confirm the vast majority of heart disease is due to preventable risk factors. For example, having an elevated blood level of "bad" LDL cholesterol is a primary risk factor for heart artery disease. Whole foods containing fiber and heart-healthy fats have been proven to decrease "bad" LDL cholesterol levels. A whole-foods diet also works to protect your heart by decreasing systemic inflammation, lowering your C-reactive protein (CRP) level, and decreasing your blood pressure.
- **Senility.** Much of what we call "Alzheimer's disease" is really mental degeneration caused by the accumulation of vascular disease within your brain. Whole foods protect against this type of dementia in the same way they protect you from heart artery disease.

(continued from page 6)

- **Arthritis.** Inflammation plays a role in the severity of your symptoms. Increased consumption of certain healthful fats such as those found in fish, flaxseeds and nuts, combined with avoidance of harmful fats significantly decreases the amount of inflammation in your body. Arthritis responds very well to a healthful whole-foods diet.
- **Fibromyalgia.** Whole foods can ease your symptoms while also improving your energy level. Fibromyalgia is another disease made worse by inflammation and is therefore a disease that responds well to dietary intervention.
- **Multiple sclerosis.** This disease is also worsened when inflammation is allowed to run unchecked. Inflammation can be thought of as the tendency of your body to attack itself. Increased consumption of whole foods containing certain healthful fats, such as those found in fatty fish, flax and nuts, combined with a reduced intake of harmful saturated fats and the elimination of processed products containing trans fats and empty carbohydrates promotes decreased inflammation and often leads to decreased severity of disease symptoms. A whole-foods diet also helps combat the fatigue that almost universally plagues MS patients.
- **Asthma.** This is another disease made worse by inflammation. Increasing good-fat intake while decreasing bad-fat consumption and reducing empty carbohydrate intake all serve to ameliorate asthma symptoms. Our clients report this is one area where nearly immediate results are appreciated.

2

Choose "Fit Foods"

Our overall philosophy regarding diet is to eat whole foods that are as natural and unrefined as possible and to eat as wide a variety of foods as possible. In this chapter we'll help you choose "Fit Foods" that have the power to dramatically improve your health while at the same time solve your weight problems.

All of the Fit Foods we mention in this chapter help control inflammation, reverse insulin resistance and combat malnutrition—three main reasons people gain weight and cannot break through their weight-loss plateaus. (In chapter 4, we give you detailed lists of these foods as well as optimum serving sizes for men and women.)

Vegetables and Fruits

It should come as no surprise that vegetables and fruits are at the very top of the Fit Foods list. Contrary to what you might have read in other diet books, all fruits and all vegetables are healthy and helpful for weight loss.

☑ **On the *Fitter, Firmer, Faster* program, you should eat either vegetables or fruits at every meal.** Why? Because vegetables and fruits are antiaging superstar foods that help you lose weight and achieve optimal health. Vegetables and fruits are nutrient-rich, calorie-poor and full of fat-fighting fiber. If you increase your intake of vegetables and fruits, you'll feel full on fewer calories and naturally lose weight. The nutrients in vegetables and fruits fight food cravings, further assisting with weight control.

Bonus health boost: Each vegetable and fruit offers its own set of health-promoting vitamins, antioxidants and phytonutrients that provide protection against degenerative diseases such as hypertension, heart disease, senility, cataracts and even certain cancers. Experts agree that it's wise to eat a vegetable and fruit "rainbow," in other words eat a wide variety of differently colored vegetables and fruits. The micronutrients found in vegetables and fruits work synergistically to improve your health, protect you from disease and strengthen your immune system. For example, yellow and red vegetables are rich in antioxidant carotenes, while dark green leafy vegetables are rich in vitamin C and calcium. Your body needs all of these nutrients in combination in order to attain and maintain optimal health.

Incorporating Veggies and Fruit into Your Life

Many people in today's busy world skimp on eating fruits and vegetables because they don't have the extra time required to shop regularly or prepare elaborate side dishes with fresh fruits and vegetables. We have good news for the time-crunched: You don't need to eat fresh fruits and vegetables in order to reap their health and weight-loss benefits. Canned and frozen fruits and vegetables are usually cheaper, more convenient and equally as healthful. Plain frozen vegetables are convenient and are almost always a good choice.

You have to be somewhat more selective with canned produce. While it's important to avoid fruits packed in sugary syrups, it's perfectly acceptable to eat canned fruit packed in all-natural fruit juice. Unsweetened frozen fruit is always a good choice as are dried fruits without added sugar.

Contrary to what you might think, fresh fruits and vegetables are not always the most nutritious. In some instances, canned and frozen fruits and vegetables are in reality more nutritious. This is because once fruits and vegetables have been picked they are no longer alive. The nutrient content begins to diminish as natural enzymes are released. One reason canned and frozen fruits and vegetables sometimes rank nutritionally superior to fresh produce is they are usually packaged close to their nutritional peak, immediately after harvest. The canning and freezing processes put a halt to enzymatic degradation and therefore preserve nearly all the nutritional benefits. The bottom line is, don't miss out on the benefits of eating a wide variety of fruits and vegetables.

Get-Real Ways to Sneak Vegetables and Fruits into Your Life

Vegetables:
- Pack raw vegetables to munch on the run or buy prechopped vegetables you can sauté or stir-fry in extra-virgin olive oil.
- Mix vegetables into sauces such as marinara sauce, or make vegetable-based soups from butternut squash or roasted red peppers.
- Snack on celery and peanut butter boats, or dip baby carrots into hummus.
- Top ¾ cup raw spinach with organic low-fat cheese, then heat in the microwave for a quick and delicious side dish or snack.
- For a tasty lunch, treat yourself to a grilled or roasted vegetable sandwich. We especially love fire-roasted canned red peppers.
- When you make meat-based sandwiches, ham or turkey, for example, be sure to include some type of vegetable such as sliced tomatoes, shredded carrots, thinly sliced cucumbers, sliced onions or spinach.
- You can eat vegetables in the morning, too! How about an omelet prepared using sautéed onions and bell peppers along with a side of fresh salsa or pico de gallo?

Fruits:
- Blend fruit into creamy smoothies made with plain, unsweetened, low-fat yogurt or kefir. These smoothies make great quick breakfasts or snacks.
- Make fruit a featured ingredient in your desserts. Try some of our signature fruit-based desserts such as Chocolate Blackberry Brownie Pudding, Palm Beach Pineapple-Walnut Bread Cake or Apple-Cranberry Torte (see recipes in chapter 9).
- Mix fruit into your cereal or use fruit to top off whole-grain pancakes and waffles.

(Continued from page 10)

- As a quick snack, try baked apples served with walnuts with a slice of low-fat cheddar cheese.
- Salsas, such as mango-avocado or pineapple-jalapeno, are another way to add fruit to your plate.
- Make fruit- and nut-based muffins, such as apple-walnut muffins, banana-pecan muffins or raisin-almond muffins.
- Try including fruit as part of your main meal. For example, add fruit to salads or grill it as a side dish. We often enjoy grilled peaches, plums and pineapples served alongside grilled chicken, pork or fish. At your next barbecue, try grilling fruit on skewers.
- Don't forget, you can eat fruit "straight up," too!

Nutrient- and Fiber-Rich Whole-Food Carbohydrates

☑ **On the *Fitter, Firmer, Faster* program, you should eat nutrient- and fiber-rich whole-food carbohydrates at every meal.** This means carbohydrate-rich whole foods such as potatoes, beans, legumes and all whole grains including oatmeal, barley and corn. Nutrient- and fiber-rich carbohydrates possess a synergistic set of antiaging, weight-reducing properties. These foods are just as important for preserving health as fruits and vegetables. You cannot enjoy optimal health choosing one over the other.

Many of these carbohydrate foods are truly rich in fiber. There are many reasons to care about significantly increasing the amount of fiber you eat. For one, fiber is probably your most reliable ally when it comes to shedding pounds and attaining a trim physique. Fiber-rich foods are slowly absorbed, so they help you feel full longer. This has been proven to result in ultimately eating fewer total calories over the course of the day. This slow absorption of fiber-rich foods has another benefit, too. The slower food is absorbed the less impact the nonfiber carbohydrate calories have on your blood sugar level, which means less of that "fat-storing" hormone insulin will be secreted. Finally, because your body has to work hard to digest fiber, many additional calories are burned through a process called thermogenesis—the generation of heat energy that occurs following digestion. In a manner of speaking, fiber consumption boosts your overall metabolism.

Bonus health boost: Fiber-rich diets have been proven to decrease your risk of colon cancer, improve your cholesterol profile, and protect you against type 2 diabetes and heart disease. Recent research suggests fiber may even help decrease inflammation.

Nonfruit, nonvegetable whole-food carbohydrates contain many other nutrients that are also important for good health and good looks. While most people think fruits and vegetables are the best sources of antiaging antioxidants, it turns out beans and whole grains are truly the "new broccoli" since they exhibit significant antioxidant activity—often greater than what can be found in fruits and vegetables. These antioxidants help conquer inflammation, which in turn helps fight obesity. Nutrient- and fiber-rich whole-food carbohydrates are rich in disease-fighting, health-enhancing vitamins, minerals and phytonutrients. Only carbohydrate foods contain phytonutrients. Phytonutrients possess protective antiaging, disease-fighting and inflammation-fighting properties that cannot be obtained anywhere else. Phytonutrient research is flourishing, and it's becoming increasingly clear that for optimal health and good looks you should obtain as wide an array of phytonutrients from as many plant-based foods as possible. Contrary to what many people think, plant-based foods include more than just fruits and vegetables; whole grains, nuts, seeds, beans and soy are all "plant-based" foods.

Go for Whole Grains

If you're looking at nutrient- and fiber-rich whole-food carbohydrates individually, whole grains belong at the top of the list. Unlike refined grains and refined flour, whole grains retain the nutrient-rich germ, which contains antioxidants, vitamins, minerals and essential fat, and the fiber-rich bran. This combination of nutrition and fiber is proven to help you gain health and lose weight. Whole grains take longer than refined carbohydrates to digest, so eating whole grains results in significantly less secretion of the "fat-storing" hormone insulin when compared with eating refined grains and sugar.

Several very large studies have examined the relationship between whole-grain consumption and weight management, and the results are consistent: People who eat whole grains weigh less than people who eat refined grains.

Bonus health boost: Eating three servings of whole grains daily can reduce your risk of developing heart disease by one third and reduce your risk of developing type 2 diabetes by about 25 percent. Whole grains also protect against certain types of cancer.

For anyone who thinks that whole-grain dining means brown rice and wheat germ, think again. The list below shows just some of the many whole grains you can enjoy on the *Fitter, Firmer, Faster* program.

Note: While for most of us there is no reason to either avoid gluten-containing whole grains, we have included this information for the benefit of our gluten-sensitive readers.

WHOLE GRAINS

Amaranth (gluten-free)   Oat
Barley   Quinoa (gluten-free)
Brown rice (gluten-free)   Rye
Buckwheat (gluten-free)   Spelt
Corn (gluten-free)   Wheat
Kamut   Wild Rice (gluten-free)
Millet (gluten-free)

In addition to the whole foods listed, appendix A gives a comprehensive shopping list of prepared convenience foods that are acceptable whole foods—foods like pizza, lasagna, bread and crackers.

Get-Real Ways to Sneak Whole Grains into Your Life

- Make your favorite pasta recipe using whole-grain pasta instead of the refined "white" stuff.
- Try a grilled portobello mushroom and cheese sandwich on sprouted whole-grain bread.
- Make French toast using whole-grain raisin bread.
- Enjoy a bowl of oatmeal topped with wheat germ and fresh strawberries.
- Add barley to vegetable based soups.
- Conjure up pilaf using buckwheat, brown rice, millet or quinoa instead of white or yellow refined rice.
- Try making fruit-and-nut-based muffins using whole-wheat flour.
- Serve whole-wheat couscous as a side dish to lamb.
- Create salads from quinoa, diced vegetables and your favorite vinaigrette.
- Combine cooked wild rice with dried cranberries, diced carrots and balsamic vinegar.
- Grill corn on the cob.
- Try remaking your favorite lasagna recipe using whole-grain lasagna noodles.

Love Your Beans and Legumes

All beans and *all* legumes, such as peas and lentils, are excellent, healthful, nutrient- and fiber-rich whole-food carbohydrates. Beans and legumes provide maximum nutritional bang for minimum calorie buck. They're crammed with protein, fiber, iron, potassium and folate. The health benefits associated with beans and legumes are numerous. Diets rich in beans and legumes improve your cholesterol profile, decrease your risk of heart disease and provide powerful protection against obesity, type 2 diabetes and even cancer. They keep you feeling full despite reduced calorie intake.

Beans and legumes are digested slowly and therefore result in less secretion of that "fat-storing" hormone insulin. They help keep your blood sugar level more stable, curb food cravings and suppress hunger.

In fact, studies show people who get most of their protein from plant-based foods such as beans have lower body weights than people who obtain most of their protein from meat.

Bonus health boost: Beans are another often-overlooked source of antiaging antioxidants. The darkest beans seem to pack the most antioxidant punch (black and red beans are best, followed by brown, yellow and white). Here are some of the delicious varieties of beans and legumes you can enjoy while on the *Fitter, Firmer, Faster* program.

BEANS AND LEGUMES

Adzuki beans	Kidney beans
Anasazi beans	Lentils
Black beans	Lima beans
Black-eyed peas	Navy beans
Brown beans	Peas
Cannellini beans	Pinto beans
Chickpeas	Split peas
Great northern beans	

Get-Real Ways to Sneak Beans into Your Life

- Use canned beans as the perfect "fast food" option. Canned beans maintain all the health benefits of their dry counterparts. Just remember to thoroughly rinse canned beans with warm water to remove any trace of "tin can" flavor.
- Try adding beans and legumes to soups, salads, casseroles and stir-fries.
- Beans provide the perfect base for veggie burgers. You can make your own, or you can look for prepared veggie burgers in the frozen foods section of your local supermarket.
- For your next party, try making bean dip using black beans, white beans, pinto beans or chickpeas.
- Split pea soup is a tasty way to get your legume fix.
- Serve thawed frozen petite peas seasoned with a dab of butter as a side to chicken or even filet mignon.
- Seek out ethnic and regional bean- and legume-based recipes. Try Cuban recipes featuring black beans or Southern-style dishes that make use of black-eyed peas. Chickpeas are often added to Spanish stews, and cannellini beans are delicious in minestrone soup. Kidney beans often take center stage in spicy Cajun dishes.

Potatoes: Undeserved Bad Rap

For the bad rap potatoes have received for being fattening, they in fact provide a strong nutritional punch in a relatively low-calorie package. (News flash: It's the butter, sour cream and bacon bits that pack on the pounds!) Whether mashed, baked or roasted, this delicious, filling comfort food is most definitely allowed and encouraged on the *Fitter, Firmer, Faster* program.

Bonus health boost: Potatoes are brimming with nutrients including vitamin C, iron, B vitamins and phytonutrients. If you eat the potato skins, you'll also enjoy a healthy dose of potassium and even a good dose of slimming fiber.

Heart-Healthy Proteins

☑ **On the *Fitter, Firmer, Faster* program, you should eat one heart-healthy protein at every meal.** Protein is an important component of every cell in your body. It's used to build and repair tissues, make enzymes and support basic life functions. Protein-rich foods provide energy for your body while keeping you feeling full and satisfied for hours. They curb your appetite and control food cravings, assisting greatly with weight management. Unfortunately, many protein-rich foods are rich in unhealthy saturated fat. You want to limit your intake of saturated fat because eaten in excess saturated fats increase inflammation, increase your risk of heart disease, and even increase your risk of developing the insulin resistance that ultimately leads to diabetes and obesity.

Fortunately, the majority of proteins are indeed heart-healthy. Lean cuts of meat; eggs; low-fat dairy products such as low-fat cheese, low-fat plain yogurt, low-fat milk and low-fat cottage cheese; fish; shellfish; soy; and skinless white-meat turkey and chicken are all heart-healthy foods.

Super Proteins

☑ **For optimum health, you should eat at** *least* **one "super" protein food at some point during the day every day.** Soy and fish are considered "super" protein foods because they are low in bad saturated fat and rich in good essential fat. Essential fats optimize your metabolism, improve your sensitivity to insulin, reduce inflammation, and support the health of your reproductive system, immune system, central nervous system and cardiovascular system.

Super Protein #1: Fish

The typical American diet is more deficient in the omega-3 fats found in fish than any other nutrient. Omega-3 fats help fight fat because they facilitate fat burning as opposed to fat storing.

Bonus health boost: The omega-3 fats in fish happen to be the most potent anti-inflammatory substances available without a prescription. This means anyone suffering with any inflammation-mediated disease such as asthma, multiple sclerosis or arthritis should be especially vigilant about eating fatty fish regularly. Anyone concerned about their heart health should also increase their consumption of fish since eating fish has been proven to reduce your risk of stroke, heart attack, congestive heart failure, heart rhythm problems and sudden cardiac death. In fact, a review study published in the *Archives of Internal Medicine* found the omega-3 fats in fish oil to be one of the most effective means to prevent heart disease with or without a prescription. Omega-3 fats directly reduce your risk of obesity and type 2 diabetes and help your body make hormones that encourage softer, smoother skin.

If you want to stay on top of your game, mentally that is, fish can help here, too. The essential fats in fish improve memory and concentration. Studies show regular fish consumption keeps you sharp mentally and significantly reduces your risk of developing senile dementia. Eating more fish can even improve your mood. Studies have linked low seafood intake to major depression and omega-3 fat deficiency to increased severity of depressive symptoms.

Get-Real Ways to Sneak Fish into Your Life

Fish is always a good choice, but the "fatty" fish are especially rich in omega-3 oils. Fatty fish include anchovies, tuna, herring, mackerel, salmon, sardines, sea bass, striped bass, shad and trout. Fish is easy to prepare healthfully.

- Even non-fish lovers will eat fish if it's hidden under a flavorful fruit or spicy salsa.
- Marinate fish in a salad dressing made with extra-virgin olive oil, then grill.
- Grilled fish kabobs are great for firm-fleshed fish like tuna and salmon.
- A tuna salad sandwich made using canned tuna, canola-oil mayonnaise to taste, canned roasted red peppers, and low-fat cheese on top of toasted whole-grain bread, or a quick pasta meal made from whole-grain pasta, canned tuna, marinara sauce and freshly shredded Parmesan cheese can be ready in less than ten minutes.
- If you are truly pressed for time consider a "seafood snack" consisting of lox, canned salmon, canned tuna, or even sardines on whole-grain crackers.

"But I Hate Fish": Help for Non-Fish-Eaters

If fish is just not your thing you should take a high-quality pharmaceutical grade fish oil supplement. We recommend non-fishy tasting name-brand supplements in chapter 11. Actually, we suggest everyone, fish eaters and non-fish eaters alike, take a fish oil supplement daily to obtain adequate amounts of omega-3 essential fats. Supplements are not a substitute for eating fish because fish has so many important nutrients, but many of the truly vital omega-3 essential fats found in fish can indeed be obtained from a pill.

Super Protein #2: Soy

Soy can help you lose weight because it is a nutrient-dense food providing lots of satiety in a low-calorie package. Some whole soy foods, especially edamame beans and soy beans, have the added benefit of being exceptionally rich in slimming fiber.

Bonus health boost: Soy is a "super food" packed with vitamins, minerals and antioxidants. Soy protein contains all of the essential amino acids found in animal protein without the artery-clogging, pro-inflammatory saturated fat you should avoid. By volume, soy contains more protein than beef and more calcium than milk. A large body of evidence indicates replacing excess animal protein with soy decreases your risk of heart disease. In the *New England Journal of Medicine* researchers report that "the consumption of soy protein rather than animal protein significantly decreased serum concentrations of total cholesterol, LDL cholesterol and triglycerides." Soy is also rich in those "good" essential fats that optimize the health of your immune system, reproductive system, cardiovascular system and central nervous system.

Whole-soy products contain disease-fighting substances called phytoestrogens believed to moderate hormonal imbalances by exerting mild estrogen-like actions that benefit men and women alike. The hormone actions of "whole-soy" phytoestrogens provide protection against prostate cancer in men and protection against many estrogen-related diseases in women such as breast cancer, endometriosis and the discomforts associated with menopause. Through a combination of mechanisms, whole-soy foods provide protection against osteoporosis.

Get-Real Ways to Sneak Soy into Your Life

Many ready-to-eat soy products are available. Suggestions include:

- **Tofu.** Extremely versatile, tofu comes in firm, soft and silken textures. Firm tofu can be grilled or baked. Firm tofu is an excellent substitute for meat in stir-fries and can be used in place of some, perhaps as much as one half, of the ground beef you would normally use in meatloaf or tacos. Soft and silken tofu are delicious in soups, lasagna and creamy desserts such as cheesecake and pudding. Soft tofu can be blended into smoothies or dips, too.
- **Soy milk.** Mild-tasting, soy milk is great alone or when used along with fruit to make smoothies. Soy milk is also perfect in just about any recipe or drink in which you would normally use milk, including, for example, cappuccino.
- **Edamame beans** (green soybeans). Look for soft, shelled edamame beans in the frozen section of your grocery store. You can also buy them frozen still in the pod. Edamame beans are delicious served plain or lightly salted as a snack or side dish. They're also great in stir-fries.
- **Soy flour.** This full-bodied flour is made from roasted soybeans that have been ground into powder. Use soy flour in baked goods for added protein and fiber.
- **Tempeh.** You can buy tempeh frozen or refrigerated in a cake-like form. Tempeh has a meaty texture and nutty flavor, so you can often use it as a substitute for meat. Tempeh is especially well-suited for stir-fries.
- **Miso.** This rich, salty condiment is essential in Japanese cooking. Miso is a delectable fermented soybean paste that can be used as a base for soups or as a seasoning in sauces, salad dressings and marinades.
- **Soy nuts.** Salted, dry-roasted soy nuts are readily available in grocery stores. If you're looking for a crunchy, salty snack try reaching for a handful of soy nuts instead of the chips or crackers you might otherwise choose.
- **Soy cheese.** Low in saturated fat yet still rich and creamy, soy cheese is an excellent alternative to dairy cheese.
- **Soy sauce.** Although soy sauce has a very salty taste it's actually lower in sodium than your typical table salt and can therefore be used as a more healthful alternative to salt in many recipes. Always buy naturally fermented soy sauce made without artificial additives.

Flavor-Enhancing Fit Fats

☑ **On the *Fitter, Firmer, Faster* program, you should eat "Fit Fats" with every meal.** Adding good fats to every meal enhances flavor and helps keep you feeling full longer, assisting greatly with weight management. The Fit Fats we recommend are anti-inflammatory foods that enhance overall health and reverse insulin resistance, protecting against heart disease, obesity and type 2 diabetes. Fit Fat foods are rich in either omega-3 essential fat or monounsaturated fat. The omega-3 essential fats are the fats we in modern society are most deficient in. Remember, these fats are the most powerful anti-inflammatory substances available without a prescription. Omega-3 essential fats play an important role in keeping you fit and trim while at the same time improving your health.

Fit Fat #1: Flaxseeds and Flaxseed Oil

☑ **You should enjoy at least one serving of ground flaxseeds or flaxseed oil every day.** Flax is your best, most readily available vegetarian source of omega-3 fat. The omega-3 fat in flax supports the health of your cardiovascular system by reducing your bad LDL cholesterol level and your triglyceride level while at the same time reducing systemic inflammation. Just like the omega-3 fats in fish, the omega-3 fats in flax serve as the building blocks for special hormones that improve the health and appearance of your skin.

Flax can help you stay trim and maintain a healthier weight for several reasons.

- Your body doesn't store omega-3 fats as body fat but instead uses these essential fats for the repair and maintenance of its tissue.
- Deficiency of omega-3 fat interferes with your natural metabolism, making it more difficult for your body to burn fat for energy.
- Omega-3 fats improve sensitivity to insulin therefore, facilitating weight loss by decreasing the amount of the "fat storing" insulin your pancreas needs to secrete.
- Flaxseeds and flax oil are slowly digested and therefore keep you feeling full and satisfied for hours.
- Flaxseeds in particular offer added weight-loss benefits because they are exceptionally rich in filling fiber.

You can choose to eat either ground flaxseeds—be sure they are indeed ground so you can more fully absorb the omega-3 fat—or flaxseed oil. Flax oil spoils quickly, so purchase it in small quantities. Be sure to keep flax oil refrigerated, and avoid buying flax oil that has not been kept refrigerated. Flaxseeds can be used in recipes requiring heat but flaxseed oil must not be used for cooking. Heat destroys the fragile omega-3 essential fats in flaxseed oil.

Oils: To Heat or Not to Heat?

Oils rich in omega-3 essential fats such as flaxseed oil and expeller-pressed canola oil cannot withstand heat, so they are best for no-heat recipes. To preserve freshness, store all omega-3-rich oils in the refrigerator. Oils rich in monounsaturated fat such as extra-virgin olive oil, high-oleic canola oil and avocado oil are heat-stable and are therefore by far the better choice for cooking. Oils rich in monounsaturated fats can be used in no-heat recipes, too. They are great for making vinaigrettes, for example.

Best Oils for Cooking: Oils Rich in Monounsaturated Fat	Best Oils for No-Heat Recipes: Oils Rich in Omega-3 Fat
Extra-virgin olive oil (the best choice)	Cold-pressed flaxseed oil
Avocado oil	Cold-pressed or expeller-pressed canola oil
Macadamia nut oil	Cold-pressed or expeller-pressed walnut oil
High-oleic canola oil	
High-oleic sunflower oil	
High-oleic safflower oil	

Note: Saturated fat rich foods such as butter and extra-virgin coconut oil are also heat-stable and therefore good for use in recipes requiring high-heat temperatures. However, because of the negative health consequences associated with eating a diet rich in saturated fat, it is important to use butter and extra-virgin coconut oil sparingly.

Besides being able to use ground flaxseeds in recipes requiring heat, flaxseeds have a slight health-promoting edge over flax oil because the seeds contain fiber and lignans, potent antioxidants that fight free radical damage and also act as phytoestrogens. As is the case with the phytoestrogens in soy, the naturally occurring lignan phytoestogens in whole-flax products provide protection from hormone-sensitive cancers such as breast cancer, ovarian cancer, uterine cancer and prostate cancer. In fact, according to the United States Department of Agriculture, flaxseeds contain twenty-seven identifiable cancer-preventing compounds.

Get-Real Ways to Sneak Flax into Your Life

One serving of flax is equivalent to one tablespoon flaxseed oil or 3 tablespoons ground flaxseeds. Remember, you need to eat one serving of flax every day. Flaxseed oil and flaxseeds can be used in a variety of ways.

- Use flaxseed oil to make vinaigrettes and salad dressings (see recipes chapter 9).
- Mix flaxseed oil with freshly grated Parmesan cheese as a dip for whole-grain bread.
- Drizzle flaxseed oil on top of warm, already-baked potatoes or any other warm side dish such as vegetables, beans or a whole-grain pilaf.
- Try using flaxseed oil in making homemade cold soups such as gazpacho or in making dips such as hummus.
- Try mixing ground flaxseeds into breads, muffins, pancake batter and even cake!
- Mix ground flaxseeds into your breakfast cereal or oatmeal.
- Add ground flaxseeds to fruit smoothies.
- Stir ground flaxseeds into low-fat plain yogurt or cottage cheese.
- Mix ground flaxseeds into meatloaf or casseroles.

Fit Fat #2: Moderately Rich Sources of Omega-3 Fats

Although flax is the *richest* vegetarian source of omega-3 essential fats, other good sourcees of this important anti-inflammatory, "slimming" fat include walnuts, pumpkin seeds, walnut oil and canola oil. All-natural, *trans fat-free* vegetable spreads including Smart Balance (especially Smart Balance Omega Plus) and Earth Balance also contain omega-3 essential fats and can be used in place of butter. These foods are all healthful and can all be included on the *Fitter, Firmer, Faster* program.

Fit Fat #3: Monounsaturated Fats

Monounsaturated fats are also Fit Fats. These heart-healthy fats improve your cholesterol profile, reduce inflammation and boost your body's ability to metabolize the essential omega-3 fats. Foods and oils rich in monounsaturated fats tend to be highly nutritious and rich in antiaging antioxidants.

Foods and Oils Rich in Monounsaturated Fat

NUTS	OILS
(must be either dry roasted or raw, no added oil) Almonds Cashews Chestnuts Hazelnuts Peanuts Pecans Pistachios Pine nuts Walnuts	Avocado oil Extra-virgin olive oil *High-oleic* canola oil (use for cooking) *High-oleic* safflower oil (use for cooking) *High-oleic* sunflower oil (use for cooking)
NUT BUTTERS	**SEED BUTTERS**
("all-natural" products; avoid brands containing any hydrogenated or partially hydrogenated oils) Almond butter Cashew butter Peanut butter	("all-natural" products; avoid brands containing any hydrogenated or partially hydrogenated oils) Tahini (sesame seed butter) Sunflower seed butter
SEEDS	**OTHER**
(choose dry roasted or raw) Pumpkin seeds Sesame seeds Sunflower seeds	Avocados Olives

What Are "High-Oleic" Oils?

High-oleic oils are sometimes called "super" oils or "high-monounsaturated" oils.

They come from grains that have been bred to contain more monounsaturated fat and less omega-6 fat than the standard grain. These oils have a light, mild taste and can be used in place of more flavorful oils such as extra-virgin olive oil or avocado oil in recipes requiring mild oil flavor. Because high-oleic oils are rich in monounsaturated fat, they are heat stable and ideal for recipes requiring high heat and a mild flavor.

High-oleic oils are not as rich in nutrients or antioxidants as less-processed monounsaturated oils such as extra-virgin olive oil or avocado oil. High-oleic canola oil also contains far less omega-3 fat than expeller-pressed canola oil, so make sure to use expeller-pressed canola oil in your no-heat recipes or you'll miss out on the omega-3 benefit. While high-oleic oils won't harm your health, they have not been clinically proven to enhance your health, either. We suggest you eat these oils in moderation. Use them only in recipes requiring high heat and a mild flavor.

Knowing When to Go the Extra Mile— and the Extra Expense—of Organic

You don't have to eat 100 percent organic to reap the benefits of the *Fitter, Firmer, Faster* program. While it would be nice if we could all eat purely organic foods all of the time, we realize this is not always practical or possible. It is better to eat a broad variety of "conventional" Fit Foods than to eat an excessively limited variety of "organic" Fit Foods. Furthermore, just because the ingredients in a product are grown "organic" is no guarantee the product is a healthy, nutrient-rich food. For example, plenty of high-sugar, highly refined flour-based foods such as cakes and cookies are "organic"; that doesn't mean eating them will improve your health. Just because butter, heavy cream and fatty pork sausages are organic doesn't mean these saturated, fat-rich foods should be consumed as a dietary staple.

What to Look for When Buying Organic, Heart-Healthy Proteins

When it comes to animal protein, organic really does make a difference. We strongly urge you to buy organically raised animal products if at all possible in order to minimize your consumption of antibiotic residues, hormones and other toxins found in conventionally raised animals. Many of the antibiotics fed to mass-produced farm animals are identical to the ones administered to humans. As has been well publicized in the media, overuse of such antibiotics leads to bacterial resistance, opening doors wider to the potential for human disease. Certified organic animals are fed only certified organic grains and grasses and are always free of hormones and antibiotics.

Organic is not the only important word to look for. Search also for the words "free range." Though the term is not strictly regulated, free-range animals are encouraged to forage for their food. These animals grow and live free from the stress of overcrowded conditions. Conventionally raised animals are kept in extremely cramped quarters. Not only is it much more humane to allow animals to move around, roaming is good exercise for the animal. Farm animals that exercise are leaner and therefore healthier than animals that don't. Farm animal fat is not healthy fat. Lean animal meat is always better.

Finally, "grass-fed" animals are better for your health than grain-fed animals. Not all organic animals are grass-fed. Grass-fed meats and the dairy products provided by grass-fed animals are the best choice for four important reasons.

1. Grass-fed animals are leaner than grain-fed animals. Ounce for ounce their meat contains fewer calories and less "bad" saturated fat.
2. Meat from grass-fed animals has two to four times more "good" essential omega-3 fats than the meat of grain-fed animals.
3. Meat from grass-fed animals is higher in the antioxidant vitamin E.
4. Meats and dairy products from grass-fed animals are the richest source of conjugated linoleic acid (CLA) in its natural form. Natural CLA has been shown to promote fat loss in overweight individuals and may even help prevent cancer. Levels of CLA are very low in the meat and milk of grain-fed animals.

Note: Although commercially produced CLA is available in supplement form, we advise against taking these supplements because they are made from sunflower or safflower seeds. They do not contain the same form of CLA that is found in natural meat sources. Some studies suggest artificial CLA can increase insulin resistance and decrease your "good" HDL cholesterol level.

Farmed or Wild Fish

If you're like most people, you're probably wondering if it's worth the extra money necessary to buy wild-caught fish as opposed to farmed fish. There are benefits to eating wild fish if it is available to you. Wild fish are not exposed to antibiotics and wild fish contain lower levels of PCBs, dioxin and mercury on the average. So if you can afford to buy wild fish go right ahead, but there is no reason to feel guilty about eating farmed fish if wild is not within your budget.

Eating fish regularly is mandatory if you want to get the omega-3 essential fats your body needs. Farmed fish contains slightly more saturated fat than wild fish. However, it still contains significantly less saturated fat than other animal products and significantly more omega-3 fat than any other commonly eaten food. So whether you choose farmed fish or wild fish you're way ahead of your non-fish-eating friends when it comes to losing weight and staying healthy.

Mercury and Fish

We know the mercury present in certain species of fish sends up red flags for many people. We want to assure you an overwhelming amount of research documents numerous overlapping benefits associated with increased consumption of fish, despite the fact that people who eat fish do indeed have higher blood levels of mercury than people who don't eat it. Multiple studies performed on people prove beyond a shadow of a doubt fish eaters live longer and suffer fewer heart attacks than non-fish eaters so long as the fish is prepared healthfully and not deep fried. To us, the prevailing issue is not how much mercury is in our blood but how long and how well we live.

If you are still worried or are unable to afford wild fish, here are some suggestions:

1. Buy canned wild salmon, always cheap and readily available.
2. Look for smaller canned fishes. Small fish accumulate less mercury than larger fish. Sardines, herring and anchovies are all healthful.
3. Avoid large predator fish, especially tilefish, shark, swordfish and king mackerel. Larger fish tend to accumulate more mercury in their flesh. These four species have been identified as being the most likely to contain high levels of mercury.
4. Supplement your diet with pharmaceutical grade fish oils that have been molecularly distilled. Fish oil supplements are made from species of fish known to contain low levels of mercury.

What to Look for in Organic Dairy Products

Spending the money to buy organic dairy products, such as organic milk, yogurt, butter and cheese, is well worth your time and effort for the same reason we urge you to buy organic meat. Organic dairy products are derived from cows raised on organically grown feed that is free from pesticides. Organic dairy cows are never exposed to growth hormones and are not routinely fed antibiotics.

We advocate *against* intentionally consuming three servings of dairy a day. While low-fat dairy foods are allowed in moderation, there is no need for you to go to any extra effort to consume three servings of dairy a day. In fact, you don't need to eat any dairy at all on the *Fitter, Firmer, Faster* program. Many people are lactose intolerant, and many people around the world are able to maintain good health without eating dairy products.

The primary reason pro-dairy nutritionists are so enthusiastic is the calcium. Yes, calcium is an extremely important mineral—especially for building and maintaining bone mass and preventing osteoporosis. It helps with blood clotting and with the transmission of nerve impulses. It has also been shown to help with weight loss. However, it's important to note long-term studies are not conclusive in determining exactly how much calcium we really need. For example, in a large Harvard study, male health professionals and female nurses who drank one glass of milk or less per week were at no greater risk of breaking their bones than persons who drank two or more glasses of milk per week. Other researchers have presented similar findings. Many factors are involved in the prevention of osteoporosis and the resulting hip and forearm fractures, including vitamin D intake, weight bearing exercise and protein intake.

And remember, plenty of nondairy sources of calcium exist, including broccoli, collards, tofu, beans, almonds and sardines. All of these foods contain more overall nutrition than milk. In conclusion, organic low-fat milk is acceptable, but there are far more healthful protein foods to choose from.

Choose Low-Fat Plain Yogurt over Milk

Yogurts and other cultured dairy products such as kefir contain more nutrition than milk. In addition to providing the calcium-related benefits that are common to all low-fat dairy products, kefir and yogurt are probiotic foods. Probiotics promote the colonization of "good" bacteria in your intestines that compete with less-beneficial "bad" bacteria that constantly threaten our health.

Although yogurts and kefirs contain different strains of beneficial bacteria, both promote proper digestion, and both increase your resistance to infection. Good bacteria keep your digestive tract healthy and play important roles in the vitality of your immune system. Yogurt and kefir can help prevent yeast overgrowth. Since many medically necessary antibiotics wipe out naturally occurring "good" bacteria along with the bad it is especially wise to eat low-fat yogurt or low-fat kefir should you require treatment with antibiotics for a medical condition.

Not all cultured dairy products are healthy. Always choose low-fat plain yogurt. Avoid yogurts laden with sugary syrups. Try to go organic if at all possible. Lactose intolerant persons are often able to tolerate kefir and yogurt. This is because the "good" bacteria in foods such as yogurt and kefir possess the ability to break down lactose into more easily digested sugars.

A Better Butter?

You can enjoy butter in moderation on the *Fitter, Firmer, Faster* program. Butter is exceptionally rich in saturated fat, but it does have redeeming qualities. Butter is a good source of the fat-soluble vitamins A, D, E and K. Butter also contains lecithin, which assists in the proper assimilation and metabolization of cholesterol. One of the main fats in butter, butyric acid, helps feed the friendly bacteria that keep your colon healthy. Butter from grass-fed cows but not from grain-fed cows contains natural CLA that may help with weight control.

If you do choose to eat butter, we suggest you eat organic butter, and we urge you to use it sparingly. Limit your use of butter to cooking and baking in recipes requiring high heat and "buttery" flavor.

Omega-3-Enriched Eggs

Eggs are "egg-ceptional" nutrient-dense powerhouse foods. Eggs contain several B vitamins, vitamins A and D, zinc, iron and the antioxidant lutein, thought to help prevent macular degeneration and cataracts. All varieties of eggs contain lecithin, a nutrient that helps protect against cardiovascular disease and may even improve brain function. Eggs also provide the raw materials your body needs to make glutathione, a powerful antioxidant and detoxifier that protects against free radical damage and fights inflammation.

When possible, we strongly encourage you to look for the new "chicks" on the block, "omega-3-enriched" eggs. They are even more desirable than conventional eggs because their yolks contain a higher percentage of those "good" omega-3 essential fats we are so deficient in. As you know by now, omega-3 fats support the health of your cardiovascular system, reproductive system, immune system and central nervous system. Omega-3 fats also support a healthy metabolism, prevent and help reverse insulin resistance, and even help you lose weight. Omega-3-enriched eggs contain less saturated fat than standard, classic eggs and more of the antioxidant vitamin E. Omega-3 eggs taste every bit as delicious, if not more delicious, than standard eggs. These new, improved eggs are popping up in supermarkets and natural foods stores across the country. We recommend specific brands in appendix A.

Choose Organic or "High-Quality" Fats

It is very important to buy only "dry-roasted" or "raw" nuts and seeds. Avoid nuts and seeds that have been roasted in oil. The oils used in roasting nuts and seeds are not healthful. All-natural nut butters and seed butters are extremely healthful. However, it is particularly important to read the labels of nut butters. Be sure the nut butters you purchase *do not* contain hydrogenated or partially hydrogenated oils. The label should specifically say "all-natural." All-natural peanut butters, almond butters, tahini (sesame seed butter), cashew nut butters and hazelnut butters are readily available, nutritious and delicious.

The best monounsaturated fat to use is extra-virgin olive oil. Extra-virgin olive oil has proven itself to be healthful and remains the best all-around oil for cooking. It's the safest, most-widely studied, most versatile oil and is a prime component of the extensively researched, extremely healthful Mediterranean Diet. It's also rich in monounsaturated fat and antioxidants. Studies have shown people who consume two tablespoons of extra-virgin olive oil daily for as little as one week show less oxidation of LDL cholesterol and higher levels of antioxidants in their blood. This antioxidant effect of olive oil is very relevant because oxidation of LDL cholesterol, more so than having high levels of LDL cholesterol, encourages artery clogging plaque deposits. Other studies have shown olive oil offers protection against heart disease by raising "good" HDL cholesterol levels. In comparison, less-healthful vegetable oils reduce "bad" and "good" cholesterol levels alike.

Oils rich in omega-3 essential fats such as flaxseed oil, canola oil, hazelnut oil and walnut oil must be of the highest quality. The essential fats in these oils are vulnerable to oxidation and easily spoil and become rancid. Consuming rancid oil does more harm than good! Unfortunately most grocery-store quality oils are refined at very high temperatures, processed with chemicals, then deodorized and "purified" to make their taste acceptable. Processed oils not only contain toxic by-products, they are also devoid of natural nutrients. The best oils are expeller pressed, and ideally, cold pressed. *Expeller pressing* is a chemical-free mechanical process that extracts oils from seeds and nuts. This method of oil extraction is a better alternative to the solvent-based extraction methods used to process many conventional oils. The temperatures reached during expeller pressing depend in part on the hardness of the nut or seed being pressed. The harder the nut or seed, the more pressure required to extract the oil, which in turn creates more friction and higher heat. While no external heat is applied during expeller pressing, harder nuts and seeds must still endure elevated temperatures. Oils that are cold pressed are expeller pressed in a heat-controlled environment to keep temperatures below about 120 degrees Fahrenheit. The very best oils are cold pressed; these are the truly "unrefined" oils you should purchase if optimal health is important to you. While standard expeller-pressed oils are also acceptable and certainly far more healthful than grocery-store quality oils, cold-pressed oils are best. This is especially important when it comes to choosing flaxseed oil. Though flaxseed oil is nature's most healthful oil, because it is so rich in heat-sensitive omega-3 essential fat it is critical that the flaxseed oil you purchase is indeed cold pressed.

Now that you know all about the healthy "fit foods" you should be eating more of, it's time to learn about all the fake and fattening foods you should eat less of.

3 Avoid Fake and Fattening Foods

Fake foods are highly processed foods. Think of highly processed "fake" foods as wasted calories that will make you gain weight. Fake foods lack the nutrients your body needs to stay full, curb food cravings and maintain a healthy metabolism.

You probably don't need us to tell you that it's better for your waist-line and your health to make a whole-grain pilaf with brown rice than it is to heat up white minute-rice, and it's better to make a bowl of old-fashioned oatmeal as opposed to processed, microwaveable instant oatmeal. The problem is convenience.

We get it. We're busy working parents ourselves. That's why this chapter is about compromise. We'll show you how you can still enjoy healthy convenience foods that still qualify as "whole foods" by apply-ing five simple rules whenever you shop. (If you're really pressed for time, and don't want to do any thinking at all, skip to appendix A where you'll find a shopping list of healthy packaged foods.)

Become Label Conscious: How to Read Food Labels

Hundreds of healthful whole foods are available at your local super-market. You need to know how to find these good packages amongst the sea of junk. This is what this chapter is all about—teaching you how to identify healthful packaged "convenience" whole foods, understand food labels and how to permanently avoid overly processed empty-calorie foods.

Our "5 Fit Food Rules" do most of the work for you. Once you know how to apply these rules you'll know whether or not foods advertised as "heart-healthy" are in fact truly what they promise. You'll know whether foods advertised as "low-carb" or "low-fat" are not just "low" but actually healthy. You'll learn whether or not foods endorsed by the svelte model on the package have any chance of making you look like her. You get the picture. Now let's get to the rules . . .

RULE #1: Put Trans Fats in the Trash Can

The unfortunate reality is that many of the foods we eat are processed in factories weeks or even months ahead of time. The potato chips you ate last night might have been packaged a year ago, or even longer! Mass-market food producers and distributors benefit from longer shelf life, thus the need for additives, preservatives and, worst of all, longer-lasting artificial fats called trans fats.

For decades trans fats have been the fats of choice for budget-minded food giants. While these artificial fats extend shelf life, they have been proven without a doubt to shorten human life and pack on the pounds. According to the Institute of Medicine there is no safe level of intake for trans fat. Why?

1. Trans fats are empty calories that have been linked with weight gain, obesity, type 2 diabetes, heart disease and cancer.
2. Trans fats contribute to insulin resistance by "desensitizing" your cells to the actions of insulin, therefore making it necessary for your body to produce more of this "fat-storing" hormone than it should.
3. Trans fats increase your "bad" LDL cholesterol level, decrease your "good" HDL cholesterol level, and increase your triglyceride level, which increases your risk of heart disease.
4. Trans fats increase your risk of developing premature senility.
5. Trans fats interfere with your body's ability to metabolize and utilize "good" essential fats. If you eat foods containing trans fats

you cancel out many of the health benefits associated with eating foods such as fish, flax and nuts that contain "good" fat.

6. Trans fats increase inflammation in your body and therefore exacerbate the symptoms of inflammation-mediated diseases such as asthma and arthritis.
7. Trans fats wreak havoc on your skin, contributing to inflammation-mediated skin conditions such as acne, eczema, psoriasis and even premature skin aging.

Where Are Trans Fats Found?

The United States FDA now requires food manufacturers to include the amount of trans fat contained in all packaged food products on their nutrition information labeling. This law, along with increased public awareness, has prompted many food manufacturers to overhaul their recipes. However, while many food manufacturers have reduced or eliminated their use of trans fat, these fats are still commonly found in many typical junk food products such as cookies, cakes, frosting, candy, doughnuts and fried foods.

Trans fats are also found in foods you may think of as being more healthful such as crackers, cereals, muffins, breads, "light" frozen food entrees, peanut butters and soups. Although some trans fats can be found in foods specifically advertised as being "cholesterol-free," make no mistake; eating trans fat raises your blood cholesterol level far more than eating cholesterol itself.

How to Avoid Trans Fats

"No" doesn't always mean "no" in the world of food labels. According to government labeling laws, foods containing one-half gram or less trans fat per serving can still list their products as having no trans fats. Because there is no safe level of trans fat intake, and one-half gram can add up over the course of the day, you must still read the ingredients list of *any* packaged food you purchase.

Avoid foods containing any partially hydrogenated or hydrogenated oils anywhere in their listing of ingredients. Any amount of hydrogenated or partially hydrogenated oil is too much. Trans fats are found in vegetable shortening and most margarines. Read the labels!

Finally, avoid eating fried foods, especially frozen fried foods available in the supermarket and any fried foods served at either restaurants or fast food chains. The oils used to create these fried foods must be assumed to contain trans fat unless specifically mentioned otherwise.

RULE #2: Stay Away from Omega-6-Rich Vegetable Oils

Now that the public is becoming more aware of just how dangerous trans fats are, food manufacturers are starting to use omega-6 vegetable oils such as corn oil, peanut oil, soybean oil, sunflower oil and "pure" vegetable oil in greater quantities than ever before. This sounds healthful enough. Omega-6 fats can be good for you in moderation; however, there are a number of reasons to avoid the routine overconsumption of omega-6 vegetable oils.

First, conventional processing techniques used to refine grains and seeds into oil damage the highly heat-sensitive omega-6 essential fats within. Omega-6 fats are by their very nature unable to withstand high-heat processing. Nevertheless, the vast majority of the vegetable oils sitting on grocery store shelves and used in the creation of processed foods are refined at excessively high temperatures. Omega-6 fats react negatively when exposed to heat. They become rancid. Vegetable oils that are not cold pressed or, at the very least, expeller pressed are highly processed, empty-calorie foods and should therefore be avoided. Refined vegetable oils are calorie rich and nutrient poor. These oils increase your risk of becoming obese.

Ever since researchers learned that diets rich in saturated fat increase your risk of heart disease, nutritionists have recommended replacing saturated fats such as butter, lard and palm oil with vegetable oils such as corn oil, soybean oil and sunflower oil. The reasoning behind this recommendation was that the omega-6 fats in vegetable oil do indeed reduce your total blood cholesterol level. However, most vegetable oils lower both your "bad" LDL cholesterol level *and* your "good" HDL cholesterol level. Consequently, these oils don't provide nearly the heart protection researchers once thought.

It's All About the Ratio

What's more, researchers now know vegetable oils are unhealthful in other ways. Vegetable oils increase your risk of developing chronic disease and exacerbate the symptoms of many degenerative diseases because they have a definite tendency to increase inflammation in your body when they are eaten in excess. By now you're familiar with the two types of essential fat, omega-3 and omega-6 fat. In order to minimize the amount of inflammation in your body and therefore minimize the symptoms of any disease related to inflammation—heart disease, asthma, arthritis and fibromyalgia—your body needs a proper balance between these two fats. An imbalance of omega-3 fat to omega-6 fat can even increase your risk of obesity and type 2 diabetes by decreasing your cells' sensitivity to insulin.

Omega-6 fats and omega-3 fats are both necessary to promote good health. It's important to obtain both of these fats in your diet; you just need to make sure you are eating these fats in the proper balance to support optimal health and an optimal metabolism. While omega-3 fats are always anti-inflammatory, if you eat the omega-6 fats in excess they have the potential to increase inflammation, increase your risk of the twin epidemics obesity and type 2 diabetes, and decrease overall health. Too much omega-6 fat is not good.

This brings us back to vegetable oil. Most of the vegetable oil used by modern food processing companies is very rich in omega-6 fat. Because of our overreliance on omega-6 vegetable oils such as corn oil, soybean oil, "pure" vegetable oil, sunflower oil and safflower oil, *the average person today eats approximately fourteen to twenty times more omega-6 fat than omega-3 fat*. To control inflammation, improve the symptoms of inflammation-mediated diseases and help reverse insulin resistance, you should eat a more balanced ratio of approximately four times more omega-6 fat than omega-3 fat.

Omega-6 Oils to Avoid

The easiest way to optimize your "omega ratio" without having to worry about calculating this ratio yourself is to eliminate common omega-6-rich vegetable oils from your diet. They can be replaced with the delicious, more healthful oils we recommend in chapter 2. No thinking. No calculating. There are plenty of better tasting, more healthful alternatives to standard grocery store vegetable oils.

Do not buy or cook with these oils and avoid packaged foods containing corn oil, soybean oil, sunflower oil, safflower oil, "pure" vegetable oil, peanut oil or cottonseed oil. *Note:* The occasional use of omega-6 oils for use in preparing homemade special recipes is acceptable. For this reason sesame oil and peanut oil may be used *in moderation* as part of a special recipe. It would be ideal if you did not heat or cook with these oils (use them in salad dressings instead, for example). Ideally, these oils should not be used regularly even if all of your meals are homemade.

RULE #3: Limit Your Intake of Saturated Fat

Some whole, natural foods do contain high levels of saturated fat, so you need to eat these foods in moderation. Diets high in saturated fat increase your risk of heart disease. Anything harmful to your heart is also harmful to your brain and diets rich in saturated fat are no exception. Eat too much saturated fat and you increase your risk of developing vascular dementia (senility) and even stroke. Eating too much saturated fat can also negatively affect your mood and worsen depression. Less publicized is the fact that saturated fats contribute to gallbladder disease and certain types of cancer.

In addition, saturated fats increase inflammation within your body. Think of inflammation as the tendency of your body to attack itself. Saturated fats interfere with your body's ability to produce natural hormones that fight inflammation. Eating too much can exacerbate symptoms of inflammation-mediated diseases such as multiple sclerosis, asthma, allergies, arthritis and fibromyalgia. It also accelerates the aging of your skin and worsens skin conditions such as acne, psoriasis and eczema.

Are "Cholesterol-Free" Foods Heart-Healthy Choices?

Not necessarily. Most of the cholesterol in your bloodstream is created by your own body from the fats you eat. Your blood cholesterol level is minimally affected by the cholesterol content of the foods you eat. In other words, the cholesterol found in cholesterol-rich foods such as eggs and shrimp has a *minimal* effect on your blood cholesterol level.

Your liver makes cholesterol from the saturated fats and trans fats you eat. Eating too many empty carbohydrates such as sugar and refined flour can increase your cholesterol level, too. This is because excess, empty carbohydrate intake stimulates your body to produce large amounts of insulin, and insulin activates an enzyme responsible for making cholesterol in your liver.

What should cholesterol-conscious people do? Eat more good fat. That means more nuts, more seeds, more extra-virgin olive oil and more fatty fish. Eat more fiber. Even more important, completely eliminate trans fats found in many margarines, vegetable shortenings and packaged foods containing hydrogenated or partially hydrogenated oils. You should also avoid or limit your intake of sugar, refined flour and saturated fats.

Don't worry about the cholesterol content in your foods. Learn to ignore claims such as "cholesterol-free" on food packaging. There is absolutely no need to eliminate otherwise healthful foods, including eggs and shrimp, just because they happen to be high in cholesterol.

Where Is Saturated Fat Found?

Unlike the case with trans fat, saturated fats are often found in foods that contain important nutrients. Therefore it's neither necessary nor desirable for you to completely eliminate foods containing saturated fat from your diet. For example, low-fat yogurt contains saturated fat, but low-fat yogurt is also an excellent source of calcium. Beef contains saturated fat, but beef is also a good source of B vitamins, iron and zinc. Pork, lamb, chicken, duck, eggs and dairy products all contain saturated fat, yet all of these foods can be part of a healthful lifestyle so long as they are eaten in moderation.

How to Control Your Saturated-Fat Intake

Healthy people should eat no more than 20 grams of saturated fat each day. If you already have a health condition related to your blood vessels, such as heart disease, or you already have a health condition related to inflammation, such as asthma, arthritis, allergies or multiple sclerosis, you should aim to eat no more than 15 grams of saturated fat per day. This is the only "counting" required in order to follow the Fitter, Firmer, Faster program.

By law, packaged food products must provide certain nutrition information, including the amount of saturated fat contained per serving. If you take the time to read the labels of the packaged foods you buy, and you know the amount of saturated fat in just a few of the following whole-foods staples, you can't go wrong.

Saturated Fat Content in Whole-Foods Staples

FOOD	SERVING SIZE	SATURATED FAT
Butter	1 tablespoon	7 grams
1% milk or yogurt	1 cup	1½ grams
2% milk or yogurt	1 cup	3 grams
Low-fat cheese	¼ cup	3 grams
Full-fat cheese	¼ cup	5 grams
"Extra-lean" cuts of pork, veal, lamb, game, beef, dark meat turkey and dark meat chicken	4 ounces	4 grams
Ostrich	4 ounces	2 grams
Buffalo (bison)	4 ounces	2 grams
Skinless white meat chicken and turkey	4 ounces	1½ grams
Eggs	1 whole egg	1½ grams
Extra-virgin coconut oil	1 tablespoon	12 grams

All of the foods listed in the table are healthful, nutrient-rich whole foods. Try to make sure all of the foods you eat that do contain saturated fat are indeed nutrient-rich, healthful foods. For example, it is much better to get 4 grams of saturated fat from a lean cut of beef as opposed to getting the equivalent amount in an ice cream sandwich.

We find it easiest to stick to our saturated fat budget when we eat only two meals a day that contain saturated fat, and we avoid foods that

How to Count Your Saturated-Fat Intake

☑ You now know it is best to limit saturated-fat intake to 20 grams total per day if you are healthy and 15 grams total per day if you suffer from any chronic medical condition. Many healthful whole-foods products do contain modest amounts of saturated fat. For example, most oils and most foods that contain any fat at all contain a combination of all four of the basic types of natural fat: saturated fat, monounsaturated fat, omega-6 fat and omega-3 fat. In other words, even heart-healthy foods such as fish and olive oil contain at least small amounts of saturated fat. However, because olive oil contains mostly monounsaturated fat, nutritionists classify it as a monounsaturated fat despite the fact that there is a small amount of saturated fat in olive oil.

☑ You *only* need to count the saturated fat in three types of food toward your daily saturated-fat budget:

1. The saturated fat in animal products such as beef, chicken, turkey, butter, eggs and dairy products (you do not have to count the saturated fat in fish)
2. The saturated fat in packaged foods, any food you eat out of the box, such as ice cream, crackers, cake mixes and frozen dinners
3. The saturated fats in tropical vegetable oils such as extra-virgin coconut oil and palm oil

☑ You *don't* need to count the small amount of saturated fat found in vegetarian foods such as nuts, seeds, olive oil, avocados, nut butters, seed butters, grains and so forth toward your daily budget. You also *don't* need to count the saturated fat in fish and shellfish. None of these foods count toward your 15 to 20 gram daily budget. The reason is these foods contain healthful fats that far outweigh the negatives associated with the small amount of saturated fat in them.

contain saturated fat in our snacks. This way we only have to do the math twice a day. We use butter sparingly, and when cooking or baking we often mix butter with high-oleic canola oil to reduce the overall saturated-fat content. We choose only white meat, skinless chicken and turkey, and we eat only low-fat dairy products. Finally, we choose the absolute leanest meats possible, and we often substitute extra lean meats such as ostrich and buffalo for beef. These meats have all the flavor and juiciness of beef but contain considerably less saturated fat. Ostrich and buffalo are readily available in the frozen section of most natural foods stores.

RULE #4: Reduce Your Sugar Intake

In addition to avoiding unhealthful fats, it's also important to learn how to avoid unhealthful carbohydrates. Sugar tops the list. Sugar is an empty-calorie food that contributes to malnutrition, excess hunger and out-of-control food cravings. It's rapidly absorbed, forcing your pancreas to produce a lot of insulin. You already know it's not desirable from a health or weight-loss standpoint for your pancreas to secrete large amounts of insulin; excess insulin dramatically increases your risk of developing type 2 diabetes and obesity.

That's two strikes for sugar. But that's not all. If you're not particularly active, and the sugars you eat are not burned off for energy right away, your body converts them into saturated fat. As you now know, saturated fats promote inflammation, worsening the symptoms of inflammation-mediated conditions such as asthma and arthritis and accelerating the aging of your skin. What's more, because high-sugar foods often replace more healthful foods, nutrition experts believe sweets indirectly contribute to diseases such as osteoporosis, heart disease and cancer. That's a lot more than three strikes against sugar.

Tipping the Scale

Although government authorities recommend eating no more than ten teaspoons of sugar per day, the average American gulps down approximately thirty-four teaspoons, more than three times the recommended limit. Thirty-four teaspoons of sugar contains 544 calories. If you eat an additional 544 calories every day for one year you will end up weighing an extra 56 pounds at the end of a year. Yikes! Of course the reverse is also true; it is possible to lose 56 pounds in one year if you are able to eliminate 544 sugar calories per day from your diet.

How to Limit Your Sugar Intake

Obviously if you stop adding sugar to your cereal and eating candy you'll decrease your sugar intake. However, many of us fail to realize how much sugar is added to an astonishing array of packaged and processed foods. Many convenience items that crowd grocery store shelves, vending machines, school cafeterias and home kitchens are loaded with sugar. Sugar hides in products including frozen entrees, soups, salad dressings, condiments, pasta sauces, cereals, protein bars and much more! If you eat these packaged foods regularly, you're almost certainly consuming much more sugar than you think. . . . It all adds up.

Beverages are one of the biggest sources of sugar in the modern diet. We suggest you completely eliminate beverages containing sugar, including soda, sports drinks, sweetened iced teas, sweetened alcoholic drinks and any fruit beverages containing less than 100 percent pure fruit juice. If you eliminate just one twelve-ounce can of soda or one twelve-ounce sports beverage every day for one year you will lose fifteen pounds!

If you are currently a heavy soda drinker, why not try fruit spritzers instead? Mix one-eighth part 100 percent real fruit juice with plain seltzer water. One small lifestyle change such as this can make a big difference if you are trying to fit back into your skinny jeans.

Become a Sugar-Savvy Shopper

To become sugar savvy, it's important to read ingredient labels. If sugar is listed as the first or second ingredient, the product probably contains too much sugar. Be aware, however, sugar is often described more subtly in the ingredients listing. You *have* to become label conscious. Look for sugar pseudonyms such as *corn syrup, dextrin, dextrose, fructose, fruit juice concentrate, high-fructose corn syrup, cane syrup, galactose, glucose, honey, maltose, lactose, maple syrup, molasses* and *sucrose*. Select items low in these added sugars whenever possible.

Here are a few more tips to help you out:

- Avoid *all* foods containing high-fructose corn syrup. The mere existence of this ingredient is a red flag that you are eating a low-quality, overly processed food.
- Buy fresh fruits and canned fruits packed in either water or fruit juice as opposed to canned fruits packed in sugar syrups.
- Avoid all beverages containing added sugar.
- Be aware: many "low-fat" foods are loaded with sugar. Sweetened yogurts are prime culprits. As a general rule of thumb, any low-fat yogurt containing more than about 130 calories per 8 ounces contains too much sugar. Look for low-fat plain, unsweetened yogurts instead. You can add the fruit and the flavor at home.
- Avoid sports bars, energy bars and protein powders. These products are notoriously high in sugar. They are almost always no better for you than candy bars. You'll often notice either the first or second ingredient in these bars is some type of sugar. Trail mix containing dried fruit, nuts, seeds and a few dark chocolate chips makes a far better "energy" snack.
- Condiments containing sugar such as barbecue sauce or ketchup are acceptable in moderation. Use sugar-containing condiments sparingly. Because these products are typically eaten in moderation this is not the best place to concentrate your sugar-busting efforts.

Kick Sugar Out of Your Kitchen

It's also important to use less sugar in the foods you prepare at home. While some sugars are more processed than others, all sugars contribute to health problems. Strive to use less of even the "healthier" less-processed sugars: brown sugar, honey, molasses and pure maple syrup. Gradually make over your favorite recipes by reducing the amount of sugar called for until you've decreased the sugar content by one-half or even more. Try these ideas:

- Experiment with spices such as cinnamon, cardamom, coriander, nutmeg and ginger to replace sugar for sweetness and flavor in foods. Spiced foods taste even sweeter when warmed.
- Sweeten plain yogurt with fresh fruit instead of sugar.
- Reach for fruit instead of sugary sweets for dessert. Snack on fruits instead of sugary junk foods.
- Use sweet condiments such as jelly and sweet sauces in moderation only (think teaspoon-size servings rather than tablespoon size).
- Add less sugar to foods such as cereal and fruit. Get accustomed to using half as much, and then see if you can eliminate sugar completely.
- Substitute sparkling non-calorie beverages such as Perrier, San Pellegrino or generic seltzer water for sugary soft drinks. Herbal teas are a great alternative to sweetened beverages.

Sugar Alternatives

It's best to wean yourself from sweets altogether as much as possible. While many sugar alternatives exist none of them enhance your health in any way. Furthermore, you might be surprised to know no scientific evidence exists to suggest using calorie-free sugar substitutes helps with weight loss. So if you decide to use sugar substitutes, we suggest you use them in moderation. The less often you use sugar substitutes the better. To keep your intake low avoid packaged foods and beverages made with sugar substitutes; instead, use these products to lightly sweeten foods such as plain yogurt, oatmeal and fruit smoothies.

Stevia is a calorie-free all-natural herb native to Paraguay that has been used for hundreds of years in South America. You can purchase stevia in natural foods stores in powder form or in liquid form as a dietary supplement. Stevia is best used to sweeten fruits, cereals and dairy. This herb is much trickier to use in baking. Although high-heat temperatures have no effect on stevia's sweetness, stevia has a different chemical makeup than sugar, and it behaves quite unlike sugar when used for baking. The number one thing to remember with stevia is not to use too much; it is extremely sweet, and it has an aftertaste when used in excessive quantities. For more details and for information on where to purchase stevia visit *www.sweetleaf.com.*

Raw honey makes a good replacement for sugar in most recipes. Although it's a concentrated source of sugar calories, and we certainly are not suggesting it be used in excess, raw honey does contain antioxidants, phytonutrients and antibacterial, antiviral substances not present in regular table sugar. To obtain the most nutrition possible from honey, buy unheated, unfiltered, unprocessed *raw* honey. The processing of honey removes many of the phytonutrients found in *raw* honey straight from the hive. When raw honey is extensively processed and heated to create refined honey, the benefits of these phytonutrients are largely lost. Since honey is sweeter than sugar, you need to use less at a time, one-half to three-quarters cup honey for each cup of sugar. For each cup of sugar replaced, you should also reduce the amount of liquid in the recipe by one-quarter cup. In addition, reduce the cooking temperature by 25 degrees since honey causes foods to brown more easily. *Note:* Never give honey to an infant under the age of one.

(continued from page 46)

Sucralose (Splenda) is an artificial sweetener made by bonding three chlorine molecules to natural sugar molecules. Don't be alarmed by the chlorine. Keep in mind the salt you use to season your food is simply chlorinated sodium. Chlorine is one of the most abundant electrolytes in your bloodstream. Sucralose passes through your digestive tract essentially unabsorbed; therefore, sucralose neither affects your blood sugar level nor adds calories to your diet. Sucralose was introduced to the American market in 1998, and the research to date shows it is safe. This doesn't mean we are suggesting you eat it by the bucketful; use it in moderation. Splenda is a helpful option for cooking and baking because it maintains its sweetness and consistency under a wide range of temperatures. We often use the Splenda branded "Sugar Blend for Baking," which is a mix of Splenda brand sweetener and pure sugar. This product provides half the calories of pure sugar yet tastes equally as sweet.

While we do want you to curb your sugar intake, this isn't an entirely black-and-white situation—shades of gray are okay, too. Sugar does not promote health but indulging in a small sweet treat every day can help you feel less deprived and might even help you stick to what would otherwise be an overly spartan lifestyle. On the *Fitter, Firmer, Faster* program you can safely enjoy one *small* sweet treat per day so long as you are making a conscientious effort to reduce your sugar intake throughout the day. On average, desserts contain about five teaspoons of sugar per small serving. Our dessert recipes in chapter 9 contain about half this amount. We'll discuss the daily "sweet treat" in more detail on page 65.

RULE #5: Avoid Foods Made with Refined Flour

This section is very important. Refined flour is equally as unhealthy as eating sugar. Eating it has the same negative health consequences and weight gain consequences as are associated with eating sugar. While refined flours are made from healthful whole grains, refined flour contains none of the health-promoting, antiaging, weight reducing properties provided by whole grains.

During the refinement process the nutrient- and antioxidant-rich "germ" and the fiber-rich "bran" found in whole grains are removed leaving only the nutrient-poor, fiber-free, calorie-rich starch behind. The calorie-rich starch is then "enriched" with small amounts of synthetic nutrients. This vitamin "enrichment" process is not helpful because all of the fiber and all of the disease-fighting phytonutrients have already been lost forever during the refinement process. Eating enriched flour is no more healthful than eating a sugar-laden lollypop infused with vitamins. "Enriched" is a code word for junk.

Enriched wheat flour is the most common variety of flour used in processed foods. Most of the standard carbohydrate-containing foods we eat are made with highly refined, enriched wheat flour. Examples include breads, cereals, pastries, crackers, pizza crusts and many other baked goods. Read the ingredients list on the back of the packaged foods you buy. Avoid foods containing enriched flour or any of the following highly refined flours: all-purpose flour, bleached flour, bread flour, cake flour, durum flour (often used to make noodles and pasta), high-gluten flour, pastry flour or semolina (often used to make pasta).

Alternatives to Refined, "Enriched" Flour

Baked goods made with whole-grain flour represent much more healthful alternatives to the highly refined flour products mentioned earlier. Whole-grain flours are healthful because they still contain the fiber-rich bran and the nutrient- and antioxidant-rich germ as well as important minerals and phytonutrients not found in refined-grain products. Whole-grain flours are more slowly digested than refined flours and therefore cause less insulin secretion. Be very careful when reading the food label. Don't confuse refined "wheat" and "multi-grain" flours with whole-wheat or other whole-grain flours. *The word "whole" must appear on the ingredients list.*

Products made from "100% whole grains" usually proudly state this fact prominently on their packaging. These are often excellent, healthful foods. Products advertised as being "made with whole grains" are typically not 100% whole-grain products. They may contain only a small percentage of their calories in whole-grain form.

Don't be tricked by the words *natural, organic, seven-grain, multi-grain,* or *enriched.* To be sure the product is in fact made with whole-grains look for the word *whole* in the listing of ingredients. Look for terms such as *whole-wheat* or *whole-wheat flour.* Another word that identifies products as being whole grain is the word *sprouted,* often found in whole-grain breads such as *sprouted* wheat bread or *sprouted* barley bread.

You can also look for one of two "seals" of approval—one seal, promoted by the FDA, links consumption of whole grains to a reduced risk of heart disease and certain cancers, and the other is a yellow and black stamp promoted by the Whole Grains Council (*www.wholegrainscouncil.org*). Their stamp stating "100% Whole Grain" strongly suggests the product is a healthy choice.

Foods with Healthy Flours

Almost any baked good typically made with highly refined flour can now be found in a whole-grain flour version. Because of the presence of bran, which reduces gluten development, baked goods made from whole-wheat flour are naturally heavier, denser and more flavorful than those made with refined flours. From pancakes and waffles to breads, pastas, cereals and crackers, healthful alternatives to your favorite baked goods are readily available. Be sure to check out appendix A for an abundance of brand-name "figure-friendly" suggestions!

Many varieties of whole-grain flours exist. You need not limit yourself to wheat. For example, whole-amaranth flour, whole-barley flour, whole-buckwheat flour, whole cornmeal, whole-oat flour, whole-brown rice flour, whole rye and whole-soy flour are all equally as healthful as whole-wheat flour. However, many of these grains lack gluten, the protein that makes flour easier to bake with. Many whole-grain flours are mixed with varying amounts of gluten-rich whole-wheat flour when they are intended to be used in baked goods. This is not a problem so long as the product is whole grain, so long as you are not gluten-sensitive.

Healthful products containing whole grains always contain at least some fiber. One way to determine if a product is "whole grain" or not when the labeling is not clear and the list of ingredients is lengthy or confusing is to look at the total carbohydrate content and the total fiber content. Healthful products contain at the very least 2 grams of fiber per 25 grams of total carbohydrate. Preferably, the packaged carbohydrate-containing foods you purchase such as cereal, bread, cake mix, crackers and snack foods, should contain at least 3 grams of fiber per 25 grams total carbohydrate. Take a look at this cereal label:

Nutrition Facts

Serving Size 3/4 cup
Servings Per Container 12

Amount Per Serving

Calories 110   **Calories from Fat 15**

	% Daily Value*
Total Fat 1.5 g	2%
Saturated Fat 0.5 g	3%
Trans Fat 0 g	
Cholesterol 0 mg	0%
Sodium 110 mg	5%
Total Carbohydrate 21 g	7%
Dietary Fiber 3 g	12%
Sugars 3 g	
Protein 3 g	

This is a healthy whole-grain product. Despite having only 21 grams of total carbohydrates per serving, there are 3 grams of fiber in each serving. In other words there are actually *more* than 3 grams of fiber in this product per 25 grams carbohydrate. Excellent choice!

One final word about flour: While whole-wheat flour is far better than highly refined "enriched" flour for both health and weight-loss purposes, whole-wheat berries are an even better choice. If weight loss is a top priority, try to eat less of your whole-grain servings in the form of whole-grain flour. All flours, even whole-grain flours, are a concentrated source of calories in comparison to the original whole-grain food. For example, one cup of corn flour contains 400 calories compared to one cup of cooked corn kernels containing just 130 calories. You'll feel more satiated and eat fewer calories if you choose the corn kernels over the corn flour. Sprouted whole-grain breads are a flourless, figure-friendly alternative to breads made with flour. It is now also possible to purchase sprouted whole-grain pastas made without flour (see appendix A for name-brand recommendations). Sprouted grains contain all of the nutrients, fiber, phytonutrients and antioxidants found in whole grains in a lower-calorie package.

Now that you have an idea of the "fake foods" to avoid, it's time to move on to exactly how you are going to reach your goal weight. So read on!

4

Plan Your Day's Meals with the "Fit-Body Plate"

B y now you have a good handle on how to identify healthful whole foods and how to read food labels. In this and the next chapter, we'll show you how to put healthful, balanced whole-foods meals together in a way that will maximize weight loss and health gain.

If you're following the *Fitter, Firmer, Faster* program to lose weight, you'll be happy to learn it is possible to achieve your weight loss goals without going to extremes. All too often excessively restrictive diets set the stage for failure. Thousands of people have successfully lost weight on our program—all without a sense of deprivation.

Calories Count, But Not All Calories Are Equal

Counting calories is definitely not the best way to lose weight for a variety of reasons. First, not all calories are equal. For example, although one-quater cup of raw nuts (a whole food) and one serving of cake (an empty-calorie food made with refined flour, partially hydro-genated soybean oil, and high fructose corn syrup) might both contain the same number of calories, your body is not going to metabolize those calories the same. The nutrients in the nuts will actually support a healthy metabolism and help your body convert the food into energy (as opposed to fat), and the cake will only provide empty calories and no nutrients. Therefore the cake calories are much more likely to make you fat. In addition, the empty calories from the cake won't make you feel as full and satiated as the nutrient-rich calories from the fibrous nuts. This means you'll end up having more food cravings and eating more calories later in the day if you've had the cake instead of the nuts.

The point is, when you choose nutrient-rich whole foods over empty-calorie foods your appetite becomes regulated *naturally* and you don't need to carry around a pocket calorie counter. This is one of the reasons we don't like people to count calories; it creates the wrong mind-set. If you're counting calories, psychologically you tend to categorize the nuts and cake as equal simply because they have the same number of calories per serving.

What Is a Calorie Exactly?

Before we go on, let's get the definition of a calorie straight. In scientific terms, the word "calorie" on food labels refers to a kilocalorie (kcal), which is the amount of energy required to raise 1 kilogram of water 1 degree Celsius. According to that definition, all calories are equal, and biochemically speaking, many experts agree that a calorie is a calorie. Yet, when you address the physiological effect of calories from different foods, the picture changes. For example, fiber-rich foods require your body to do a lot of work to process the fiber. All of this work burns calories, and so some of the calories in fiber-rich food are actually "lost" during the digestive process.

When you eat food a large number of complex chemical reactions take place in your body—these reactions depend on many factors, including the nutrient content of the food you eat. Did the food you eat contain a lot of sugar or a lot of refined flour? If so, your blood sugar levels will spike, and your body will need to produce a lot of "fat-storing" insulin to help transport that sugar into your cells. And did the food you eat contain trans fats (such as partially hydrogenated soybean oil)? If so, those trans fats are going to interfere with your body's ability to burn fat for energy.

Whole Foods Burn More Calories

Even eating an excess amount of omega-6 fats (such as eating too much refined vegetable oil) in relation to omega-3 fats (found in foods like fish and flax) can interfere with your metabolism and increase your risk of becoming overweight. However, if the food you ate was rich in phytonutrients, omega-3 essential fats, antioxidants, fiber and other nutrients, then your body is going to process those calories differently than it would process empty-calorie junk food. Your body is going to be able to extract the energy (calories) it needs from the nutrient-rich food, and it's going to be able to use the nutrients to support a healthy metabolism and burn fat for energy, fight free radicals, produce anti-inflammatory hormones, repair muscle, and so on. Choosing a food based on how many calories it contains does not take the fiber or nutrient content of the food into consideration and therefore doesn't accurately represent how the calories from different foods are going to be used and metabolized once eaten.

Building Balanced Whole-Foods Meals

By eating the proper balance of nutrients at every meal, you'll be able to reap the benefits of improved blood sugar control, reduced insulin secretion and appetite suppression. It's important to eat healthful whole-food sources of carbs, fats and protein. This means at breakfast, lunch and dinner you'll need to eat at least one serving from each of the following:

- **Nutrient- and Fiber-Rich Whole-Food Carbohydrates:** such as whole-grain pasta, whole-grain bread, brown rice, beans, corn, lentils, peas, potatoes, oatmeal, etc.
- **Vegetables and Fruits:** all vegetables and all fruits are healthy.
- **Flavor-Enhancing Fit Fats:** such as the monounsaturated fats found in extra-virgin olive oil, nuts, seeds, nut butters, olives and avocados, and the essential fats found in flaxseeds, flaxseed oil, walnuts, and canola oil.
- **Heart-Healthy Protein:** that is low in saturated fat. Heart-healthy

protein is found in lean cuts of meat, eggs, low-fat dairy, fish, soy and skinless white meat turkey and chicken.

The Benefits of Eating Whole-Foods Meals

Balanced whole-foods meals are guaranteed to keep your insulin secretion minimal, your blood sugar level stable and your hunger suppressed. The fats, proteins and fiber in balanced whole-foods meals slow down digestion of the carbohydrate-containing foods you eat while allowing you to enjoy the nutritional benefits and the antioxidants and phytonutrients found exclusively in whole-food carbohydrates. However, if you eat a carbohydrate such as a potato all by itself, the carbohydrate will be rapidly absorbed, which will result in a spike in your blood sugar level followed by a surge of insulin secretion. The surge of insulin will not only put your body in "fat storing mode," it will also lower your blood sugar so much that you will soon feel hungry again—which is not desirable if you are trying to control your weight. For example, if you add some fats, proteins, and fiber-rich vegetables to your potato—such as some chicken and broccoli with extra-virgin olive oil—you'll slow the digestion of your potato and reduce its ability to spike your blood-sugar level and cause the release of too much insulin. You'll also feel full longer on fewer calories and curb food cravings.

By following our balanced meal planning guidelines and eating only whole foods, you'll be able to enjoy numerous health and weight-loss benefits. Balanced whole-foods meals promote:

- Improved appetite control and reduced food cravings
- Increased sensitivity to the actions of insulin and therefore a reduced risk of developing type 2 diabetes or pre-diabetes, obesity and heart disease
- Reduced cholesterol levels; remember, insulin stimulates cholesterol production
- Improved management of type 2 diabetes
- Decreased triglyceride levels
- Enhanced ability to burn fat for energy

The Fit-Body Plate

To help you visualize what a balanced meal should look like we've devised a Fit-Body Plate based on nutrient- and fiber-rich whole-food carbs, heart-healthy protein, and vegetables/fruits. You'll then enhance the flavor and satiety of your meal by adding Fit Fats. We don't want you to get hung up on exact measuring; instead, just use the plate as a visual guidance. Because men need more total calories than women, men get a larger portion size than women (sorry, ladies).

Note: In addition to eating three balanced meals a day, you'll also be able to enjoy snacks, one small sweet treat, wine, coffee and tea.

The Fit-Body Plate

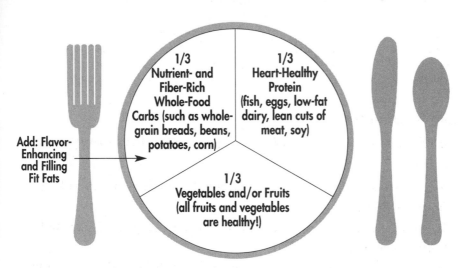

Vegetables and Fruits

For vegetables (see the list below), serving size is really not important. Since veggies are all low-calorie foods, you can eat as many and as much of them as you want.

For fruit (see the list below), follow these serving suggestions:
- Men: A fresh fruit serving is roughly the size of your closed fist. For dried fruit, one serving is ¼ cup.
- Women: A fresh fruit serving is roughly the size of your closed fist. For dried fruit, one serving is 2 tablespoons.

VEGETABLES/FRUITS

Vegetables		Fruits	
Artichoke	Green beans	Apples	Kiwi
Asparagus	Kale	Apricots	Lemons
Bell peppers	Leeks	Bananas	Limes
Bok choy	Mushrooms	Berries	Mango
Broccoli	Onions	(strawberries,	Nectarines
Broccoli rabe	Parsnip	blueberries,	Oranges
Brussels sprouts	Salad greens	raspberries,	Papaya
Butternut	(the darker	blackberries,	Peaches
squash	the better)	etc.)	Pears
Cabbage	Snap peas	Cantaloupe	Pineapple
Carrots	Snow peas	Cherries	Watermelon
Cauliflower	Spinach	Cranberries	
Celery	Squash	Dried fruit	
Collards	Tomatoes	(prunes, raisins,	
Eggplant	Tomato sauce	apricots, etc.)	
Fennel	Zucchini	Grapefruit	

Whole-Food Carbs

For whole-food carbs (see the list on page 58), follow these serving suggestions:

- **Men:** One serving is 1 cup cooked whole grains or 1½ cups high-fiber dry cereal.
- **Women:** One serving is ½ cup cooked whole grains or 1 cup high-fiber dry cereal.

For beans and legumes (see the list below), follow these serving suggestions:

- **Men:** One serving is 1 cup cooked beans or lentils.
- **Women:** One serving is ½ cup cooked beans or lentils.

NUTRIENT- AND FIBER-RICH WHOLE-FOOD CARBS

Whole-Grain Carbs	Bean/Legume Carbs
Amaranth	Adzuki beans
Barley	Anasazi beans
Brown rice	Black beans
Buckwheat	Black-eyed peas
Bulgur	Brown beans
Corn	Cannellini beans
Cracked wheat	Chickpeas
High-fiber dry cereal	Great northern beans
Kamut	Kidney beans
Millet	Lentils
Oats	Lima beans
Plain popcorn (1 serving = 2 cups for women and 3 cups for men)	Navy beans
	Peas
	Pinto beans
Polenta (whole grain only)	Split peas
Quinoa	
Rye berries	
Wheat berries	
Wheat germ	
Whole-grain pasta	
Whole wheat	
Whole-wheat couscous	
Wild rice	

For breads and crackers (see the list on page 59), follow these serving suggestions:

- **Men:** One serving is approximately 2 slices bread, 1 large pita, 4 tortillas or a large handful of crackers.
- **Women:** One serving is approximately 1 slice of bread, ¾ pita, 3 tortillas or a small handful of crackers.

For potato carbs (see list below), follow these serving suggestions:

- **Men:** One serving is 1 medium-sized potato, sweet potato or yam
- **Women:** One serving is ½ a medium-sized potato, sweet potato or yam.

NUTRIENT- AND FIBER-RICH BREADS, CRACKERS AND POTATOES

Breads & Crackers	Potatoes
Sprouted whole-grain bread	Potatoes
Stone-ground whole-wheat pita	Sweet potatoes
Stone-ground corn tortillas	Yams
Whole-grain bread (such as whole wheat)	
Whole-grain crackers	

Heart-Healthy Proteins

The fat in animal protein (not fish) consists mostly of bad saturated fat, so always purchase the leanest cuts (see the list on page 60) available. Always choose white-meat chicken and turkey as opposed to dark meat, and trim off all visible fat and skin—kitchen shears make snipping fat a snap. Remember: You don't want to eat more than 15 to 20 grams of saturated fat per day. Follow these serving suggestions for lean meats:

- **Men:** One lean animal protein is the size and thickness of your palm.
- **Women:** One lean animal protein is the size and thickness of your palm.

For fish and shellfish, follow these serving suggestions. *Note:* The fish with the asterisk (*) in the list on page 60 are the ones richest in omega-3 essential fats.

- **Men:** One serving fish or shellfish is the size and thickness of your palm.
- **Women:** One serving fish or shellfish is the size and thickness of your palm.

LEAN MEATS AND FISH

Lean Animal Protein	Fish and Shellfish
Beef (tenderloin, filet mignon, sirloin, eye of round, chuck, arm pot roast)	Anchovy*
	Black cod*
	Bluefin tuna*
Bison (buffalo)	Clams
Chicken (white meat, no skin)	Crab
Deer	Dolphin (mahimahi)
Elk	Flounder
Extra-lean chicken sausage	Grouper
Extra-lean ground turkey	Halibut
Lamb (the foreshank, leg, shanks half, stew meat, loin, shoulder, arm)	Herring*
	Lobster
	Mackerel*
Ostrich	Mussels
Pork (ham [boiled or cured] Canadian bacon, pork tenderloin, center cut pork loin chop, pork loin, pork sirloin chop and roast, top loin)	Orange roughy
	Oysters
	Sablefish*
	Salmon*
	Sardines*
Turkey (white meat, no skin)	Scallops
Turkey bacon	Sea bass*
Veal (leg, top round, loin, shoulder arm, sirloin)	Shrimp
	Snapper
	Striped bass*
	Tilapia
	Trout*
	White (albacore) tuna*

Choose "Extra-Lean" Over "Lean" Beef When Possible

Be extra careful to choose the leanest animal proteins possible (see next page) because there can be a significant difference in the amount of saturated fat in a lean cut as compared to a high-fat cut.

"Lean" and "Extra-Lean" Beef

"Lean"	"Extra-Lean"
One 4-ounce serving = 10 grams total fat and 4.5 grams saturated fat	One 4-ounce serving = 5 grams total fat and 2 grams saturated fat
Arm pot roast	Bottom round roast
Chuck shoulder roast	Eye of round roast
95% lean ground beef	Mock tender steak
Rib eye steak	Top round steak
Round tip roast	
Shoulder steak	
Strip steak	
Tenderloin steak	

Dairy and Soy

Choose these dairy and soy products (see below), noting that serving sizes vary by gender for each product.

Serving Sizes for Dairy Products

Men	Women
Eggs, omega-3 enriched eggs when possible, 2 whole eggs plus 2 egg whites = 1 serving	Eggs, omega-3-enriched eggs when possible, 2 whole eggs = 1 serving
Low-fat yogurt or low-fat kefir (plain, no sugar added), 1½ cups = 1 serving	Low-fat yogurt or low-fat kefir (plain, no sugar added), 1 cup = 1 serving
Low-fat milk, 1½ cups = 1 serving	Low-fat milk, 1 cup = 1 serving
Low-fat cheese, ½ cup = 1 serving	Low-fat cheese, ¼ cup = 1 serving
Low-fat cottage cheese, ¾ cup = 1 serving	Low-fat cottage cheese, ½ cup = 1 serving

Serving Sizes for Soy Products

Men	Women
Tofu, the size and thickness of your palm = 1 serving	Tofu, the size and thickness of your palm = 1 serving
Tempeh, the size and thickness of your palm = 1 serving	Tempeh, the size and thickness of your palm = 1 serving
Veggie burgers (made with soy protein), 2 burgers = 1 serving	Veggie burgers (made with soy protein), 1 burger = 1 serving
Textured vegetable protein (made from soy), 1 cup = 1 serving	Textured vegetable protein (made from soy), ½ cup = 1 serving
Soy milk, 1½ cups = 1 serving	Soy milk, 1 cup = 1 serving
Shredded veggie cheese, ¾ cup = 1 serving	Shredded veggie cheese, ½ cup = 1 serving
Edamame beans, 1 cup = 1 serving	Edamame beans, ½ cup = 1 serving
Soy nuts (also known as "dry roasted soybeans"), ½ cup = 1 serving	Soy nuts (also known as "dry roasted soybeans"), ¼ cup = 1 serving

Adding Flavorful and Filling Fit Fats to Your Fit-Body Plate

In addition to eating nutrient- and fiber-rich whole-food carbs, heart-healthy proteins, and vegetables and/or fruits at each and every meal, you'll also want to add some monounsaturated fats or essential fats (see the list on page 63) to your Fit-Body Plate to enhance the flavor and satiety of your meal.

Avoid nuts and seeds that have been roasted in oil. Only purchase raw nuts or dry roasted nuts. For nuts, seeds and nut butters follow these serving suggestions:

- **Men:** One serving of nuts or seeds is 3 tablespoons. One serving of nut butter is 1½ tablespoons.
- **Women:** One serving of nuts or seeds is 2 tablespoons. One serving of nut butter is 1 tablespoon.

For oils, follow these serving suggestions:
- Men: One serving is 1½ tablespoon.
- Women: One serving is 1 tablespoon.

FIT FATS AND OILS

Nuts, Seeds and Nut Butters	Oils
Almonds or all-natural almond butter (to repeat, all-natural means no hydrogenated oils and no partially hydrogenated oils, period)	Avocado oil, use for either no-heat recipes or high-heat recipes
Cashews or all-natural cashew nut butter	Expeller-pressed canola oil, use for no-heat recipes
Chestnuts	Expeller-pressed walnut oil, use for no-heat recipes
Hazelnuts or all-natural hazelnut butter	Extra-virgin coconut oil, use for either no-heat or high-heat recipes
Peanuts or all-natural peanut butter	Extra-virgin olive oil, use for either no-heat or high-heat recipes
Pecans, Pine nuts, Pistachios	Flax oil, use for no-heat recipes
Pumpkin seeds, dry roasted or raw	High-oleic canola oil, use for cooking
Sesame seeds, dry roasted or raw	High-oleic safflower oil, use for cooking
Sunflower seeds, dry roasted or raw	High-oleic sunflower oil, use for cooking
Tahini (sesame seed butter)	
Walnuts	

Healthy Vegetable Spreads	
Smart Balance	Earth Balance

High-Fat Condiments

Use these high-fat foods (see page 64) as condiments (serving sizes for each product vary by gender).

Serving Sizes for Condiments

Men	Women
Avocado, ¼ avocado = 1 serving	Avocado, 2–3 tablespoons = 1 serving
Butter, 2 teaspoons = 1 serving	Butter, 1 teaspoon = 1 serving
Ground flaxseeds, 3 tablespoons = 1 serving	Ground flaxseeds, 3 tablespoons = 1 serving
Olives, 15 small olives = 1 serving	Olives, 10 small olives = 1 serving
Canola oil–based mayonnaise, 1½ tablespoons = 1 serving	Canola-oil–based mayonnaise, 1 tablespoon = 1 serving
Hummus, ¼ cup = 1 serving. (Be sure the hummus you buy is made with either olive oil or expeller-pressed canola oil.)	Hummus, 2 tablespoons = 1 serving (Be sure the hummus you buy is made with either olive oil or expeller-pressed canola oil.)
Full-fat cheese (such as Gorgonzola or feta cheese), ¼ cup = 1 serving	Full-fat cheese (such as Gorgonzola or feta cheese), 3 tablespoons = 1 serving

Are You Really Hungry? Or Are You Just Thirsty? Or Bored?

If you feel as though you are hungrier than you really should be you might be mistaking thirst for hunger. Or maybe you are just bored. In either case, a beverage such as hot herbal tea or even broth can be a powerful appetite suppressant. If you drink a cup of hot herbal tea and wait ten minutes, you'll almost always suppress your appetite (you might also try adding just a little milk and a dash of honey). If tea doesn't work for you, drink organic vegetable (or chicken) broth. However, if after drinking the beverages and waiting ten or fifteen minutes you find you are still hungry, then eat! Just be sure to eat something healthy.

Indulging in Your "Vices"

Earlier we mentioned our lifestyle plan allows for coffee, tea, wine and even a daily sweet treat. We know these are all too often the first "vices" to go on many diet plans but not on our plan. Why? We live this lifestyle, and we realize no plan can work long-term for us or for anyone else if it's impossible to follow.

Furthermore, many of the "bad guy" vices have seen their images rehabilitated of late. As new research has dispelled worries and even pointed to potential health benefits, nutritionists are now welcoming favorite indulgences back into our kitchens. But before loosening your belt too far in eager anticipation, read on; moderation is essential if you want to "cheat" yet still succeed in gaining health and losing weight.

Enjoying Sweet Treats

It is acceptable to include one *small* "sweet treat" as part of your daily meal plan if desired. We define a "sweet treat" as a food made primarily from sugar and flour—in other words, something that we normally discourage on the *Fitter, Firmer, Faster* program. Your "sweet treat" can also include all-natural sources of saturated fat such as eggs, milk and butter . . . but these saturated fat grams do count toward your daily allotment!

Ideally, sweet treats should contain nuts and fruit whenever possible. But remember: Desserts absolutely *must* be all-natural, and they may never contain trans fats. A sample list of acceptable, all-natural desserts is included below.

ACCEPTABLE SWEET TREATS

All-natural ice cream
Bread puddings
Cakes made without vegetable
   shortening
Carrot cake
Cheesecake
Crème brûlée
Custards
Good-quality dark chocolate
   (made without hydrogenated
   or partially hydrogenated oils)

Homemade cookies
Mousse
Pastries (made without vegetable
   shortening)
Pumpkin pie
Soufflé
Strawberry shortcake
Sweet (dessert) wines
Sweet liqueurs, ports, brandies,
   sherries

Obviously the vast majority of desserts contain a significant amount of sugar. On average, a *small* serving of dessert contains four to five teaspoons of sugar. Many desserts are also made with refined, enriched flour. If you have the inclination to make your own desserts at home, why not make them more healthful by using at least some whole-wheat flour in place of the refined flour? Why not also try to reduce the sugar in your homemade desserts? Our dessert recipes (chapter 9) have about half the amount of sugar of regular desserts, plus they are made with whole-grain flours, and they are low in saturated fat and still delicious.

Size Does Matter

We allow this small dessert each day because total deprivation is not necessary or realistic . . . or fun. A small sweet treat a day is not going to ruin your health, make you fat or keep you from getting trim. However, "small" is an important word, especially when it comes to dessert. It is important to be clear here. As a general rule of thumb, rich desserts such as cheesecake, crème brûlée, brownie, pie or cake should be no larger than about *one inch thick* and half the size of your palm, not including your thumb and fingers. Servings of ice cream, puddings, mousse and soufflé should be no larger than half a cup, that's just *four ounces*. Lighter desserts made with fruit and flour only, containing a minimal amount of fat and cream, such as angel food cake, can be about *one inch thick* and the size of your palm but no more!

A final few words on the "sweet treat": Overweight people will see quicker weight loss if these treats are skipped (no surprises here). Also, no matter how much or how little you weigh, it is important from a health standpoint to eat *no more than one small dessert per day*. If you're too thin and you need to gain weight, add more healthful, nutrient-rich foods such as dried fruits and nuts, not more empty-calorie sweets.

Ivy has a definite sweet tooth. She's found she can satisfy her sweet tooth with just two or three small bites of a decadent dessert as opposed to an entire low-quality packaged dessert. Try a few bites of high-quality all-natural dark chocolate before reaching for your favorite low-quality processed dessert. Dark chocolate (only) contains high concentrations of cocoa, exceptionally rich in disease-fighting phytonutrients and antioxidants.

The Coffee Buzz

Coffee, when consumed in moderate amounts, is not harmful to your health. Besides helping you wake up to face the day with more enthusiasm than you might otherwise have, coffee offers potential health benefits. In fact, a Japanese study shows coffee consumption was associated with a decreased risk of death from all causes. Other benefits include a reduced risk of developing type 2 diabetes, Parkinson's disease and Alzheimer's disease.

There is no reason to switch from regular coffee to decaffeinated coffee in an attempt to improve your cardiovascular health. Coffee consumption at reasonable levels is unrelated to heart risk. Large population studies strongly suggest there is no relationship between caffeinated coffee consumption and heart disease. Although the caffeine in coffee can *temporarily* raise blood pressure, several extensive studies have shown coffee drinkers are no more likely than nondrinkers to suffer from chronic high blood pressure. Finally, some studies suggest decaf coffee may increase cholesterol levels in your blood. If you are going to drink coffee, we suggest you drink (and enjoy) the real thing, with one caveat: If you are sensitive to caffeine and have difficulty sleeping at night after having coffee later in the day, we suggest you limit your caffeine-containing coffee to the mornings only.

Black and Green Tea

Tea is a great-tasting alternative if you don't drink coffee. Teas are rich in antiaging antioxidants called flavonoids, special phytonutrients shown to be helpful in deactivating free radicals and fighting inflammation. Tea flavonoids have been shown to prevent the oxidation of "bad" LDL cholesterol, which could decrease your tendency to develop artery disease.

Some researchers believe the flavonoids in tea may interfere with one or more of the cell-damaging processes that ultimately lead to cancer. Other studies have shown green tea, but not black tea, to have thermogenic properties that could be helpful in fighting obesity.

Cheers to Wine

Here's something to raise your glass to: Alcohol, in moderation, does fit into the *Fitter, Firmer, Faster* program (assuming you are over the age of twenty-one). Moderation means no more than 1½ drinks per day for women and no more than 2½ drinks per day for men. One drink is equivalent to one 5-ounce glass of wine, one shot (1½ ounces) of hard liquor, or one 12-ounce beer. We strongly encourage wine over hard liquor and beer because wine contains antioxidants and is very low in sugar (hard liquor is low in sugar but contains no antioxidants; beer contains antioxidants yet most varieties contain a good deal of empty-calorie sugar). *Note:* Low-carb beers do contain significantly less sugar than regular beer, but they also contain significantly less antioxidants.

Here's the real kicker: Moderate wine consumption is not associated with weight gain. In April 1997, the *Journal of the American College of Nutrition* reported on a twelve-week crossover study. Fourteen men were given two glasses of wine to drink every day for six weeks, and then they were asked to abstain for six weeks. The men did not gain weight while they were drinking nor did they lose weight upon stopping. Two glasses of wine contain about two hundred calories. Over a six-week period these men should have gained about two and a half pounds, yet they did not. Researchers theorize the alcohol may enter a futile cycle where it is not metabolized in the same way as carbohydrates, fat or protein.

A more recent study showed that women who routinely drank moderate amounts of alcohol, totalling about one drink per day, carried almost ten pounds less body fat than women who did not drink at all. Prior to this, researchers at the Centers for Disease Control showed that, over a ten-year study period, drinking alcohol seemed to have very little effect on body weight. However, in this study, drinkers tended to gain less weight when compared with people who abstained from alcohol. In a similar ten-year study, drinkers actually displayed a slight tendency to *lose* weight.

What's more, many studies show *moderate* consumption of wine as part of an otherwise healthful lifestyle causes no negative health consequences and, for many people, provides health benefits. Studies in the medical literature such as the Copenhagen City Heart Study and the Framingham Heart Study have found that consuming wine in *moderation* is associated with an increased life expectancy. Wine can decrease arterial inflammation, reduce your risk of developing cardiovascular disease, and reduce your risk of stroke, Alzheimer's disease, and type 2 diabetes. Studies also suggest light-to-moderate drinkers are relatively more insulin sensitive than nondrinkers.

We certainly are not trying to suggest drinking alcohol is a smart way to shed pounds, but if you currently avoid drinking wine because you fear the calories, you can relax. Research shows wine does not lead to weight gain. Cheers!

Adjusting Your Meal Plan Based on Gender and Activity

By using the Fit-Body Plate and snack suggestions already mentioned, you should have a good idea of how to create balanced meals. In this section, we'll show you exactly what a day's worth of meals and snacks would be based on your gender and activity level. If your activity level varies from day to day, you'll want to adjust your meal plan accordingly. For example, on Monday you may fit into the "light activity" category if you sit at a computer all day, but on Tuesday you may fit into the "very active" category if you exercise by doing an hour-long workout; this means you'll need to eat more food on Tuesday than you need on Monday. Refer to the previous sections for suggested serving sizes based on your gender.

Women's and Men's Basic Meal Plan
for Very Light Activity

"Very Light" activity involves sitting at a desk the majority of the day, driving your car to work, reading and typing.

Breakfast
☐ 1 serving Fruits and/or Vegetables (unlimited vegetables are allowed)
☐ 1 serving Heart-Healthy Protein
☐ 1 serving Whole-Food Carbs
☐ 1 serving Fit Fats

Snacks
Note: The snack can be eaten at any time of the day.
☐ 1 serving Soy/Dairy

Lunch and Dinner
☐ 1 serving Fruits and/or Vegetables (unlimited vegetables are allowed)
☐ 1 serving Heart-Healthy Protein
☐ 1 serving Whole-Food Carbs
☐ 1 serving Fit Fats

Sweet Treat: You are allowed one *small* sweet treat a day. Please refer to pages 65–66 for a definition of "small" and an explanation of acceptable sweet treats.

Wine: Women are allowed 1 glass of wine and men are allowed 1½ glasses of wine with lunch or dinner.

Reminders
☐ One of your fat servings at some point during the day must be either flaxseeds or flaxseed oil.
☐ One of your protein servings at some point during the day must be either fish or soy.
☐ Limit your intake of saturated fat to 20 grams a day if you are healthy, 15 grams if you have an inflammatory or heart condition.

Women's and Men's Basic Meal Plan for Light Activity

"**Light**" activity would include shopping, running errands, child care, cooking and light housework. One trip to the grocery store is still considered very light activity, but several hours spent shopping or running errands bumps you up into the light category.

Breakfast
☐ 1 serving Fruits and/or Vegetables (unlimited vegetables are allowed)
☐ 1 serving Heart-Healthy Protein
☐ 1 serving Whole-Food Carbs
☐ 1 serving Fit Fats

Snacks
Note: The snack can be eaten at any time of the day.
☐ 1 serving Soy/Dairy
☐ 1 serving Fruit

Lunch and Dinner
☐ 1 serving Fruits and/or Vegetables (unlimited vegetables are allowed)
☐ 1 serving Heart-Healthy Protein
☐ 1 serving Whole-Food Carbs
☐ 1 serving Fit Fat

Sweet Treat: You are allowed one *small* sweet treat a day. Please refer to pages 65–66 for a definition of "small" and an explanation of acceptable sweet treats.

Wine: Women are allowed 1 glass of wine and men are allowed 1½ glasses of wine with lunch or dinner.

Reminders
☐ One of your fat servings at some point during the day must be either flaxseed or flaxseed oil.
☐ One of your protein servings at some point during the day must be either fish or soy.
☐ Limit your intake of saturated fat to 20 grams a day if you are healthy, 15 grams if you have an inflammatory or heart condition.

Women's and Men's Basic Meal Plan
for Moderate Activity

"**Moderate**" activity includes light daily activity plus a 30 to 35 minute moderate to high intensity exercise routine such as one of our *Fitter, Firmer, Faster* workouts. Several hours of outdoor work, such as light yard work, would also qualify as moderate activity so long as you are on your feet most of the time.

Breakfast
☐ 1 serving Fruits and/or Vegetables (unlimited vegetables are allowed)
☐ 1 serving Heart-Healthy Protein
☐ 1 serving Whole-Food Carbs
☐ 1 serving Fit Fats

Snacks
Note: The foods listed as snacks can be eaten at any time of the day.
☐ 1 serving Soy/Dairy
☐ 1 serving Fruit
☐ 1 serving Nuts/Seeds (choose from the Fit Fats category)

Lunch and Dinner
☐ 1 serving Fruits and/or Vegetables (unlimited vegetables are allowed)
☐ 1 serving Heart-Healthy Protein
☐ 1 serving Whole-Food Carbs
☐ 1 serving Fit Fat

Sweet Treat: You are allowed one *small* sweet treat a day. Please refer to pages 65–66 for a definition of "small" and an explanation of acceptable sweet treats.

Wine: Women are allowed 1 glass of wine and men are allowed 1½ glasses of wine with lunch or dinner.

Reminders
☐ One of your fat servings at some point during the day must be either flaxseed or flaxseed oil.
☐ One of your protein servings at some point during the day must be either fish or soy.
☐ Limit your intake of saturated fat to 20 grams a day if you are healthy, 15 grams if you have an inflammatory or heart condition.

Women's and Men's Basic Meal Plan for the Very Active

"Very Active" activity includes light daily activity plus a 30 to 35 minute moderate to high intensity *Fitter, Firmer, Faster* workout plus an extra 20 to 25 minutes of aerobic exercise. Alternatively, all-day heavy outdoor labor would qualify as very active.

Breakfast
☐ 1 serving Fruits and/or Vegetables (unlimited vegetables are allowed)
☐ 1 serving Heart-Healthy Protein
☐ 1 serving Whole-Food Carbs
☐ 1 serving Fit Fats

Snacks
Note: The foods listed as snacks can be eaten at any time of the day.
☐ 1 serving Soy/Dairy
☐ 1 serving Fruit
☐ 1 serving Nuts/Seeds (choose from the Fit Fats category)
☐ 1 serving Whole-Food Carbs

Lunch and Dinner
☐ 1 serving Fruits and/or Vegetables (unlimited vegetables are allowed)
☐ 1 serving Heart-Healthy Protein
☐ 1 serving Whole-Food Carbs
☐ 1 serving Fit Fats

Sweet Treat: You are allowed one *small* sweet treat a day. Please refer to pages 65–66 for a definition of "small" and an explanation of acceptable sweet treats.

Wine: Women are allowed 1 glass of wine and men are allowed 1½ glasses of wine with lunch or dinner.

Reminders
☐ One of your fat servings at some point during the day must be either flaxseed or flaxseed oil.
☐ One of your protein servings at some point during the day must be either fish or soy.
☐ Limit your intake of saturated fat to 20 grams a day if you are healthy, 15 grams if you have an inflammatory or heart condition.

Don't Get Hung Up on Rigid Serving Sizes

We provide guidelines for serving suggestions as a convenience to get you started, but we don't want you to get hung up on rigid guidelines. In the long run, consistently choosing healthful whole foods and eating balanced meals has much more to do with weight loss and health improvement than obsessing over serving sizes. Inflexibility regarding portion sizes can set you up for failure. Instead, learn to listen to your body. Eat when you are hungry; stop when you are full. No diet plan will be optimally effective if you eat for reasons other than for hunger. Fuel up primarily, ideally exclusively, on healthful, nutrient-rich foods. Limit the portion size of your "sweet treats" not the portion size of your balanced meals.

Now that you have and idea of how to fill your plate with suitable foods on the *Fitter, Firmer, Faster* program, you can look at our next chapter for two weeks of delicious menus!

5

Putting It All Together: Two Weeks of *Fitter, Firmer, Faster* Menus

The following *Fitter, Firmer, Faster* sample menus were created based on the approximate energy requirements for a moderately active woman. Please note these meal plans are intended as *guidelines* only. It is impossible to create a one-size-fits-all meal plan because calorie needs from individual to individual vary so greatly depending on a wide number of factors. If you are a very active woman or man, you'll need to eat more food than we suggest here. On the other hand, if you are sedentary, you'll need to eat less. We'd like you to look over the suggested menus so you can become acquainted with what a balanced whole-foods meal looks like. For the sake of convenience, you'll notice we've mixed in some healthful prepared foods. If you combine these meals with those provided in our earlier book, *The Gold Coast Cure,* you've got an entire month's worth of no-repeat whole-foods dining.

Day 1

Breakfast

1 toasted Van's All Natural "Wheat Free Gourmet Flax Waffle" topped with:

- 2 tablespoons chopped walnuts
- 1 teaspoon pure maple syrup
- ½ diced apple (softened in microwave for 45 seconds)
- Cinnamon, to taste

1 cup soy milk (such as Silk brand)

Coffee with organic half-and-half cream (or Silk brand soy milk creamer), or green tea with soy milk

Lunch

Toasted salmon sandwich with roasted red peppers:

- 2 pieces *sprouted* whole-grain bread, toasted
- ½ of a 7-ounce can Sockeye salmon
- 1 tablespoon canola oil mayonnaise
- Roasted red peppers (canned)

Snack

1 cup low-fat plain yogurt mixed with ½ cup fresh blueberries

Dinner

(Recipe for the following thirty-minute meal in chapter 10)

- Pasta a la Vodka
- Seared Chicken
- Salad of mixed greens with Italian dressing

1 glass of wine (optional)

Optional Sweet Treat

Strawberry ice cream cone (use 3 ounces Breyers "All Natural Strawberry" ice cream in an all-natural, trans-fat-free, cake-style cone such as Let's Do Organic brand)

Day 2

Breakfast

French toast with fresh blueberries and pure maple syrup:

- Spray a large nonstick skillet with canola oil cooking spray, and heat over medium-high heat.
- Meanwhile, in a medium-sized bowl, beat together 1 omega-3-enriched egg, a dash of pure vanilla extract, cinnamon to taste and 1 tablespoon organic, low-fat milk.
- Dip both sides of 2 pieces *sprouted* whole-grain bread into the egg mixture. Transfer bread to the heated skillet, and brown both sides.
- Top French toast with blueberries plus 1 teaspoon pure maple syrup and serve at once.

Coffee with organic half-and-half cream (or Silk brand soy milk creamer), or green tea with soy milk

Lunch

1 Kashi all-natural entree "Lemon Rosemary Chicken"
1 side salad with flaxseed oil and balsamic vinegar

Snack

Soy milk cappuccino (made from Silk brand unsweetened soy milk)
Small bowl of raspberries

Dinner

Grilled filet mignon
½ baked sweet potato (season with 1 teaspoon Smart Balance, a dash of nutmeg and 1 teaspoon honey)
Broccoli sautéed with garlic and extra-virgin olive oil
1 glass of wine (optional)

Optional Sweet Treat

Mixed berries with 1 tablespoon Kahlúa liqueur and 1 dollop fresh whipped cream

Day 3

Breakfast

Cinnamon-Blueberry Smoothie:

- Blend 1 cup soy milk (such as Silk brand), ½ cup frozen blueberries, 1 teaspoon cinnamon and 3 tablespoons ground flaxseeds in a blender, and process until smooth and creamy.
- Sweeten to taste with Splenda or stevia.

Coffee with organic half-and-half cream (or Silk soy milk creamer), or green tea with soy milk

Lunch

Butternut squash soup (such as Pacific Foods "Creamy Butternut Squash Soup")
Cobb Salad:

- Use 2 cups baby spinach leaves then top with 1 chopped hard-boiled omega-3-enriched egg, 2 ounces chopped ham, chopped roasted red peppers (look for high-quality canned roasted peppers) and 2 tablespoons crumbled low-fat feta cheese.
- Toss with 1 tablespoon dressing (such as Annie's Naturals "Roasted Red Pepper Vinaigrette").

Snack

1 slice toasted sprouted whole-grain bread topped with:

- 1 tablespoon all-natural peanut butter
- 1 teaspoon raw honey

Dinner

Side salad of mixed greens dressed with balsamic vinaigrette (made with flaxseed oil and balsamic vinegar) and cherry tomatoes
Mixed Mushroom and Rigatoni Bake with Gruyère (recipe in chapter 9)
1 glass of wine (optional)

Optional Sweet Treat

Mini banana split:

- Slice ½ banana lengthwise.
- Top with 2 tablespoons all-natural chocolate ice cream and 1 tablespoon finely chopped peanuts.

Day 4

Breakfast

¾ cup Kashi "Good Friends" cereal with:

- 1 tablespoon ground flaxseed (such as Barlean's brand)
- 1 cup low-fat plain kefir or yogurt
- Fresh blueberries

Coffee with organic half-and-half cream (or Silk brand soy milk creamer), or green tea with soy milk

Lunch

1 cup whole-grain pasta (choose *sprouted* whole-grain pasta if available) with:

- ½ cup prepared marinara sauce (such as Emeril's "Roasted Red Pepper Pasta Sauce")
- ½ cup organic low-fat mozzarella cheese

Snack

½ cup edamame (soybeans) or Smart Balance Popcorn (1½ cups)

Dinner

Grilled chicken with barbecue sauce
Corn on the cob
Grilled zucchini and mushroom kabobs
1 glass of wine (optional)

Optional Sweet Treat

Chocolate Blackberry Brownie Pudding (recipe in chapter 9)

Day 5

Breakfast

Tofu Vegetable Scramble (recipe in chapter 9)

1 slice *sprouted* whole-grain bread, toasted, topped with 1 teaspoon Earth
Balance or Smart Balance spread

Coffee with organic half-and-half cream (or Silk brand soy milk creamer), or
green tea with soy milk

Lunch

Tabbouleh salad

Sliced red peppers dipped in 2 tablespoons hummus (look for hummus made
with extra-virgin olive oil)

Rotisserie chicken breast (remove skin)

½ cup pineapple chunks

Note: The tabbouleh, hummus and rotisserie chicken can be found in the deli
section of your supermarket.

Snack

1 sliced Anjou pear

1 wedge soft, light Swiss cheese (such as The Laughing Cow "Light Swiss
Original")

Dinner

Salad of mixed greens with Creamy Tarragon Dressing (recipe in chapter 9—
contains flaxseed oil)

Turkey burger (use extra-lean ground turkey) with:

• Thinly sliced avocado *or* Roasted Red Pepper and Walnut Tapenade
(tapenade recipe in chapter 9)

• 1 Alvarado Street Bakery "*Sprouted* Wheat Burger Buns" (toasted)

1 glass of wine (optional)

Optional Sweet Treat

Fresh strawberries drizzled with hot chocolate sauce (to make chocolate
sauce: in a microwave-safe dish combine 1 tablespoon dark gourmet
chocolate mini chips with 1 teaspoon light cream, and microwave on high
for 30 seconds, or until chocolate melts) and 2 tablespoons finely chopped
walnuts

Day 6

Breakfast
Almond-Flax Pancakes with Raspberries (recipe in chapter 9—contains flaxseeds)
Coffee with organic half-and-half cream (or Silk brand soy milk creamer), or green tea with soy milk

Lunch
Amy's frozen "Santa Fe Enchilada Bowls"
Chopped tomato salad with extra-virgin olive oil and balsamic vinegar

Snack
Reese Cup Baked Apple:

- Core an apple and split it in half lengthwise; place apple in a bowl, cut-side up, and spread both apple halves with 1 tablespoon all-natural peanut butter.
- Arrange 4 or 5 "mini" dark chocolate chips on top of each apple half. Microwave on high for 1½ minutes or until apple is soft and chocolate is melted.

Dinner
Pan-seared tilapia
Brown rice pilaf with garlic, shallots and parsley (use extra-virgin olive oil)
Green beans (try Birds Eye "Herb Garden Collection: Green Beans with Thyme")
1 glass of wine (optional)

Optional Sweet Treat
1 square dark chocolate

Day 7

Breakfast

Hot cereal (place the following ingredients in microwave-safe bowl and heat for 1½ minutes or until creamy):

- ½ cup old-fashioned oats
- ¾ cup soy milk (such as Silk brand)
- 2 tablespoons chopped walnuts
- 1 tablespoon ground flaxseed (such as Barlean's brand)
- ½ chopped apple
- Cinnamon, to taste

Coffee with organic half-and-half cream (or Silk brand soy milk creamer), or green tea with soy milk

Lunch

Almond butter (or peanut butter) sandwich on toasted *sprouted* whole-grain bread:

- 2 tablespoons all-natural almond butter (or all-natural peanut butter)
- 2 slices toasted whole-grain bread (such as Food for Life "Ezekiel 4:9 Sprouted Grain Bread")

1 cup organic low-fat yogurt or kefir
Carrot sticks

Snack

Kashi "Honey Almond Flax Chewy Granola Bars"
or 2 cups Smart Balance Popcorn

Dinner

Baked salmon brushed with gourmet fruit-flavored mustard (such as Napa Valley "Apricot-Ginger Mustard" or Terrapin Ridge "Orange Cranberry Mustard")
Millet
Roasted red peppers (use extra-virgin olive oil)
1 glass of wine (optional)

Optional Sweet Treat

1 small serving chocolate pudding (such as Kozy Shack "Real Chocolate Pudding")

Day 8

Breakfast

1 slice toasted Hemp Sprouted Bread (by French Meadow Bakery) topped with
    1 tablespoon apple butter
2 hard- or soft-boiled omega-3-enriched eggs (such as Eggland's Best)
Fresh sliced peaches
Coffee with organic half-and-half cream (or Silk brand soy milk creamer), or
    green tea with soy milk

Lunch

Stuffed baked potato with:

- ¼ cup diced extra-firm tofu
- ½ cup tomato sauce (such as Amy's "Premium Organic Puttanesca Sauce")
- ¼ cup shredded low-fat organic cheese

Note: Place baked potato in the microwave to melt cheese

Snack

1 whole-grain cracker (such as Ryvita Rye Crackers) topped with:

- 2 ounces smoked salmon (lox)
- 1 teaspoon organic Neufchatel cheese (such as Organic Valley)

½ cup fresh berries

Dinner

Gazpacho (recipe in chapter 9)
Grilled shrimp and vegetable kabobs
Whole-grain dinner roll (such as Alexia Whole Grain) dipped in:

- Flaxseed oil (such as Barlean's brand)
- Parmesan cheese
- Freshly ground pepper

1 glass of wine (optional)

Optional Sweet Treat

1 oatmeal cookie (such as Barbara's Bakery "Old Fashioned Oatmeal Crisp
    Cookies")

Day 9

Breakfast

1 slice toasted French Meadow Bakery brand "Women's Bread" or "Men's
 Bread" topped with:

- 1 tablespoon all-natural peanut butter
- ½ banana

1 cup organic plain low-fat yogurt or kefir
Coffee with organic half-and-half cream (or Silk brand soy milk creamer), or
 green tea with soy milk

Lunch

Spinach salad with flax oil and balsamic vinegar
Amy's frozen entrée "Tofu and Vegetable Lasagna"

Snack

Tortilla chips (such as Kettle Organic Tortilla Chips "Blue Corn")
Salsa

Dinner

(Recipe for the following thirty-minute meal in chapter 10)

Parmesan Fish Bake
Lemony Corn Chowder
Tomato Salad with Balsamic Vinaigrette

1 glass of wine (optional)

Optional Sweet Treat

1 small brownie (use an all-natural mix such as Hodgson Mill "Brownie Mix
 with Whole Wheat Flour and Milled Flaxseed") topped with fresh
 raspberries

Day 10

Breakfast

½ toasted whole-grain English muffin (such as Thomas' English Muffins Hearty Grains "100% Whole Wheat") topped with 1 tablespoon all-natural nut butter
Sliced oranges
½ cup organic low-fat cottage cheese
Coffee with organic half-and-half cream (or Silk brand soy milk creamer), or green tea with soy milk

Lunch

Turkey and black bean chili (such as Shelton's "Turkey Chili with Beans")
Sliced tomatoes drizzled with flaxseed oil and seasoned with salt and shredded Parmesan cheese

Snack

1 sliced apple spread with The Laughing Cow "Light Soft Gourmet Swiss Cheese"

Dinner

Indonesian Baked Tofu with Peanut Sauce (recipe in chapter 9)
Brown rice
Roasted asparagus (with extra-virgin olive oil)
1 glass of wine (optional)

Optional Sweet Treat

1 small serving flan (such as Kozy Shack "Crème Caramel Flan")

Day 11

Breakfast

Ricotta with cherries:

- ½ cup low-fat organic ricotta
- ½ cup pitted cherries (use fresh or frozen)

1 slice toasted sprouted whole-grain bread dipped in 1 teaspoon flaxseed oil
(such as Barlean's brand)

Coffee with organic half-and-half cream (or Silk brand soy milk creamer), or
green tea with soy milk

Lunch

Salad of mixed greens topped with:

- ½ package of StarKist Tuna Creations "Sweet and Spicy Flavor"
  mixed with 1 tablespoon Hellmann's canola oil mayonnaise

Split pea soup (such as Tabatchnick "Split Pea Soup")

Snack

1 cup low-fat plain kefir or yogurt

½ cup fresh strawberries

2 tablespoons ground flaxseed (such as Barlean's brand)

Dinner

Pork chops with chutney (look for high-quality prepared chutney such as
Silver Palate "Spiced Cranberry Apple Chutney" or "Mango Chutney")

Baked sweet potato fries (such as Alexia "Sweet Potato Hanna Gold Julienne
Fries")

Leeks sautéed with garlic and extra-virgin olive oil

1 glass of wine (optional)

Optional Sweet Treat

Tart Persian Lime Custard (recipe in chapter 9)

Day 12

Breakfast
Muesli cereal with fresh strawberries:
- ⅔ cup no-sugar added muesli (such as Alpen "No Sugar Added Muesli")
- 1 cup low-fat plain yogurt or kefir
- ¾ cup fresh sliced strawberries
- 2 tablespoons ground flaxseed (such as Barlean's brand)

Coffee with organic half-and-half cream (or Silk brand soy milk creamer), or green tea with soy milk

Lunch
Creamy carrot soup (such as Pacific Foods "Creamy Roasted Carrot Soup")
Chicken Sausage in a bun:
- Han's All-Natural "Gourmet Sausage Apple-Spokane Chicken"
- *Sprouted* whole-grain hot dog bun (such as Alvarado Street Bakery "Sprouted Hot Dog Buns" or Food for Life "Sprouted Wheat Hot Dog Buns")

Snack
Small handful of almonds
Sliced plum

Dinner
Pan-Roasted Red Snapper with Jalapeno-Pineapple Salsa (recipe in chapter 9)
Quinoa
Sautéed broccoli rabe (sauté in extra-virgin olive oil and garlic)
1 glass of wine (optional)

Optional Sweet Treat
Peanut butter cookie (use an all-natural mix such as Arrowhead Mills "Peanut Butter Cookie Mix")

Day 13

Breakfast

1 cup low-fat plain kefir or yogurt with:

- 1 cup fresh blueberries
- 3 tablespoons ground flaxseed (such as Barlean's brand)
- Cinnamon, to taste

Coffee with organic half-and-half cream (or Silk brand soy milk creamer), or green tea with soy milk

Lunch

Chicken, cheese and vegetable roll-up—use a whole-grain tortilla (such as Food for Life "Ezekiel 4:9 Sprouted Grain Tortillas") and stuff with the following:

- 3 ounces chicken breast
- 1 ounce organic low-fat shredded cheese
- Baby spinach leaves
- Diced red peppers

Snack

Lemon-Peach Pie Smoothie (recipe in chapter 9—contains soy)

Dinner

Spice-Rubbed Lamb Kabobs with Tahini Sauce (recipe in chapter 9)
Whole-wheat couscous
Grilled Vegetables
1 glass of wine (optional)

Optional Sweet Treat

1 small slice pumpkin pie (make your own, or try Wholly Healthy "Truly Natural Pumpkin Pie")

Day 14

Breakfast

Baked apple with macadamia nuts and cheese:

- Core a Granny Smith apple and split it in half lengthwise. Place apple in a microwave-safe bowl, cut side up, and sprinkle with a generous amount of cinnamon.
- Place 2 tablespoons finely chopped macadamia nuts in both sides of the hollowed apple halves and top with ¼ cup shredded low-fat organic cheddar cheese. Microwave on high for 2 minutes.
- Optional: Top with 1 teaspoon pure maple syrup.

Coffee with organic half-and-half cream (or Silk brand soy milk creamer), or green tea with soy milk

Lunch

Bowl of vegetable and bean soup (such as Wolfgang Puck's "Thick and Hearty Lentil and Vegetable")
Side salad of mixed greens with:

- Balsamic vinegar, to taste
- 1 tablespoon flaxseed oil (such as Barlean's brand)
- 2 ounces chopped ham

Snack

1 hard-boiled omega-3-enriched egg (such as Eggland's Best)
Whole-grain crackers (such as Dr. Kracker "Pumpkin Seed and Cheese")

Dinner

Tofu Parmesan (recipe in chapter 9)
Creamed spinach (such as Tabatchnick "Creamed Spinach")
Corn (use frozen thawed corn kernels seasoned with extra-virgin olive oil, salt and coarsely ground black pepper)
1 glass of wine (optional)

Optional Sweet Treat

Fresh mixed berries with a tablespoon of mini dark chocolate chips and a dollop of fresh whipping cream

6

Get Your Kids on the Fit Track

I t's never too late, or too early, to start eating healthfully. The growing bodies and brains of children need nutrient-rich foods just as much, if not more so, than adults. On top of that, the demographics of disease are changing. Children are growing up sicker and heavier at younger and younger ages. Yes, children still enjoy innate protection from some degenerative conditions such as senility and heart disease, but they are not immune from obesity, type 2 diabetes, high cholesterol, and inflammation-mediated conditions such as asthma and allergies—all of which can be prevented or greatly improved by following our lifestyle program.

The *Fitter, Firmer, Faster* program is designed for your entire family to follow together. Keep in mind that the earlier you introduce a healthy, whole-foods diet to your child the more receptive he will be. We firmly believe teaching your child how to live healthfully is one of the greatest gifts you as a parent can give. Proper nutrition in childhood establishes lifelong habits that contribute to his health and overall well-being for decades to come.

Many children living in today's "Fast Food Planet" are being shortchanged when it comes to good nutrition. The president of the Robert Wood Johnson Foundation, Risa Lavizzo-Mourey, M.D., M.B.A., was recently quoted as saying, "We are in danger of raising the first generation of American children who will be sicker and die younger than the generation before them." That's a dismal statement. Certainly there is reason for concern, but not despair. With proper parental intervention, it is still possible to raise fit and healthy children.

Leading by Example

As parents ourselves, we know helping children with lifestyle changes, especially when it comes to the foods they consume, is often easier said than done. But we have learned it is possible. Parents have more control than they realize. First, don't go out of your way to look for trouble. Don't wait for your child to throw a temper tantrum when you serve grilled chicken instead of tater tots and chicken wings. Expect more. You'll be amazed to see the powerful influence you have on your children's food choices. Research shows children are often more willing to eat nutritious foods and be active if they see their parents and other family members embrace a healthful lifestyle. Just remember, foundation is everything.

Parents are almost always responsible for buying and storing the family's food supply. If you simply refuse to buy junk food, your kids will already be way ahead of the game. By default they're going to eat healthfully the vast majority of the time, at least at home. Sure, they might sneak junk when you're not looking, but how much junk can they realistically sneak . . . if there isn't any junk in the house?

Top Seven Nutrition Tips for Kids

The guidelines regarding nutrition are the same for children as they are for adults. Here we've included seven kid-friendly tips. Try having your children adopt just one of the following nutrition tips every day for seven days. By the end of the week they'll be well on their way to eating healthfully for life.

Top #1: Toss the Soda, Limit the Juice

Soda is obviously not a healthful choice for kids. We don't need to spend time explaining why your child can do without an additional

10 teaspoons of sugar—the amount contained in one 12-ounce can of soda—added to her diet. However, many parents think juice is a healthy alternative to soda. A word of caution is in order here. Many products marketed to children as "juice" are not 100 percent juice; they're nothing more than sugar water. Be sure to read the list of ingredients! You only want to purchase 100 percent juice; *any* amount of added sugar is too much.

Nevertheless, any way you pour it, juice provides a much more concentrated source of calories with fewer nutritional benefits as compared to whole fruit. It's also very easy to overconsume juice because it is fiber-free and therefore less filling than the whole fruit. Fruit juice is especially undesirable for overweight children. Try to get your kids in the habit of drinking water. If they hate the taste of plain water, try diluting juice with water by combining 1 part 100 percent juice with 3 parts water. This mixture can be stored in a large pitcher in your fridge and can last several days.

Tip #2: Get Them on the Whole-Grain Train

Whole-grain foods provide the vitamins, essential fats, fiber and antioxidants needed by the growing bodies of children. By increasing your child's intake of whole grains you'll cut their risk of obesity and type 2 diabetes and provide them with protection against certain types of cancer in adulthood. Only purchase 100 percent whole-grain breads (or sprouted whole-grain bread), buns, cereals and crackers and switch to whole-grain pasta. Use brown rice instead of white rice and whole-grain flours when baking. Don't forget about the "classic" whole grains most kids love: oatmeal, barley, corn and even popcorn. These high-energy foods should be encouraged, not limited.

Tip #3: Increase "Good" Essential Fats

The essential fats are the good fats, and they're necessary for the proper development and function of your child's brain and immune system. These good fats have been shown to improve mood and decrease childhood behavior problems such as hyperactivity and attention deficit disorders.

As you'll recall from chapter 3, you need a balance of both omega-3 and omega-6 fats to support optimal health and to help prevent the insulin resistance that can pave the way for obesity and type 2 diabetes. Omega-3 fats are found mostly in fish, ground flaxseed and flaxseed oil, walnuts, and omega-3-enriched eggs. As parents we understand it's not always easy, or even possible, to get kids to eat fish so we do recommend a high-quality fish oil supplement in chapter 11. Don't worry, all of the supplements we suggest are very high quality and they don't taste the least bit fishy. You can tell your kids it is vitamin "X"; they won't know the difference. Omega-6 fats are found in nuts, seeds, soy products and even whole grains.

We've had great success sneaking "Kids Power Powder" into our son's food. Mix it up ahead of time, then store it in the refrigerator in a covered container for up to a week. Add a tablespoon or two to your children's cereals, waffle and pancake mixes, yogurts, and smoothies for an essential-fat boost they'll love. Here's how you make it:

Kids Power Powder

Makes eight 2-tablespoon servings

¼ cup sunflower seeds	¼ cup wheat germ
¼ cup sesame seeds	2 teaspoons brown sugar
¼ cup ground flaxseed	½ teaspoon cinnamon

Directions: Mix all of the ingredients in a coffee grinder or food processor, then store in a sealed container in the refrigerator for up to seven days.

Nutrition Information: 100 calories, 1 g saturated fat, 6 g carbohydrate, 3 g dietary fiber, 4 g protein

---

Tip #4: Say Goodbye to Trans Fat

There is no safe level of intake for these deadly, empty-calorie trans fats. These fats are much more harmful than the natural saturated fat found in foods such as butter. Trans fats increase your child's risk of obesity and type 2 diabetes and exacerbate inflammation-related conditions such as asthma and allergies.

Because trans fats greatly increase artery inflammation, children who start eating a steady diet of processed foods loaded with these artificial processed fats can be expected to develop heart problems as adults at a much younger age than kids who eat a trans fat–free diet. Researchers have shown children as young as ten years old can develop the cholesterol plaques that eventually clog arteries. As a parent you can take steps to clear trans fats from your kids plates. Take a look back in chapter 3 for how to avoid these dangerous fats.

Tip #5: Serve Three Fruits and Two Veggies Every Day

Most kids love fruit, so you shouldn't have too much of a problem getting them to eat it. We find it easiest for our own son to meet his "three fruits" daily quota by always serving it with his breakfast and including it as part of his dessert after dinner. It's easy to fit the third piece in either for lunch or as a snack.

We often rely on thawed frozen fruits for convenience—especially for smoothies and for snazzing up cold cereal, yogurt and oatmeal. We also give our son "no-sugar-added" applesauce and canned fruit packed in water for his school lunch. Frozen grapes, frozen bananas and frozen watermelon are another big hit.

Since many kids don't like anything green, you might need some creativity when serving up kid-friendly veggies. Try these ideas:

1. **Tree Tops with Cheese:** Use a small handful of thawed frozen broccoli tops then top with ¼ cup organic shredded cheese. Melt in the microwave for 1½ minutes or until the cheese melts. Season with salt to taste, then serve.

2. **Honey-Glazed Matchstick Carrots:** Place a handful of ready-to-eat matchstick carrots in a microwave-safe bowl, then dot with a dab of butter and ½ teaspoon honey. Microwave on high for 1½ to 2 minutes or until soft. Season with salt to taste, and serve.

3. **Home-Run Pasta Sauce:** In a large saucepan, heat 2 tablespoons extra-virgin olive oil. Add 1 chopped garlic clove, 1 cup chopped onion, 1 cup chopped red pepper, and 1 cup ready-to-eat matchstick carrots. Sauté until vegetables are soft-tender. Mix in a

25-ounce bottle of a mild prepared tomato sauce (such as Emeril's "Mushroom and Onion Pasta Sauce") plus 2 teaspoons brown sugar. Cover and simmer for 5 minutes. Allow sauce to cool, then transfer to a food processor or blender and puree in small batches until smooth and creamy. (*Note:* This is a great way for kids to enjoy the benefits of a number of different vegetables all at once. You can freeze this sauce in small batches or store it in a covered container in the refrigerator for up to seven days.)

4. **Cucumber Salad:** In a small bowl whisk together 2 teaspoons flaxseed oil, 2 teaspoons apple cider vinegar, 1 teaspoon brown sugar, and ⅛ teaspoon salt. Peel and then thinly slice one cucumber; toss the cucumber slices and the dressing in a zipper-top plastic bag. Marinate in the refrigerator for 15 minutes. Serve cold.

5. **Popeye's Favorite Creamed Spinach:** Heat 2 teaspoons butter and 1 teaspoon extra-virgin olive oil in a medium-sized skillet. Add ¼ cup diced onion, then sauté until the onion is tender. Remove skillet from heat, and stir in 1 tablespoon whole-wheat flour. Transfer onion mixture to a blender or food processor and add ¼ cup whole milk plus one 10-ounce package thawed frozen spinach, drained and patted dry with paper towels. Puree spinach and the onion together until smooth and creamy. Return spinach to the skillet and heat through. Add salt to taste plus a dash of nutmeg and serve.

Tip #6: Don't Deny Dessert, but Make It Healthy

Kids, like adults, should be allowed to enjoy a treat now and then. While sweets are not health food, there are ways to make your kids "sweet treats" more nutritious.

For example, sneak in some fruit in the form of a blueberry cobbler (recipe in chapter 9) or an ice-cream sundae made with bananas and strawberries. Mix some nuts or nut butter into your child's dessert by making peanut butter cookies or try our recipe for Palm Beach Pineapple-Walnut Bread Cake in chapter 9. You can even add whole grains to desserts if you substitute whole-grain flour for the white refined stuff.

Tip #7: Choose Low-Fat Animal Foods

While kids don't need to be on a low-fat diet, they do benefit from a "good" fat diet. Animal fats are not the "good" fats. Animal fat is mostly saturated fat, the type of fat that's bad for your heart and increases inflammation, therefore exacerbating conditions such as asthma and allergies.

Replace animal fat with the good monounsaturated fats in nuts, seeds, avocados, olives and nut butters as well as the essential fats found in fish, flax, walnuts and omega-3-enriched eggs. Here are the three most important steps you can take to reduce the amount of animal fat (saturated fat) in your child's diet:

1. Use butter in moderation. Cook with extra-virgin olive oil or high-oleic canola oil. Use whipped butter or trans-fat-free spreads such as Earth Balance to top your children's whole-grain toast.
2. Choose low-fat (1% or 2%) cheese, milk, yogurt and kefir. Try to choose organic dairy foods when possible.
3. Choose only the leanest cuts of meat, then meticulously trim all the visible fat.

Use the Fit-Body Plate to Build Healthy Family Meals

An easy way to make sure your child is eating a balanced meal is to use the guidelines for our Fit Body Plate in chapter 4. Children need the same basic balance of nutrient- and fiber-rich whole-food carbs, fruits, vegetables, heart-healthy protein and fit fats as adults; they just might need smaller or larger quantities depending on their age, activity level and gender.

For example, active teenage boys in particular can require a surprisingly tremendous number of calories a day to fuel both growth and activity. But the bottom line is children and teenagers require the same balanced intake of whole foods as do adults to stay healthy, perform their best, have energy and reduce their risk of developing chronic diseases.

Don't Be Overly Portion-Savvy with Kids

As a general rule you should *not* limit the portion sizes of the healthy nutrient-rich whole foods your child eats. Instead, provide him with three healthful balanced meals a day and allow for healthy snacks. However, you *should* limit the portion size of junk food or "sweet treats." Like adults, children shouldn't eat more than one "sweet treat" a day, even if they are not overweight. If your child is underweight he should eat more calorie-dense high-nutrient foods such as nuts, seeds and dried fruit. No junk food would be best, but we realize this isn't very realistic.

Note: In some instances it may be necessary to be somewhat stricter with portion size if your child or teenager is very obese. Consult with a trained medical professional who is certified in bariatric medicine before limiting the calories in your child's diet.

Eight-Minute "Happy Morning" Breakfasts

The following five breakfasts take about eight minutes to make, from start to finish. If you set your alarm just eight minutes earlier, you'll be on your way to making sure your kids get their best possible start for their day. Studies show children who eat breakfast have better test scores, improved behavior and increased attention spans at school. Children who eat a healthy breakfast are also more likely to meet their daily nutritional needs, maintain healthy body weights, and have lower blood cholesterol levels. Each of our breakfast suggestions provides a kid-friendly balanced meal packed with protein, fiber, essential fats and fruit—can't beat that combination as a great way to start the day!

Toasted Whole-Grain Waffle

(Such as Van's "All Natural Wheat Free Gourmet Waffles" in "Apple Cinnamon," "Blueberry" or "Flax") topped with:

- 2 tablespoons chopped nuts (such as walnuts or pecans)
- 1 teaspoon pure maple syrup
- ½ cup thawed frozen fruit (such as blueberries or peaches)

Power Oatmeal with Apple Tidbits

Combine the following ingredients in a microwave-safe bowl, stir, then heat in the microwave for 1½ minutes:

- ⅓ cup old-fashioned oats
- 2 tablespoons Kids Power Powder (see page 93)

- ⅓ cup chopped dried apples (you can also substitute chopped dried apricots, raisins, etc.)
- ½ cup soy milk (such as Silk brand) or organic low-fat milk
- Cinnamon, to taste
- 1 teaspoon pure maple syrup (optional)

French Toast with Peaches and Honey

1. Spray a large nonstick skillet with canola oil cooking spray and heat over medium-high heat.
2. Meanwhile, in a medium-sized bowl, beat together 1 whole omega-3-enriched egg, a dash of pure vanilla extract, cinnamon to taste and 1 tablespoon organic low-fat milk.
3. Dip both sides of 2 pieces whole-grain bread in the egg mixture. Transfer bread to the heated skillet and brown on both sides.
4. Top French toast with thawed frozen peaches plus 1 teaspoon raw honey. Serve at once.

Scrambled Eggs, Toast and Fruit

1. Beat together two omega-3-enriched eggs with 1 tablespoon low-fat cottage cheese, 1 tablespoon of milk and salt to taste.
2. Spray a large nonstick skillet with canola oil cooking spray and heat over medium-high heat. Scramble the eggs until cooked through.
3. Serve with whole-grain toast (such as Alvarado Street Bakery "Ultimate Kids Bread") and fruit. For convenience, serve thawed frozen fruits such as blueberries, raspberries or peaches.

Blueberry Surprise Smoothie

Combine the following ingredients in a blender, then process until smooth and creamy, about 1 minute:

- 1 cup soy milk (such as Silk brand) or organic low-fat milk
- ¾ cup frozen blueberries
- 1 to 2 teaspoons raw honey
- 1 tablespoon ground flaxseeds (such as Barleans)
- 1 tablespoon wheat germ

Mix-and-Match Lunch Box Ideas

Don't rely on the school to provide your child with a healthful lunch. Anyone who has seen the documentary *Super Size Me* can attest to the atrocities of school-supplied "nutrition." Instead, use our helpful "Mix-and-Match" guide below you so you can put together a tasty, nutritious lunch you and your child can both be happy about. Just choose one item from each of the four categories.

Beverages/Fruits & Vegetables

Category #1: Beverages	Category #2: Fruits and Vegetables
Boxed, long-life "Chocolate Soy Milk" (by Silk)	Del Monte "Pineapple Tidbits in 100% Juice" (packaged in plastic cups)
Boxed, long-life "Organic Low-fat Milk" (by Horizon Organics)	Del Monte "Diced Peaches in 100% Juice" (packaged in pull-top cans)
Boxed, long-life "Plain Soymilk" (by Edensoy)	Mott's "Healthy Harvest Apple Sauce" with no sugar added (flavors include "Country Berry," "Summer Strawberry" and "Peach Medley")
Thermos with ¼ cup 100% juice and ¾ cup water	Fresh apple slices (To prevent the apples from turning brown, sprinkle with a ½ teaspoon of sugar and 2 teaspoons of lemon juice, then place them in a sealed plastic bag.)
One bottle of Fruit Water by Glaceau (all-natural, low-sugar, fruit-flavored water with no artificial sweeteners or chemical preservatives— flavors include lemon, peach, raspberry and grape)	Edamame beans (put them in your child's lunchbox while still frozen and sprinkle them with a little bit of salt)

Main Dishes & Treats

Category #3: Main Dishes	Category #4: Treats
2 hardboiled eggs with whole-grain crackers (Try "Triscuit Reduced Fat Whole Grain Crackers.")	Kashi chewy or crunchy granola bars
PB&J sandwich (Use all-natural peanut butter or almond butter, whole-grain bread such as Alvarado Street Bakery "Ultimate KIDS Bread," and an all-fruit spread such as Smucker's "Simply 100% Fruit Spread.")	All-natural pudding or flan—Kozy Shack (flavors include "Crème Caramel Flan," "Original Rice Pudding," Old Fashioned Tapioca," "Real Chocolate Pudding," "Natural Vanilla Pudding," "Dulce de Leche," "Creamy Banana," and "Cinnamon Raisin Rice")
Pita Pocket stuffed with turkey and cheese (Use a whole-grain pita such as Toufayan "Oat Bran Pita" or "Whole Wheat Pita" and low-fat organic cheese.)	Garden of Eatin' "Black Bean Chips" and hummus (pack prepared hummus in a small, covered plastic container for dipping)
Chicken and corn pasta salad (Fill a thermos with thawed frozen corn kernels, rotisserie chicken, whole-grain pasta shells, and some extra-virgin olive oil and salt.)	Trail Mix (made with 2 tablespoons dried cranberries, 1 tablespoon mini chocolate chips and 2 tablespoons nuts such as cashews, walnuts or slivered almonds)
Tuna salad roll-up (Use a whole-wheat tortilla roll-up such as Tamxico's "100% Whole Wheat Tortilla Wrap-itz"; for the tuna salad, mix 3 ounces canned tuna with 1 tablespoon canola-oil mayonnaise, 2 tablespoons diced celery and salt to taste.)	½ of a Double Chocolate Walnut Muffin (see chapter 9 for recipe)

After-School Snack Attack

Unless dinner is served at 4:00 P.M., most kids need an afternoon snack. The first thing a hungry child is going to do is tear open the pantry to look for a quick bite. Big surprise: Kids will gravitate towards the nearest junk food in sight. Here we've included some of our favorite quick, yummy and nutritious snack suggestions guaranteed to satisfy those hungry little tummies until dinner time:

1. **Cinnamon Raisin Toast:** (such as Food for Life "Ezekiel 4:9 Cinnamon Raisin) with organic low-fat cream cheese (such as Organic Valley Neufchatel)
2. **Cottage Cheese:** (such as Organic Valley "Low Fat Cottage Cheese") topped with peaches (use thawed frozen peaches), 1 teaspoon colored sprinkles, and 1 tablespoon all-natural whipped cream
3. **Plain Low-Fat Yogurt:** (such as Stonyfield Farm "Low Fat Yogurt") with 1 tablespoon all-fruit jelly and 2 tablespoons wheat germ
4. **Banana-Mango Smoothie:** (In a blender combine 1 cup low-fat milk or soy milk, ½ banana, ½ cup frozen mango, 1 tablespoon honey. Puree until smooth and creamy, about 1 minute.)
5. **Cinnamon Milk and Honey:** (Mix 1 cup low-fat organic milk with a dash of raw honey and cinnamon. For an extra-special treat squirt one tablespoon whipped cream on top.)
6. **"Reese's Cup" Toast:** (Spread 1 tablespoon all-natural peanut butter on 1 slice whole grain toast. Top with six to eight all-natural "mini" dark chocolate chips—such as Ghirardelli brand—then pop in the microwave and heat on high for fifteen seconds or until the chocolate just begins to melt. Spread the chocolate over the toast with a spoon and serve immediately.)
7. **Black on White Toast:** (Spread 1 tablespoon whipped cream cheese on 1 slice whole grain toast. Sprinkle on 1 teaspoon unsweetened cocoa—such as Ghirardelli brand—and 1 teaspoon brown sugar. Microwave on high for 20 seconds. Remove from microwave then smooth cocoa over the cream cheese with the flat part of a spoon. Serve at once.)

8. **Peanut Butter and Chocolate Ice Cream Toasted Pita Sandwich:**
   (Toast ½ of an oat-bran or whole-wheat pita bread—such as
   Toufayan brand. Transfer toasted pita to freezer to cool for several minutes. Remove the pita from your freezer, then spread with
   1 tablespoon all-natural peanut butter and 2 tablespoons all-
   natural chocolate ice cream—such as Breyer's. Serve at once.)

We hope our ideas about how to get your children on the fit track
have sparked your imaginative alter-ego and will inspire you to create
your own original and healthy kids' food concoctions. Do strive to
expand you children's palates beyond mac and cheese. Expose them to
more sophisticated tastes from an early age. If they don't like the food
the first time around, keep trying and keep introducing new flavors.
But whatever you do, don't act like the food police around your kids.
Overly neurotic parenting behavior—especially when it involves
food—will backfire, so do your best to be vigilant but not obsessive
about your child's diet. Finally, remember, you, not the kids, are in
charge of the food you buy and the food you make. Buy good, healthy
food, and make good, healthy food, and your kids will eat it with all
reasonable certainty. They won't really have any other choice!

Resistance Circuit Training: The Secret to Getting Fitter, Firmer, Faster

Let's start with a pop quiz. Of the three ways your body burns calories, which one do you think accounts for the greatest percentage of calories you burn during the course of a day?

A) The calories you burn by exercising and moving

B) The calories you burn digesting breakfast, lunch and dinner

C) The calories you burn supporting basic body functions such as pumping blood, thinking and keeping warm

Most people answer "A" but "C" is the correct answer. The truth is about 70 percent of the calories you burn each day are burned solely to support basic body functions. In other words, more than two-thirds of your energy (calorie) intake is used solely to exist. Scientists call this type of metabolism your "basal" metabolism. Another 15 percent of the calories you burn are due to exercise and movement, and the remaining 15 percent of the calories your body burns are used to digest the food you eat.

Based on these percentages, it should be obvious that the smartest, most efficient way to lose weight is to increase your basal metabolism. A small change in 70 percent is a heck of a lot more significant than a small change in 15 percent. Your exercise program can be designed to increase the amount you move and therefore improve upon the 15 percent number, but even better if weight loss is important, your exercise program can be designed to increase your basal metabolism. In this book we train your body to become *Fitter, Firmer, Faster* by increasing both the calories you burn while you exercise and your basal metabolism with a resistance circuit training workout program. Women, we'll show you how to get an hourglass figure without spending hours. Men, we'll show you how to get a low-maintenance midriff that looks high maintenance. If you don't want to read all about the in-depth science behind how our exercise program works, you can skip to chapter 8 and get right to exercising. Otherwise, stay tuned and we'll explain more about how the *Fitter, Firmer, Faster* workout program can get you in the best shape of your life in the least amount of time. . . .

A Get-Fit-Quick Solution

Resistance circuit training combines the best features of resistance training and circuit training into one super-charged workout. Resistance training is strength training, any type of exercise in which your muscles have to exert force against resistance. The process of muscle healing and regrowth that follows an intense resistance training workout leads to greater strength and, ultimately, a fitter, firmer body . . . faster!

Circuit training is a method of physical conditioning in which you move from one exercise to another without stopping to rest. Resistance circuit training simultaneously improves your strength, tones your muscles, enhances your cardiovascular fitness, boosts your endurance and increases your basal metabolism in as little time as possible. Think of resistance circuit training as a form of multi-tasking. Bar none this is the best workout for the time-crunched.

Burn More Fat Than Aerobics

Many people who are exercising to lose weight dismiss resistance circuit training in favor of aerobic exercise. The logic is that it's *sometimes* possible to burn more calories during your workout doing aerobic exercise such as biking, running, swimming, rowing or elliptical training if the intensity is high enough.

With resistance circuit training, you'll indeed burn calories during your workout just like you would with an aerobic workout. However, the real weight-loss benefit of resistance circuit training exercise comes from the increase in your basal metabolism you obtain when you increase your lean muscle mass. This increase in your basal metabolism can be significant. For example, if you increase your lean muscle mass by just four pounds you will burn the caloric energy equivalent of running approximately one and a half miles every day. In addition, *intense* resistance training increases the "afterburn" or EPOC (excess post-exercise oxygen consumption), which revs your metabolism for up to 48 hours after your workout. Resistance circuit training temporarily damages your muscle fibers by overloading them, so after you complete an intense workout your body is forced to repair these "damaged" muscle fibers, a process that requires calorie energy. What this all boils down to is resistance circuit training can make over your metabolism and turn your body into a fat-burning, calorie-eating machine twenty-four hours a day.

Quality, Not Quantity

Those of you familiar with our *Gold Coast Cure* book know getting fit and maintaining a superior level of fitness requires neither a lifestyle overhaul nor major time investment. As is the case with highly restrictive diets, exercise-fanatic regimens requiring hours of your free time set the stage for failure. In the "real world," we know most people are not going to take up marathon running in order to lose weight. Of course, there are also the few people who actually stay committed to a rigorous exercise regimen yet still manage to not *look* fit. How many people do you know who exercise regularly yet still fail to lose those last fifteen to twenty pounds no matter how many hours they seem to spend at the gym or how many hours they spend pounding the pavement in their running shoes? Is this a mystery to you? Do you wonder why everyone who exercises regularly is not fit and firm?

Here's the deal: What matters most with exercise is *quality*, not quantity. A time-efficient resistance circuit training workout is far more effective than lesser-quality workouts lasting several times as long. A short but intense workout helps you gain more muscle and burn more calories not only during your workout but also during the "afterburn" we talked about earlier.

One reason intense workouts are so effective for weight loss is because an intense workout is going to require you to consume a lot of oxygen. When you do intense exercise and force your body to breathe in a lot of oxygen, you enhance the ability of your mitochondria (the energy makers within your cells) to process oxygen and therefore increase your body's ability to burn fat for energy. *In simple terms, oxygen in equals fat out.* The more oxygen you train your body to consume, the more calories and fat you will burn at rest. Working out hard by doing resistance exercises that require you to consume a lot of oxygen (such as push-ups or squats) and incorporating *high-intensity* aerobic-type intervals that also require a lot of oxygen intake is the most time-efficient way to burn mega calories.

Studies show you can reap significantly greater fat loss and significantly more metabolism-boosting muscle gain by performing short, high-intensity workouts as opposed to longer-duration, lower-intensity workouts. Higher-intensity workouts keep your body in fat-burning mode for an extended period of time.

More Secrets to Getting Fitter, Firmer, Faster

In chapter 8, we've included a stay-at-home "3-Day-a-Week 30-Minute *Fitter, Firmer, Faster* Workout" you can do without ever joining a gym. In our *Fitter, Firmer, Faster* workout we utilize a combination of nine unique training principles explained below to help you achieve your best body in the least amount of time possible. We've outlined the nine principles so you can better understand how our exercise program works and possibly even custom design your own workouts.

Principle #1: Get Warm, Then Get On with It

The myth that stretching prevents injuries still prevails, so many fitness buffs continue to waste a lot of time stretching before their workout has begun. After analyzing the results of six controlled research studies scientists at the Centers for Disease Control could find no relationship between pre-exercise stretching and injury prevention. In fact, vigorous stretching *before exercise,* when muscles are cold and therefore less supple produces less benefit and may even leave your tendons more susceptible to injury. Besides, if you waste fifteen minutes preparing for your workout with an elaborate stretching routine you've lost out on fifteen minutes that could have been spent getting fit!

The best, most efficient way to prevent injury is to gradually increase blood flow to all your major muscle groups with semi-challenging dynamic movements that increase your heart rate and prepare your muscles for the hard-core exercise to follow. Examples of efficient, effective warm-up exercises include leg squats without weights, side to side leg lunges combined with upper-body reaching motions, walking down to a pushup position, jumping rope, and so forth. You'll notice our *Fitter, Firmer, Faster* workout in chapter 8 begins with a brief warm-up of dynamic movements and ends with a recommended full-body stretching routine.

Principle # 2: Go Super-Slow

Super-slow resistance training is one of the safest, fastest ways to build strength and boost metabolism at the same time. Emphasizing the slow, downward (eccentric) phase of each exercise builds strength fast because this training technique recruits more muscle fibers per movement as compared with lifting and lowering your weights at a more rapid tempo.

According to a study published in the *Journal of Sports Medicine and Physical Fitness,* exercisers who took fourteen seconds to complete each exercise movement gained an impressive 50 percent more strength than those who spent only seven seconds completing each exercise movement even though the "seven second" exercisers performed twice as many repetitions! For maximum results it's a good idea to mix in at least two or three super-slow exercises to any workout program. The *Fitter, Firmer, Faster* workout utilizes the super-slow training method.

Principle #3: Focus on Major Muscles

On a percentage basis, your chest, back and legs are the biggest muscle groups in your body. Focusing the majority of the time you spend exercising on these muscle groups will give you the most bang for your efforts and allow you to reshape your body in the least possible amount of time. Exercises involving your chest, back and legs burn a lot of calories. Even more important, exercising these major muscles results in the greatest possible increase in your basal metabolism.

Try to think in percentage terms again. If you increase your strength in your back by 25 percent that's going to have a much greater effect on your basal metabolism than increasing the strength in your right bicep muscle by 25 percent. We're not telling you to ignore your arms. The point is you want to focus most of your best efforts on your major muscles. We're talking exercises like push-ups, lunges, squats and bent-over rows. Our workout routine in chapter 8 incorporates a variety of exercises targeting major muscles.

Principle #4: Build Muscular Strength, Then Go for Muscular Endurance

Most exercise trainers advise moderate repetition training for general fitness. "Moderate" means perhaps ten to fifteen repetitions of each exercise motion. While this is indeed a good rule of thumb we support high repetition training, perhaps 20, or even 30 repetitions for advanced exercisers to improve fitness, increase muscular endurance and optimize fat loss. High repetition training stimulates the mitochondria within your muscle cells, helping increase their ability to process oxygen, and helping increase your body's fat-burning capacity.

Unless you are trying to become an athlete who requires maximum muscular strength, or you want to compete in a bodybuilding contest you'll probably be more satisfied with your body shape if you build a baseline of functional strength first and then go for muscular endurance. This is especially true for many women who say they want a toned and firm body and who want to avoid a muscular or "bulky" look. Men may be more satisfied "bulking" up a bit, but we've found most men would be perfectly happy losing their spare and looking, fit, firm and buff without a lot of bulk. If you are looking to shed maximum inches and get a toned body with a tight midriff then you need to build up just enough muscular strength to support a speedy metabolism, but after that you need to focus on muscular endurance. Our workout formula in chapter 8 will help you safely build a baseline of muscular strength and then help you increase muscular endurance.

Principle #5: Do Just One Set

"Sets" refers to the number of times you perform a specified number of repetitions of one exercise before moving on to do a completely different exercise. For example, if you do fifteen push-ups, then rest for thirty seconds, and then do fifteen more push-ups, you have completed two "sets" of push-ups. Performing three sets of each exercise is fairly common in the world of weight training.

However, one set is sufficient to gain strength or maintain strength so long as you are exercising your muscles to fatigue. One set routines allow you to reach up to 80 percent or so of your genetic strength potential, which is perfectly fine if your goal is general fitness. Unless you are an athlete in training, stick with doing "one-set" workouts like the exercise routine in chapter 8.

Principle #6: Perform Peripheral Action Heart Training

Peripheral action heart training is a resistance training technique that conditions your cardiovascular system while simultaneously strengthening major muscles. By alternating between upper- and lower-body exercises your heart is forced to work extra hard to pump blood continuously to opposite ends of your body. For example, you might perform an exercise for your chest, then move immediately to an exercise focusing on your lower body before going back to your upper body for your next exercise. Our workout routine in chapter 8 incorporates peripheral action heart training.

Principle #7: Work Your Core

Core training exercises tone the "core" muscles of your hips, back and abdomen. Exercising these muscles helps stabilize your spine and improves your posture. When you train your core muscles you bring better alignment to the joints in your spine, warding off back pain and preventing low back injury. Core training also allows you to achieve the flattest abdomen possible because when you strengthen the muscles in your lower back your entire midsection is pulled inward. Finally, training the deep muscles in your abdomen helps your entire body feel noticeably firmer and look significantly trimmer. The workout in chapter 8 includes a number of different exercises for the core muscles of your hips, back and abdomen, including balancing poses that force your core muscles to work hard at keeping you upright.

Principle #8: Mix in Some Yoga

Look at the formidably toned bodies of avid yoga enthusiasts, and you'll notice they stand and walk with poise, balance and grace. Most of the poses in yoga are isometric contractions, a type of exercise in which your muscle exerts force yet does not change in length. For example, holding a lunge position is the yoga isometric equivalent to repeating a series of lunges. Looks can be deceiving here! Isometric contractions are not easy. In addition to toning muscles, burning calories and increasing strength, many isometric yoga poses have the added benefits of improving balance and flexibility. We include a few yoga moves in the *Fitter, Firmer, Faster* workout.

Principle #9: Train Yourself to Be Fit Enough to Jump Rope

We estimate that *at least* 75 percent of American adults wouldn't be fit enough to start an exercise program that involves jumping rope. Rope jumping is *intense* exercise, and you have to be fit to do it. However, being able to jump rope for just a few minutes at a time is a goal to strive toward. Contrary to what many people think, rope jumping is actually a very safe and low-impact exercise if it is done with proper form. In fact, it is much easier on your knees, hips and back to jump rope with proper form than it is to go jogging or running.

If you are jumping rope properly, your feet should only leave the ground about an inch. Even though it's not high impact, jumping rope requires a lot of oxygen and burns mega calories. In fact, you can burn two and a half times the amount of calories jumping rope as you would burn doing brisk walking or stationary biking. Jumping rope increases your cardiovascular strength, improves your endurance, improves balance, coordination and agility, and tones both your upper and lower body simultaneously.

However, we don't recommend jumping rope for beginners. You really do need to be in good physical condition and at close to your ideal weight before you can start jumping rope safely. Beginners can work up to jumping rope by decreasing their body fat percentage, doing the resistance training exercises we recommend in our 30-Minute Workout and doing high-intensity cardio intervals on a stationary bike. *Note:* If you don't own a jump rope or feel you are not coordinated enough to jump rope you can substitute real jump-roping for "pretend" jump-roping. (See instructions in chapter 8 for how to "pretend" jump rope.)

Real Results!

We wanted to see just how quickly and how well resistance circuit training really works in real life. To quantify the benefits we recently conducted a four-week "Fitter, Firmer, Faster Challenge" involving forty-three men combining our whole foods diet with a resistance circuit training workout. The men exercised at a Cuts Fitness for Men franchise (*www.cutsfitness.com*) along Florida's Gold Coast for thirty minutes, three times a week while following our whole-foods dietary guidelines. In just four weeks we obtained truly phenomenal results (see page 112).

Individual Profiles

David N. Age: 37	Bill O. Age: 38	Joe M. Age: 62
• Lost a total of 6 pounds • Decreased body fat 13% • Lost a total of 6 inches from hips and waist • Increased strength 36%	• Lost a total of 17½ pounds • Decreased body fat 6% • Lost a total of 11 inches from hips and waist • Increased strength 46%	• Lost a total of 9 pounds • Decreased body fat 9% • Lost a total of 7½ inches from hips and waist • Increased strength 32%
Dan H. Age: 29	Don L. Age: 74	Mark K. Age: 50
• Lost a total of 20 pounds • Decreased body fat 14% • Lost a total of 8 inches from hips and waist • Increased strength 30%	• Lost a total of 12 pounds • Decreased body fat 3.5% • Lost a total of 5 inches from hips and waist • Increased strength 25%	• Lost a total of 7 pounds • Decreased body fat 10% • Lost a total of 4½ inches from hips and waist • Increased strength 27%

Adding Aerobic Interval Training to Your Workout

Is there any role for aerobic exercise? Absolutely. The point of our workout philosophy is that if you are only going to exercise for thirty minutes, three times a week resistance circuit training is definitely your best bet for overall body shaping, fat loss and general health. However, if you want to accelerate fat loss, or if you want to dedicate more time to your fitness regimen, you should add aerobic exercise two or three days a week in addition to performing our basic workout.

Adding aerobic exercise improves the health of your heart and lungs and improves your overall physical fitness. It burns calories and speeds along the weight loss obtained performing resistance exercises. If you decide to add aerobic exercise to your resistance circuit training workouts try to mix and match a variety of motions to beat boredom and work as many different muscles as possible. For example, cycling is great for your hips while swimming helps tone your back and shoulders, and walking works your calf muscles and thighs. If you mix and match aerobic exercise you will enjoy greater overall results.

In addition, the intensity with which you exercise aerobically does make a difference. If your goal is to simply burn a few extra calories, have fun and relieve stress you can exercise aerobically at a low to moderate intensity. Recreational sports such as tennis are also great for this purpose. We really want to stress any exercise is better than no exercise.

However, if your goal is to become as fit as possible doing the least amount of exercise, aerobic interval training is the best and most time-efficient approach. Aerobic interval training consists of short bouts of intense exercise separated by less intense "rest" periods of low intensity exercise lasting perhaps two or three minutes. Aerobic interval training is a more efficient strategy for producing gains in aerobic power and endurance normally associated with longer duration training sessions.

For maximum fitness and weight loss, we encourage you to add aerobic interval training to the basic 30 minutes, 3 days a week resistance circuit training workout we recommend in chapter 8. It is best to save aerobic interval training for your days off from resistance circuit training so as not to burn yourself out—if you burn yourself out with excessively long workouts you won't be able to exercise intensely! We include an example of an aerobic interval training workout on page 114. You can do this workout outside or on a treadmill. *Note:* Don't get all hung up on trying to time the intervals precisely. The concept of interval aerobic training is simply to exercise very intensely for a short period of time, then "recover" by doing less intense aerobic exercise, and then repeat the cycle. Once you understand the concept you can apply aerobic interval training to just about any aerobic activity, such as swimming, stationary biking, elliptical training and so on.

Sample 20-Minute Interval Training Workout

Warm-Up	Interval Training (Repeat this cycle 4 times)	Cool Down
• 2 minutes, easy pace warm-up walk	• 2 minutes, light jog • 1 minute, fast run • 1 minute, brisk "power" walk	• 2 minutes, easy pace cool-down walk

Now that you know all about how our exercise program works, it's time to put that knowledge to use with our 3-day-a-week, 30-minute workout!

8

The 3-Day a Week, 30-Minute *Fitter, Firmer, Faster* Workout

Our four-phase workout is designed to first build a baseline of functional muscular strength to supercharge your metabolism and shape your body. After that you'll begin to work toward building muscular endurance, which will quickly maximize muscle tone and create a firm and sleek body. Best of all, you'll reach your fitness goals exercising just thirty minutes, three times a week!

The *Fitter, Firmer, Faster* Workout Formula

In creating our four-phase workout formula, we've taken into consideration that men and women often have slightly different goals when it comes to how they want their bodies to look. We've custom-tailored our workout to suit the aesthetic fitness goals of both genders.

Our women's four-phase formula starts by building functional muscular strength and then shifts gears to focus on maximizing muscle tone without creating any muscle bulk whatsoever. Our approach is a little unconventional because we incorporate high repetition training; this works very well for creating the long, lean muscles many women can't get following traditional workout routines.

Our men's four-phase formula also builds functional muscular strength from the get-go. However, unlike the women's formula, the men's formula goes a step beyond functional strength and builds more muscle definition and "bulk" before transitioning into a routine that maximizes muscular endurance.

Women's *Fitter, Firmer, Faster* Workout Formula

Note: If you are an experienced and advanced exerciser you may be able to skip Phase 1 or 2 (below) and go directly to Phase 3 or possibly Phase 4 (see page 117).

Women's Phase 1 and Phase 2

Phase 1	Phase 2
Stay in Phase 1 for 2–3 weeks	Stay in Phase 2 for 2–3 weeks
Use 3-pound dumbbells for all exercises requiring weights	Use 5-pound dumbbells for all exercises requiring weights
Perform each exercise using dumbbells for 12 repetitions	Perform each exercise using dumbbells for 12 repetitions
In each exercise using dumbbells go super-slow. Count to 7 while lifting the weight and count to 7 while lowering the weight.	In each exercise using dumbbells go super-slow. Count to 7 while lifting the weight and count to 7 while lowering the weight.
For the cardio intervals, either march in place vigorously, step up and down off a bench or stairs, or ride a stationary bike.	For the cardio intervals, either step up and down off a bench or stairs, ride a stationary bike, or jump on a mini trampoline.

Women's Phase 3 and Phase 4

Phase 3	Phase 4
Stay in Phase 3 for 2 weeks.	Stay in Phase 4 indefinitely; but if you want to build stronger muscles, go back to Phase 1 and start with 7 pounds.
Use 5-pound dumbbells for all exercises requiring weights.	Use 5-pound dumbbells for all exercises requiring weights.
Perform each exercise using dumbbells for 20 repetitions.	Perform each exercise using dumbbells for 30 repetitions.
In each exercise using dumbbells, count to 3 while lifting the weight and count to 3 while lowering the weight.	In each exercise using dumbbells, count to 3 while lifting the weight and count to 3 while lowering the weight.
For the cardio intervals, either do real or "pretend" jump roping (shown later).	For the cardio intervals, either do real or "pretend" jump roping (shown later).

Men's Fitter, Firmer, Faster Workout Formula:

Note: If you are an experienced and advanced exerciser you may be able to skip Phase 1 or 2 (below) and go directly to Phase 3 or possibly Phase 4 (see page 119).

Men's Phase 1 and 2

Phase 1	Phase 2
Stay in Phase 1 for 2–3 weeks	Stay in Phase 2 for 2–3 weeks
Use 7-pound dumbbells for all exercises requiring weights.	Use 10-pound dumbbells for all exercises requiring weights.
Perform each exercise using dumbbells for 12 repetitions.	Perform each exercise using dumbbells for 12 repetitions.
In each exercise, go super-slow (count to 7 while lifting the weight and count to 7 while lowering the weight).	In each exercise, go super-slow (count to 7 while lifting the weight and count to 7 while lowering the weight).
For the cardio intervals, either march in place vigorously, step up and down off a bench or stairs, or ride a stationary bike	For the cardio intervals, either step up and down off a bench or stairs, ride a stationary bike, or jump on a mini trampoline.

Men's Phase 3 and 4

Phase 3	Phase 4
Stay in Phase 3 for 2 weeks	Stay in Phase 4 indefinitely; but if you want to build stronger muscles, go back to Phase 1 and start with 20 pounds.
Use 12-pound dumbbells for all exercises requiring weights.	Use 15-pound dumbbells for all exercises requiring weights.
Perform each exercise using dumbbells for 15 repetitions.	Perform each exercise using dumbbells for 15–20 repetitions.
In each exercise using dumbbells, count to 3 while lifting the weight and count to 3 while lowering the weight.	In each exercise using dumbbells, count to 3 while lifting the weight and count to 3 while lowering the weight.
For the cardio intervals, either do real or "pretend" jump roping (shown later).	For the cardio intervals, either do real or "pretend" jump roping (shown later).

Consider Hiring a Professional

Personal trainers help prevent injury by demonstrating proper exercise motions, many of which are unfamiliar to beginning exercisers. A good trainer can teach you proper form in three to four sessions so long as you take his or her advice seriously and practice a bit in front of a mirror. When choosing your personal trainer, be sure he or she is properly trained. Request qualifications! A bachelor's degree in an exercise-related field with certification by the American College of Sports Medicine (ACSM), the National Strength and Conditioning Association (NSCA) or the American Council on Exercise (ACE) would be ideal. You can contact these associations to find personal trainers in your area via the Internet.

- Reach the American College of Sports Medicine at *www.acsm.org.*
- Contact the National Strength and Conditioning Association at *www.nsca-lift.org.*
- Learn about the American Council on Exercise at *www.acefitness.org.*

Rate Your Intensity

As you recall from chapter 7, it's important to exercise intensely if you want to see maximum results. However, high intensity means different things to different people. Some of us start out in better shape than others. Learn to estimate *your* rate of perceived exertion using the chart below as a guideline. You should feel as though you are exercising at an intensity level of 7 or 8 throughout your *entire* 30-minute workout.

Perceived Rate of Exertion

- 0 means no exertion at all, sitting in a chair, for example.
- 1 to 2 is very light exercise, standing in place, perhaps.
- 3 to 4 is moderately difficult exercise that causes you to breathe heavier than usual, walking up one flight of stairs, for example.
- 5 to 6 is difficult exercise, perhaps you feel this way after you've been jogging for ten minutes or so.
- **7 to 8 is very difficult exercise that forces you to breathe heavily. (This is the intensity zone you want to be working at for maximum results.)**
- 9 to 10 is all-out exertion; you're out of breath; you can only keep up this pace for a minute or two.

The 3-Day-a-Week
30-Minute *Fitter, Firmer, Faster* Workout

This routine will take you a little more than thirty minutes to complete the first few times, once you are familiar with the exercises you will be able to complete the workout in no more than thirty minutes. If you have time for more exercise, try adding ten to twenty minutes of moderate-intensity aerobic exercise such as walking, swimming or biking. You can add this onto the end of our resistance circuit training workout or save purely aerobic exercise for the days you would otherwise not be exercising.

As another, even more effective alternative, try twenty minutes of high-intensity interval aerobic training or our twenty-minute *"Fitter, Firmer, Faster* Park and Beach Workout." These higher-intensity aerobic workouts should be performed only on those days you are not doing resistance circuit training. You need to give your muscles time to repair.

Exercise #1: Alternating High Knee Raises with Alternating Arm Raises

- Phases One and Two: 30 reps
- Phases Three and Four: 50 reps

1. Stand with your feet hip-width apart and your arms down at your sides. Contract your abdominal muscles.
2. Briskly bring your left knee up in front of your chest and lift your right arm straight up in the air.
3. Keep alternating sides for 1 minute. Move briskly and lift your knees as high as possible for the recommended number of reps.

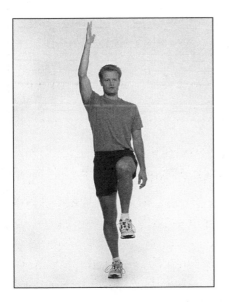 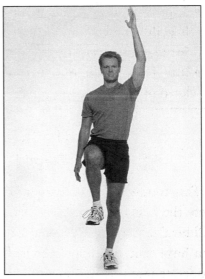

Exercise #2: Side-to-Side Lunges with Opposite-Hand Reach

- Phases One and Two: 20 reps total
- Phases Three and Four: 30–40 reps total

1. Stand with your feet more than hip-width apart, feet slightly turned out.
2. Lunge to the left by bending your left knee and simultaneously reaching your right arm across your body so that your right hand touches your left foot (if you cannot reach that far without discomfort then just do what you can).
3. Quickly rise back to the start position and switch sides. Continue lunging side to side for the recommended number of reps.

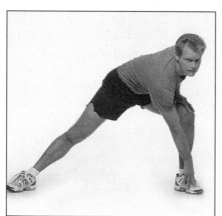 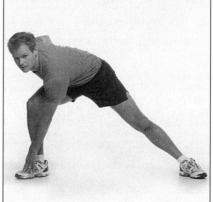

Exercise #3: Push-Ups

- Modified Push-Ups for Phases One and Two: 10–15 reps
- Full Push-Ups for Phases Three and Four: 15–25 reps

Modified Push-Ups:

1. Start with your palms and knees on the ground, shoulder-width apart. Keep your head, neck, spine and hips in a straight line. Contract your abdominal muscles.
2. Slowly bend your elbows and lower your body down. Hold this position for a count of 2. Slowly push back up, then repeat.

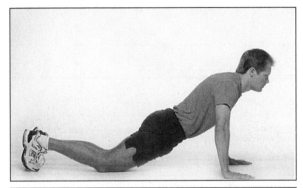

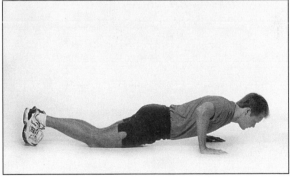

Full Push-Ups:

1. Place your hands shoulder-width apart with your fingers pointing forward. Keep your legs and torso straight and pull your abdominal muscles inward. Only your palms and toes should touch the ground.
2. Slowly bend your elbows and lower your body down. Slowly push yourself back up to the start position and repeat.

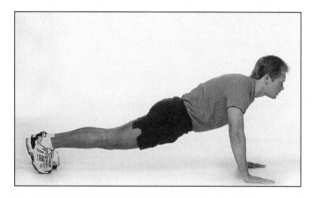

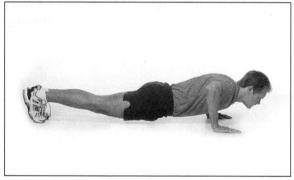

Exercise #4: Side Bends

Women:
- Phase One: 3 pounds/12 reps "super-slowly" each side
- Phase Two: 5 pounds/12 reps "super-slowly" each side
- Phase Three: 5 pounds/20 reps each side
- Phase Four: 5 pounds/30 reps each side

Men:
- Phase One: 7 pounds/12 reps "super-slowly" each side
- Phase Two: 10 pounds/12 reps "super-slowly" each side
- Phase Three: 12 pounds/15 reps each side
- Phase Four: 15 pounds/15–20 reps each side

1. Stand with your feet shoulder-width apart; keep your knees slightly bent and your abdominal muscles contracted. Hold the dumbbell in your right hand and place your left hand behind your head.
2. Keep your abdominal muscles contracted and slowly bend to the right until you feel a slight stretch or pull on the left side of your waist. Pause briefly. Reverse the movement. Repeat all reps on one side, and then switch sides.

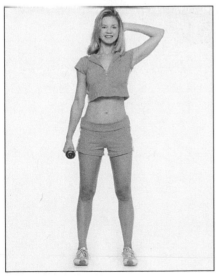 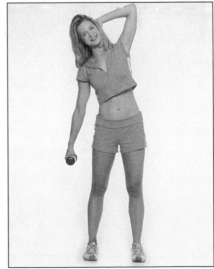

Exercise #5: Standing Knee to Opposite Chest

- Phases One and Two: 15–20 reps each leg
- Phases Three and Four: 30–40 reps each leg

1. Stand with your feet shoulder-width apart, your knees slightly bent and both hands behind your head.
2. Briskly bring your left knee up toward your right shoulder, keeping your back straight and your abdominal muscles contracted. Then briskly lower your foot back to the starting position.
3. Keep your weight on your supporting leg at all times. Do all reps with your left leg, and then switch legs and repeat.

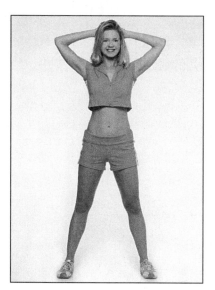 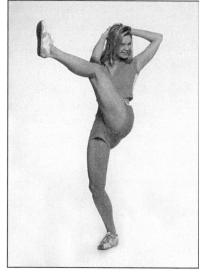

Exercise #6: Full Crunches

- Phases One and Two: 20 reps
- Phases Three and Four: 30–40 reps
1. Lie on your back with your legs in the air, knees bent, and hands behind your head with your elbows out to the side.
2. Curl your legs and pelvis toward your rib cage while simultaneously curling your shoulders forward and keeping your elbows out to the side (make sure the movement comes from your abdominal muscles—not your neck or shoulders). Repeat the movement for the recommended number of reps.

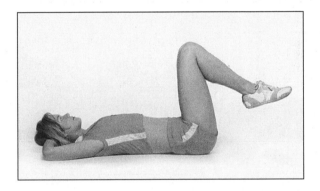

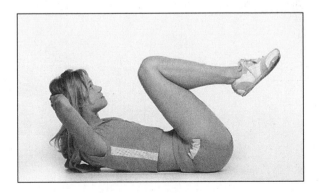

Exercise #7: Two-Minute Intense Cardio Intervals

Phases One and Two: (Choose one of the following.)
- March in place vigorously
- Step-ups onto a bench or stairs, with or without light dumbbells
- Ride a stationary bike at 70–90 rpm (revolutions per minute)
- Jump on a mini trampoline

Phases Three and Four: (Choose one of the following.)
- Jump rope
- "Pretend" jump rope

Step-Ups:

1. Use an 8- to 10-inch-tall step or bench (or staircase at home). Step up carefully with your right foot, followed by your left foot. Then, step down your right foot, followed by your left foot.
2. Continue leading with your right foot for 1 minute then switch sides and lead with your left foot for 1 minute. (To increase the intensity, hold a pair of 1–3 pound dumbbells in your hands.)

Pretend Jump Rope:

1. Keep your feet together and jump 1 inch off the ground.
2. Pretend you are holding a jump rope, and rotate your hands in small circles while keeping your upper arms and elbows stable.

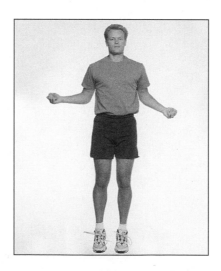

READER/CUSTOMER CARE SURVEY

We care about your opinions! Please take a moment to fill out our online Reader Survey at **http://survey.hcibooks.com.**
As a **"THANK YOU"** you will receive a **VALUABLE INSTANT COUPON** towards future book purchases as well as a **SPECIAL GIFT** available only online! Or, you may mail this card back to us and we will send you a copy of our exciting catalog with your valuable coupon inside.

(PLEASE PRINT IN ALL CAPS)

First Name _____ MI. _____ Last Name _____

Address _____ City _____

State _____ Zip _____ Email _____

1. Gender
☐ Female   ☐ Male

2. Age
☐ 8 or younger
☐ 9-12   ☐ 13-16
☐ 17-20   ☐ 21-30
☐ 31+

3. Did you receive this book as a gift?
☐ Yes   ☐ No

4. Annual Household Income
☐ under $25,000
☐ $25,000 - $34,999
☐ $35,000 - $49,999
☐ $50,000 - $74,999
☐ over $75,000

5. What are the ages of the children living in your house?
☐ 0 - 14   ☐ 15+

6. Marital Status
☐ Single
☐ Married
☐ Divorced
☐ Widowed

7. How did you find out about the book?
(please choose one)
☐ Recommendation
☐ Store Display
☐ Online
☐ Catalog/Mailing
☐ Interview/Review

8. Where do you usually buy books?
(please choose one)
☐ Bookstore
☐ Online
☐ Book Club/Mail Order
☐ Price Club (Sam's Club, Costco's, etc.)
☐ Retail Store (Target, Wal-Mart, etc.)

9. What subject do you enjoy reading about the most?
(please choose one)
☐ Parenting/Family
☐ Relationships
☐ Recovery/Addictions
☐ Health/Nutrition
☐ Christianity
☐ Spirituality/Inspiration
☐ Business Self-help
☐ Women's Issues
☐ Sports

10. What attracts you most to a book?
(please choose one)
☐ Title
☐ Cover Design
☐ Author
☐ Content

TAPE IN MIDDLE; DO NOT STAPLE

||||||

BUSINESS REPLY MAIL
FIRST-CLASS MAIL PERMIT NO 45 DEERFIELD BEACH, FL

POSTAGE WILL BE PAID BY ADDRESSEE

Health Communications, Inc.
3201 SW 15th Street
Deerfield Beach FL 33442-9875

|ₙllₙₙllₙlₙlₙlₙlₙlₙₙlₙlllₙlₙₙlₙₙlₙlₙₙₙlₙlₙlₙlₙl|

FOLD HERE

Comments

Exercise #8: Overhead Press

Women:
- Phase One: 3 pounds/12 reps "super-slowly"
- Phase Two: 5 pounds/12 reps "super-slowly"
- Phase Three: 5 pounds/20 reps
- Phase Four: 5 pounds/30 reps

Men:
- Phase One: 7 pounds/12 reps "super-slowly"
- Phase Two: 10 pounds/12 reps "super-slowly"
- Phase Three: 12 pounds/15 reps
- Phase Four: 15 pounds/15–20 reps

1. Stand with your feet hip-width apart. Hold a dumbbell in each hand with your elbows bent, palms facing forward and elbows slightly below shoulder level. Contract your abdominal muscles.
2. Keep your abdominal muscles contracted, and press the dumbbells directly overhead; be careful not to lock your arms straight.
3. Lower the dumbbells to the start position, and repeat the movement for the recommended number of reps.

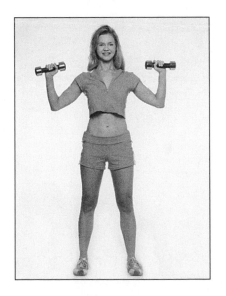 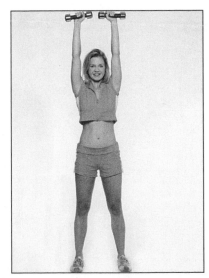

Exercise #9: Good Morning Bends

- Phases One and Two: 10–12 reps
- Phases Three and Four: 20–25 reps

1. Stand with your feet slightly wider than shoulder-width apart and your hands behind your head with your elbows out to your sides.
2. Bend forward from the waist, keeping your legs straight and your gaze straight ahead. Keep your back flat.
3. Once your body is perpendicular, rise back up to the starting position. Repeat the movement for the desired number of repetitions.

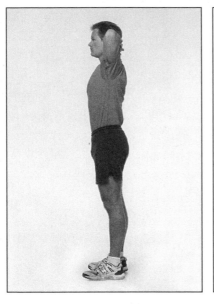 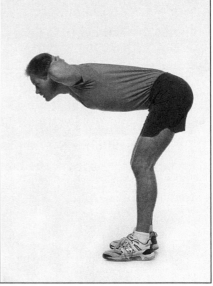

Exercise #10: Standing Alternating Side Leg Lifts

- Phases One and Two: 16–20 reps total
- Phases Three and Four: 30–40 reps total

1. Stand up straight with your abdominal muscles contracted, your legs hip-width apart and your hands on your hips.
2. Shift your weight onto your left leg, and raise your right leg out to the side as high as you comfortably can, while still keeping your right knee and foot facing forward.
3. Lower your right leg to the ground; shift your weight from your left leg to your right leg, then raise your left leg.
4. Continue alternating raising your right leg and your left leg for the recommended number of reps.

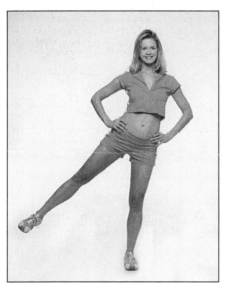 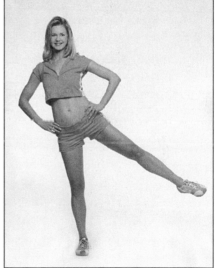

Exercise #11: Two-Minute Intense Cardio Intervals

See Exercise #7 for recommended exercises.

Exercise #12: On Your Toes Yoga "Chair Pose"

Both women and men:
- Phase One: Hold for 20 seconds
- Phase Two: Hold for 30 seconds
- Phase Three: Hold for 40 seconds
- Phase Four: Hold for 50 seconds

1. Stand with your feet hip-width apart, and balance on your toes with your arms straight up overhead. Keep your chest lifted and abdominal muscles pulled inward.
2. Bend your knees and lower your hips to the floor until your knees are bent at almost a 90-degree angle, pitching forward with your torso ever so slightly.
3. Slowly inhale and exhale, holding the pose for the recommended number of seconds.

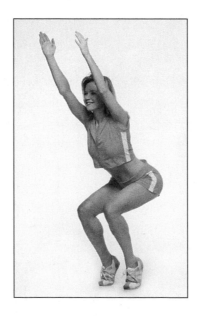

Exercise #13: Upright Rows

Women:
- Phase One: 3 pounds/12 reps "super-slowly"
- Phase Two: 5 pounds/12 reps "super-slowly"
- Phase Three: 5 pounds/20 reps
- Phase Four: 5 pounds/30 reps

Men:
- Phase One: 7 pounds/12 reps "super-slowly"
- Phase Two: 10 pounds/12 reps "super-slowly"
- Phase Three: 12 pounds/15 reps
- Phase Four: 15 pounds/15–20 reps

1. Stand with your feet hip-width apart, knees slightly bent and back straight. Hold a pair of dumbbells in front of you so that your palms face back toward your thighs.
2. Pull the dumbbells up to chest height, leading with your elbows. Slowly lower the dumbbells and return to the start position. Repeat the movement for the recommended number of reps.

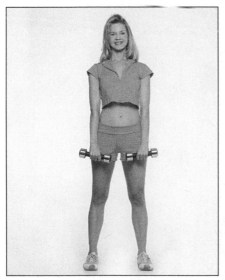 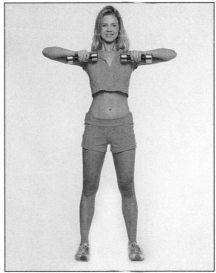

Exercise #14: Dead-Lifts

Women:
- Phase One: 3 pounds/12 reps "super-slowly"
- Phase Two: 5 pounds/12 reps "super-slowly"
- Phase Three: 5 pounds/20 reps
- Phase Four: 5 pounds/30 reps

Men:
- Phase One: 7 pounds/12 reps "super-slowly"
- Phase Two: 10 pounds/12 reps "super-slowly"
- Phase Three: 12 pounds/15 reps
- Phase Four: 15 pounds/15–20 reps

1. Stand with your feet slightly wider than shoulder-width apart. Hold a pair of dumbbells in front of your thighs, contract your abdominal muscles, and pull your shoulders back.
2. Shift your weight into your heels, and lower the dumbbells until your torso is parallel to the floor, keeping your gaze straight ahead. (Be sure to keep your back as flat as possible.)
3. Rise back up to the start position, and repeat the movement for the recommended number of reps.

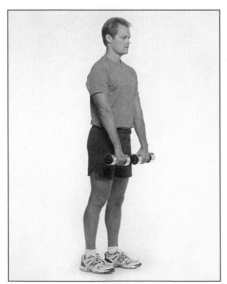 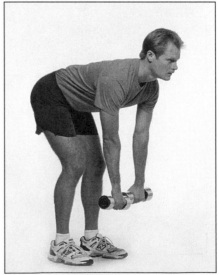

Exercise #15: Tricep Extensions

Women:
- Phase One: 3 pounds/12 reps "super-slowly"
- Phase Two: 5 pounds/12 reps "super-slowly"
- Phase Three: 5 pounds/20 reps
- Phase Four: 5 pounds/30 reps

Men:
- Phase One: 7 pounds/12 reps "super-slowly"
- Phase Two: 10 pounds/12 reps "super-slowly"
- Phase Three: 12 pounds/15 reps
- Phase Four: 15 pounds/15–20 reps

1. Stand with your feet shoulder-width apart and your abdominal muscles contracted. Hold two dumbbells overhead, with your elbows facing forward and your palms facing in toward each other.
2. Keep your elbows facing forward, and close to your head while you lower the dumbbells behind your head.
3. Return to the start position, and repeat the movement for the recommended number of reps.

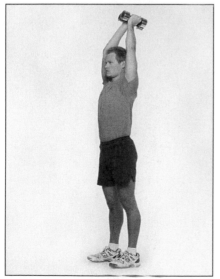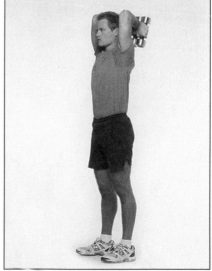

Exercise #16: Two-Minute Intense Cardio Intervals

See Exercise #7 for recommended exercises.

Exercise #17: Bent-Over Rows

Women:
- Phase One: 3 pounds/12 reps "super-slowly"
- Phase Two: 5 pounds/12 reps "super-slowly"
- Phase Three: 5 pounds/20 reps
- Phase Four: 5 pounds/30 reps

Men:
- Phase One: 7 pounds/12 reps "super-slowly"
- Phase Two: 10 pounds/12 reps "super-slowly"
- Phase Three: 12 pounds/15 reps
- Phase Four: 15 pounds/15–20 reps

1. Stand with your feet shoulder-width apart and your knees slightly bent. Bend over so that your back is almost parallel to the floor. Hold a dumbbell in each hand, and let your arms hang down toward the floor.
2. With your palms facing back toward your body, pull the dumbbells up toward your chest while keeping your back flat. Lower the dumbbells to the ground, and repeat the movement for the recommended number of reps.

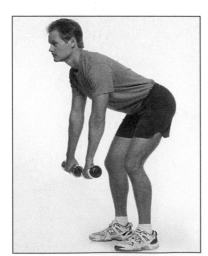 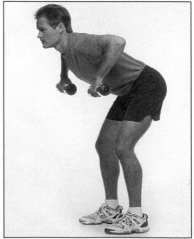

Exercise #18: Plié Squat with Biceps Curl

Women:

- Phase One: 3 pounds/12 reps "super-slowly"
- Phase Two: 5 pounds/12 reps "super-slowly"
- Phase Three: 5 pounds/20 reps
- Phase Four: 5 pounds/30 reps

Men:

- Phase One: 7 pounds/12 reps "super-slowly"
- Phase Two: 10 pounds/12 reps "super-slowly"
- Phase Three: 12 pounds/15 reps
- Phase Four: 15 pounds/15–20 reps

1. Stand with your feet outside shoulder-width and your toes turned out at a 45-degree angle. Contract your abdominal muscles while keeping your back straight. Hold the dumbbells down in front of your body with your palms facing outward.
2. Slowly bend your knees to lower your body toward the ground while simultaneously curling both dumbbells up to chest level. Lower the dumbbells back down as you straighten your legs back to a standing position. Repeat the movement for the recommended number of reps.

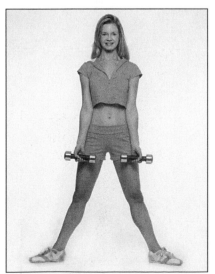 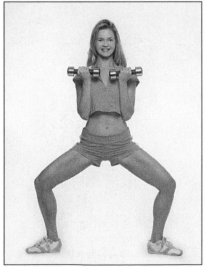

Exercise #19: Standing Backward Leg Lifts

- Phase One: 12 reps each leg
- Phase Two: 15 reps each leg
- Phase Three: 20 reps each leg
- Phase Four: 25 reps each leg

1. Stand about a foot away from the back of a sturdy chair with your chest lifted and your abdominal muscles pulled inward. Bend forward at your hips, and rest your forearms lightly on the back of the chair.
2. Shift your weight onto your right leg, keeping your right knee slightly bent. Slowly raise your left leg straight behind you while keeping your left knee facing the floor.
3. Lower your leg to the start position, and repeat for the recommended number of reps, then switch legs.

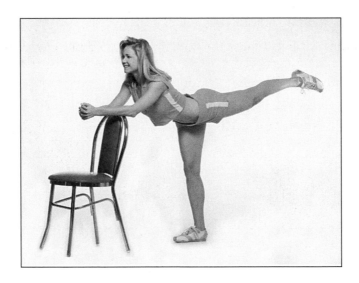

Exercise #20: Two-Minute Intense Cardio Intervals

See Exercise #7 for recommended exercises.

Exercise #21: Body Raise

- Phase One: 12 reps each leg
- Phase Two: 15 reps each leg
- Phase Three: 20 reps each leg
- Phase Four: 25 reps each leg

1. Lie on your back in front of a chair with your knees bent and your heels on the seat of the chair. Your knees should be directly above your hips, and your arms should be straight at your sides with your palms pressing into the floor.
2. Press your heels down into the chair as you simultaneously squeeze your glutes and raise your hips as high as you can off the floor.
3. Pause briefly at the top movement, and then lower your hips back to the ground. Repeat for the recommended number of reps.

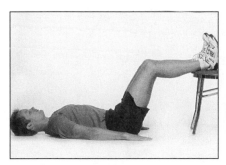 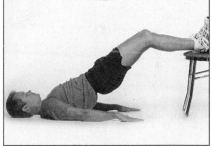

Exercise #22: Lying Down Leg Press

- Phase One: 12 reps
- Phase Two: 15 reps
- Phase Three: 20 reps
- Phase Four: 25 reps

1. Lie on your back with your legs extended straight up in the air (your toes should be turned out and your heels should be touching). Place your palms behind your head with your elbows out. Pull your abdominal muscles inward.

2. Bend your knees, keeping your heels together and toes turned out, and lower your legs and feet toward the ground. Squeeze your inner thighs as you press your heels back up to the starting position. Repeat the movement for the recommended number of reps.

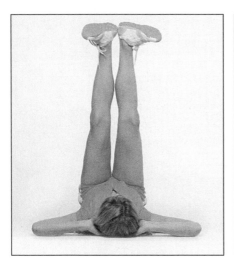 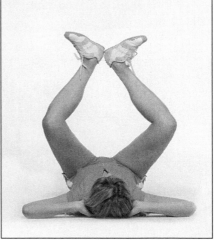

Exercise #23: Yoga Locust Pose

Both women and men:

- Phase One: Hold for 15 seconds
- Phase Two: Hold for 25 seconds
- Phase Three: Hold for 30 seconds
- Phase Four: Hold for 40 seconds

1. Lie on your stomach with your arms and legs extended, feet hip-width apart and arms stretched forward alongside your ears.
2. Keeping your gaze straight ahead, lengthen your body, and lift your arms, upper body and legs up off the floor as high as you comfortably can. Aim for length rather than height.
3. Hold the pose for the recommended number of seconds.

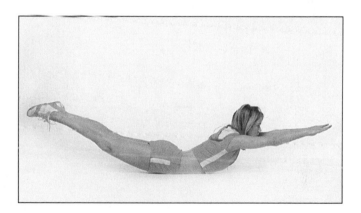

Exercise #24: Core Stabilizer

- Phase One: Hold for 10–12 seconds
- Phase Two: Hold for 20 seconds
- Phase Three: Hold for 30 seconds
- Phase Four: Hold for 40 seconds

1. Position yourself so your toes are on the ground and your elbows are on the ground directly beneath your shoulders. Raise yourself up, keeping a straight line from your shoulders to your ankles, so that your elbows and toes support your body.
2. Contract your abdominal muscles and squeeze your glutes and inner thighs together. Hold the pose for the recommended number of seconds.

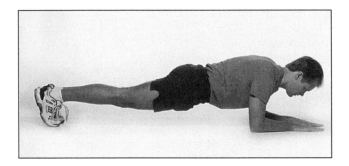

Fit-Body Post-Workout Stretches

While we discourage warm-up stretching, post-workout stretching does have an important place in a well-rounded fitness routine. Stretching maintains circulation around your joints, improves flexibility and allows your body to move more efficiently. Studies also suggest stretching can help improve your strength. Not to mention stretching after a workout simply feels good!

The best time to stretch is after your workout. Your muscles are warmer and more supple at this time, making it easier to lengthen them. As a general rule it's best to start your workout with relatively less-intense warm-up exercises that get the blood flowing to all your major muscle groups; follow up with your usual workout routine; then finish off with your stretching routine.

Two stretching mistakes to avoid:

1. **Don't bounce.** Using momentum to increase your stretch can activate protective reflexes that cause your muscles to contract as opposed to stretch.

2. **Don't stretch to the point of pain.** While you may experience a little discomfort if a muscle is tight, pain is your body's way of letting you know something is wrong. There is no benefit to stretching to the point of pain.

Stretch #1: Hip Flexor Stretch

1. Kneel on both knees. Extend your left foot forward, keeping your right knee on the floor. Place your hands on each side of your front foot. Slide your back leg out behind you until you feel the stretch in the front of your hip.
2. Push your hip forward slightly, straighten your body and place your hands on your front knee to intensify the stretch. Hold the stretch for 10–15 seconds and then switch sides.

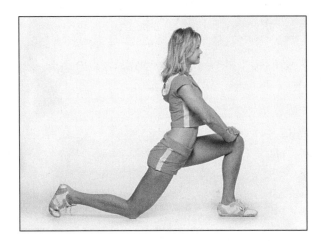

Stretch #2: Standing Chest Stretch

1. Stand with your feet hip-width apart and knees slightly bent. Contract your abdominal muscles, and keep your head, neck and shoulders relaxed.
2. Clasp your hands behind your back, and, keeping your back straight, lift your arms behind you until you feel the stretch across your chest. Hold the stretch for 10–15 seconds.

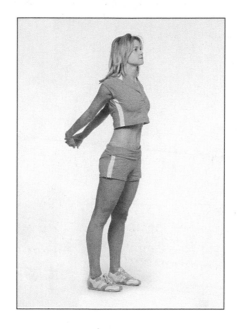

Stretch #3: Back Extension

1. Lie down on your stomach, and place your hands under your shoulders with your palms pressing down into the ground and your elbows in close to your body.
2. Keeping your hips on the floor, push your torso up by straightening your arms (contract your glutes and keep your neck relaxed). Hold the stretch for 10–15 seconds.

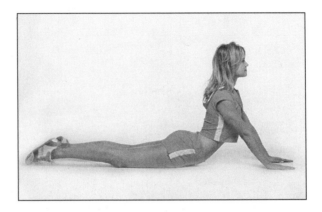

Stretch #4: Hamstring Sit and Reach

1. Sit on the floor with your right leg extended straight in front of you and your left leg bent (the sole of your left foot should be resting against your right inner thigh).
2. Keep your back as straight as possible, and reach toward your right foot until you feel a stretch in the back of your leg and lower back. Hold the stretch for 10–15 seconds, then switch sides and repeat.

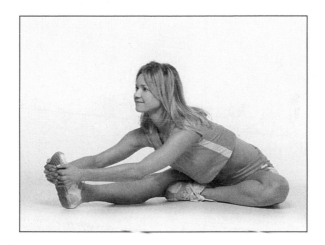

Stretch #5: Lying Down Glute Stretch

1. Lie on your back with your knees bent.
2. Cross your right foot over your left knee, and pull your left thigh in toward your chest with both hands (you should feel the stretch along the right glute). Hold the stretch for 10–15 seconds, then switch sides and repeat.

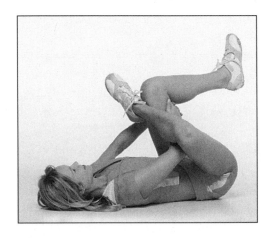

Stretch #6: Seated Spine Twist

1. Sit on the floor with your legs extended straight in front of you. Bend your right knee, and place your right foot on the floor near the outside of your left knee.
2. Place your right hand on the floor behind you, and reach across your body as far as possible with your left arm while keeping your right foot on the floor (you should feel the stretch in your back). Hold the position for 10–15 seconds then switch sides and repeat.

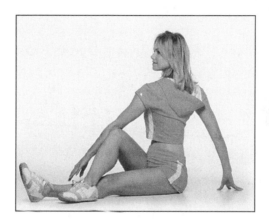

Stretch #7: Lower Back Stretch

1. Lie on the floor and place one hand behind each knee.
2. Keep your knees separated and pull both knees into your chest while keeping your head on the ground. Hold the position for 10–15 seconds.

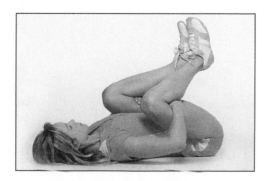

The 20-Minute *Fitter, Firmer, Faster* Park and Beach Workout

This workout was originally designed to help parents such as ourselves fit in a quick workout while the kids play at the beach or park. However, it's also great for sunny days when you just want to get outside and enjoy a breath of fresh air.

Our *Fitter, Firmer, Faster* Park and Beach Workout incorporates calisthenic-type exercises and high-intensity cardiovascular interval training. This is a full-body muscle conditioning workout that places more emphasis on high-intensity aerobic conditioning in comparison to our 3-Day-a-Week, 30-Minute *Fitter, Firmer, Faster* Workout.

Our 20-minute Park and Beach Workout can be used on alternate days in addition to our 30-Minute Workout or even substitute for it on occasion if you happen to be especially time-crunched. You'll need a stopwatch, and remember, this routine is high-intensity and should not be done on the same day as our 30-Minute Workout.

Exercise #1: Walk at a moderate pace: Two minutes

Exercise #2: Light Jog: One minute

Exercise #3: Fast Run: One minute

Exercise #4: Walking Lunges with Torso Twist

- Phase One: 10 reps total
- Phase Two: 14 reps total
- Phase Three: 18 reps total
- Phase Four: 22 reps total

1. Stand with your feet hip-width apart with your hands clasped and your elbows at shoulder height.
2. Step forward with your left foot one long stride, lower your right knee toward the ground, while simultaneously twisting your torso to the left (be careful not to let your left knee extend forward beyond your left foot at any time during the exercise).
3. Then, without pausing to return to the starting position, rise and take a long stride forward with your right foot, lower your left knee to the ground and twist your torso to the right.
4. Repeat the lunges for the recommended number of reps. The lunges should be continuous and fluid.

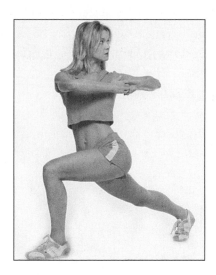

Exercise #5: One-Minute "Pretend" Jump Rope

See photo and description #7 in 30-Minute Workout.

Exercise #6: Push-Ups

See photo and description #3 in 30-Minute Workout.

Exercise #7: Jumping Jacks

Note: Try to complete at least 25–30 reps even if you have to rest in between jumping jacks.

Exercise #8: Tricep Dips

- Phase One: 10 reps
- Phase Two: 14 reps
- Phase Three: 18 reps
- Phase Four: 24 reps

1. Sit on a bench (if you are at the beach, use the stairs) with your hands on the front of the bench, your fingers facing forward and your elbows just barely bent. Start the exercise by walking your feet forward so your hips are in front of the bench (or stairs) and your knees are bent at a 90-degree angle.
2. Lower yourself down toward the ground until your elbows are bent at 90-degree angles, hold the position briefly, then push yourself back up to the starting position. Repeat the movement for the recommended number of reps.

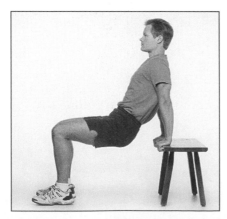 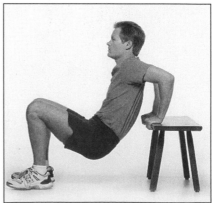

Exercise #9: Jog Backward: One Minute

Exercise #10: Squat Jumps

- Phase One: 8 jumps
- Phase Two: 10 jumps
- Phase Three: 14 jumps
- Phase Four: 18 jumps

1. Stand with your feet shoulder-width apart. Squat down slightly while keeping your chest lifted, your abdominal muscles contracted and your shoulders back. Hold your arms straight down at your sides.
2. Use your glute and thigh muscles to jump up into the air while simultaneously thrusting your arms up toward the ceiling. Land on your heels, then roll forward onto your toes and repeat. (*Note:* You do not need to jump very high for this exercise to be effective.) Repeat the jumps the recommended number of times.

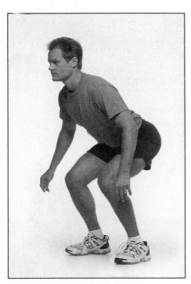
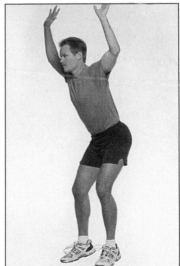

Exercise #11: Walking Lunges

- Phase One: 16 reps total
- Phase Two: 20 reps total
- Phase Three: 30 reps total
- Phase Four: 40 reps total

1. Stand with your feet hip-width apart and your knees slightly bent.
2. Step forward about 1 stride length from your back foot. In the same movement, lower your body down toward the ground. Pause briefly, then raise your body and step forward with the other leg to repeat the lunge on the other side.
3. Continue alternating lunges as you "walk" forward.

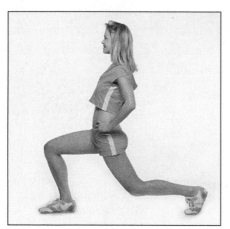 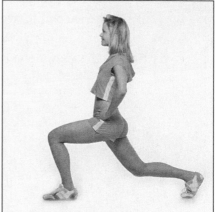

Exercise #12: Kickboxing

1. Stand with your arms in front of your body at shoulder height and your elbows slightly bent at least 90 degrees. Your knees should be facing forward. Shift your weight onto your left leg with your left knee slightly bent; pull your abdominal muscles inward.
2. Lean your torso slightly to the left while you lift and kick your right leg directly out to the side with your kneecap facing *forward*. Return to the start position and touch only your toe to the ground then quickly repeat the kicks, keeping the pace brisk, for a total of 15 reps.
3. Switch legs and do another 15 reps.

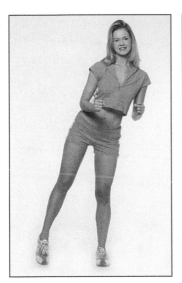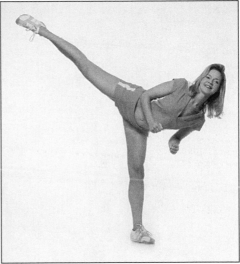

Exercise #13: Shuffle Side to Side: One Minute

Note: Make sure your feet are a little more than shoulder-width apart and your knees are slightly bent. Quickly shuffle 8 times to the left and then 8 times to the right, keeping your knees bent and staying on your toes. Repeat shuffling for 1 minute.

Exercise #14: Brisk Step-Ups

1. Stand facing a bench or two stairs. Briskly step up with your right foot, placing your entire right foot flat on the bench or top stair and keeping your back straight and abdominal muscles contracted.
2. Then briskly step up with your left foot so that both feet are flat on the step. Step down one foot at a time, right foot first.
3. Repeat 20 reps with your right foot leading, then switch sides for another 20 reps with your left foot leading (40 total reps).

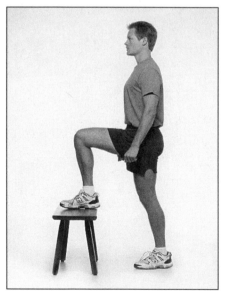 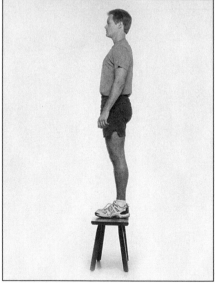

Exercise #15: Standing Oblique Exercise

- Phase One: 16 reps total
- Phase Two: 20 reps total
- Phase Three: 30 reps total
- Phase Four: 40 reps total

1. Stand with your feet hip-width apart and your hands clasped behind your head. Your elbows should be sticking out level with your ears.
2. Slowly lift your left knee up and out to the side while simultaneously bending your waist and lowering your left elbow to touch your knee.
3. Return to starting position, and alternate sides for the recommended number of reps.

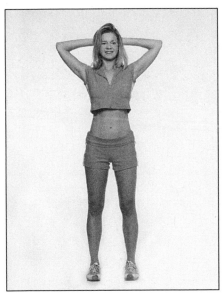 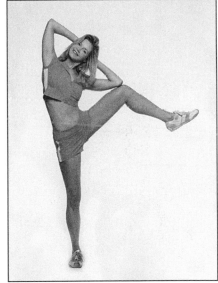

Exercise #16: The Tic-Toc Hop

1. Stand with your feet shoulder-width apart, knees slightly bent and your hands on your hips.
2. Balance on your right foot and raise your left leg out to the side (both knees should face forward); hop up while simultaneously switching feet so you are now balancing on your left foot with your right leg out to the side.
3. Continue hopping up and switching feet briskly for a total of 70 reps (each time one foot touches the ground counts as one rep).

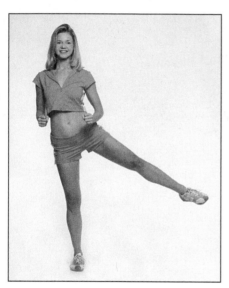 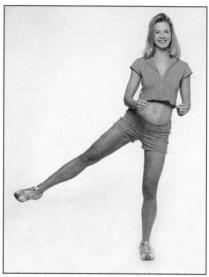

Exercise #17: Crab Walks

- Phases One and Two: 20 reps
- Phases Three and Four: 30 reps

1. Sit on the ground with your knees bent and your hands on the ground behind you, fingers pointing forward.
2. Raise your hips off the ground and begin walking backward on all fours for 20–30 "steps." (*Note:* Keep your elbows bent.)

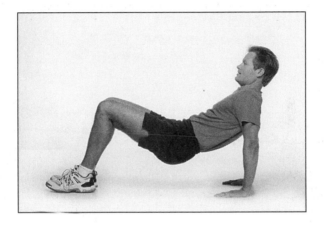

Exercise #18: Standing Bent-Knee Outer Thigh Blasters

- Phases One and Two: 12–15 reps
- Phases Three and Four: 20 reps

1. Stand and balance on your right leg with your right knee slightly bent, your hands on your hips and your left leg bent at the knee. Contract your abdominal muscles, and pull your shoulders back.
2. While keeping your abdominal muscles contracted and your torso upright, raise your left leg out to the side as high as you comfortably can while keeping both knees facing forward.
3. Hold the top position for a count of 2, and then lower your leg and repeat. Complete all reps with left leg, and then switch to your right leg.

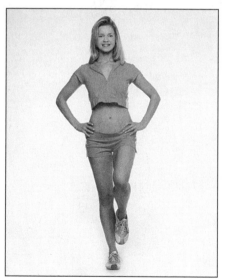 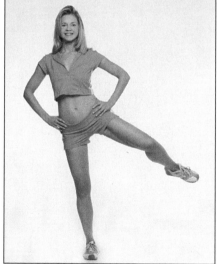

Exercise #19: Scissor Jumps

- Phases One and Two: 10–16 reps (Each time you switch feet counts as one rep.)
- Phases Three and Four: 20–30 reps (Each time you switch feet counts as one rep.)

1. Stand with your right foot forward, both knees slightly bent.
2. Contract your abdominal muscles and keep your back straight while you jump up slightly to switch legs so that your left foot is forward; land softly on your feet, keeping your knees bent.
3. Continue jumping up and switching legs briskly while pumping your arms naturally for the recommended number of reps.

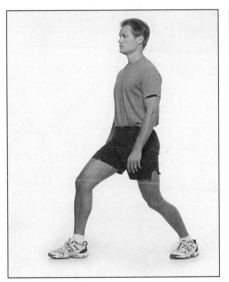 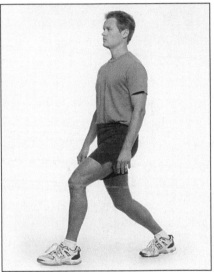

Exercise #20: Good Morning Bends

See photo and description #9 in 30-Minute Workout.

9

Enjoy Fit and Fabulous Whole-Foods Recipes

Who doesn't love to eat a great meal? Indulging in good food makes life more fun, at least we think so! However, one not-so-little snafu often stands in the way of a good home-spun meal . . . the cooking. We understand the concerns of fellow foodies who dread the thought of chopping, sautéing and simmering their way to mealtime bliss. However, you don't need to be Mrs. Cleaver to feed yourself and your family well. Truth be told, good food doesn't have to be difficult to cook, and it certainly doesn't need to take hours to prepare. We live in the real world, and we realize it's not reasonable to expect you to come home from work to spend hours stressing and fussing in the kitchen with twenty dirty pots and pans spread out all over the place all in the name of getting a great meal on the table. Thanks, but no thanks. To save you stress, a big mess, time and the fat-clogged take-out trap, we've put together fuss-free recipes that will bring to your table good food fast. We hope you enjoy our easy-does-it recipe collection as much as Ivy has enjoyed tinkering with them and Andy has enjoyed being the official taste-tester.

Breakfast and Brunch

Almond-Flax Pancakes with Raspberries

Serves: 2

These are "weekend morning" pancakes the kids will be crazy about! Moms and dads will be happy to know these jacks are loaded with antioxidants, fiber, disease-fighting lignans and anti-inflammatory omega-3-enriched essential fats, so there is no need to feel guilty about indulging.

2 omega-3-enriched eggs (such as Eggland's Best)
¼ cup low-fat plain yogurt or kefir
½ cup water
¼ teaspoon pure almond extract
¼ cup plus 2 tablespoons ground flaxseed (we recommend Barlean's "Forti-Flax")
¼ cup wheat germ
2 tablespoons quinoa flour (or whole-wheat flour)
¼ teaspoon baking powder
dash of salt
Canola oil cooking spray
1 cup fresh raspberries (you may also substitute frozen raspberries)

1. In a small bowl, beat the eggs and then slowly add the yogurt, water and almond extract. In another bowl, mix together the flaxseed, wheat germ, flour, baking powder and salt. Add the wet ingredients to the dry ingredients and mix gently until just evenly moistened.
2. Spray a nonstick skillet with canola oil cooking spray and heat the skillet over medium-high heat. Pour about 2–3 tablespoons of batter per pancake and cook until bubbles begin to form; flip and brown the other side. (*Note:* To be sure the pancakes are cooked through without burning, you may need to flip them a third time.)
3. Serve hot and top with fresh raspberries.

Nutrition Information: 260 calories, 1 g saturated fat, 30 g carbohydrate, 10 g dietary fiber, 11 g protein

Double Chocolate Walnut Muffins

Serves: 10

Serve these muffins for breakfast with a glass of organic milk or soymilk. They are simple to make, delicious to eat and healthful to boot! Although you'd certainly never know it from their name, these muffins are low in refined sugar, a great source of fiber and also provide a wide variety of nutrients.

Canola oil cooking spray
1½ cups whole-wheat flour
¼ cup wheat germ
½ cup ground flaxseed (we recommend Barlean's "Forti-Flax")
¼ cup unsweetened cocoa (such as Ghirardelli brand)
2 teaspoons baking powder
¼ teaspoon salt
2 ripe bananas, mashed (about 1 cup)
2 omega-3-enriched eggs (such as Eggland's Best) beaten
¼ cup high-oleic canola oil
⅓ cup brown sugar
⅓ cup low-fat plain yogurt
1 teaspoon pure vanilla extract
½ cup walnuts, finely chopped
¼ cup dark mini chocolate chips (such as Ghirardelli "Double-Chocolate Chip")

1. Preheat oven to 350 degrees. Coat a 10-muffin tin with cooking spray and set aside.
2. In a large bowl, stir together the flour, wheat germ, flaxseed, cocoa, baking powder and salt. In a medium bowl, stir together the bananas, eggs, canola oil, brown sugar, yogurt and vanilla.
3. Pour the liquid ingredients over the dry ingredients, and stir until just moistened. Stir in the walnuts and chocolate chips. Spoon the batter into the muffin tins and bake for 17 minutes, or until the muffins are light golden and a toothpick inserted in the center comes out clean.
4. Cool the muffin tins on a rack for 5 minutes. Remove the muffins from the tins and cool an additional 5 minutes before serving.

Nutrition Information: 300 calories, 2.5 g saturated fat, 36 g carbohydrate, 6 g dietary fiber, 9 g protein

Mexican Egg Casserole

Serves: 6

Mexican-food lovers will be especially pleased with this spicy and flavorful dish—one that's sure to wake up any grumpy, groggy person any day of the week! It's rich in calcium, protein and antioxidants, including lycopene. It's incredibly easy to make and perfect for brunch or even a simple dinner. Serve with roasted red peppers and black beans or whole-grain corn bread. (You can find a delicious corn bread recipe in our Gold Coast Cure *book.)*

  1 teaspoon extra-virgin olive oil
  2 cans (4-ounces each) chopped green chiles, drained
  1 can (15-ounces) Hunts tomato sauce
  1 cup water
  6 omega-3-enriched eggs (such as Eggland's Best)
  2 omega-3-enriched egg whites
  5 ounces light jalapeno cheese (such as Cabot brand), cut into small squares

1. Preheat oven to 350 degrees.
2. Heat oil in a large skillet over medium-high heat; add chiles and sauté for 1 minute. Pour tomato sauce and water into the skillet and simmer for 2–3 minutes.
3. In a medium-sized bowl, add eggs and egg whites; beat well. Stir cheese squares into the egg mixture.
4. Pour tomato sauce mixture into an 8 x 8-inch casserole. Carefully pour the egg and cheese mixture into the center of the sauce. Transfer casserole to the oven and bake for 1 hour.
5. Remove casserole from the oven and allow it to cool on a wire rack for 15 minutes before serving. Serve warm.

Nutrition Information: 180 calories, 4 g saturated fat, 9 g carbohydrate, 2 g dietary fiber, 16 g protein

Lemon-Peach Pie Smoothie

Serves: 2

Smoothies are one of the best ways to introduce (or sneak!) tofu into your diet. This smoothie is rich and creamy and packed with nutrients, including antiaging antioxidants vitamins C and A plus potassium, essential fats, protein and fiber.

1½ cups frozen peaches
1 cup silken tofu
½ cup low-fat plain kefir or yogurt
½ teaspoon pure lemon extract
1 tablespoon plus 1 teaspoon honey

Place all ingredients in a blender and whip until smooth and creamy, about 1 minute.

Nutrition Information: 160 calories, 0 g saturated fat, 7 g carbohydrate, <1 g dietary fiber, 5 g protein

Tofu Vegetable Scramble

Serves: 2

If you have 10 minutes to spare in the morning you can quickly whip up this dish. Tofu Vegetable Scramble is an excellent way to get your soy serving for the day right off the bat. So start your day on the fit track with a healthy dose of essential fats, phytoestrogens and antioxidants. P.S. The eggs rule in this dish, so you won't even taste the tofu.

1 cup crumbled extra-firm tofu, drained and patted dry
2 omega-3-enriched eggs (such as Eggland's Best)
⅛ teaspoon turmeric
Salt, to taste
Ground black pepper, to taste
2 teaspoons extra-virgin olive oil
2 minced garlic cloves
1 cup diced onion
½ cup diced red bell pepper
Fresh salsa (available in the deli section of your supermarket)

1. Combine crumbled tofu and eggs in a blender and blend until creamy, about 30 seconds. Season with measured turmeric and salt and pepper to taste.
2. Heat the oil in a nonstick medium-sized skillet over medium-high heat; add the garlic, onion and red pepper and sauté until vegetables are soft (1–2 minutes). Add the tofu and egg mixture and scramble until heated through (about 1 minute). Serve at once with fresh salsa.

Nutrition Information: 210 calories, 2.5 g saturated fat, 15 g carbohydrate, 2 g dietary fiber, 12 g protein

Sugar Plum French Toast Pudding

Serves: 9

We often serve this make-ahead breakfast treat on Christmas morning, when reindeers are dashing through the snow and childhood dreams of sugarplums are dancing in our heads. And despite its sinfully rich-sounding name, this recipe is actually very low in sugar, plus it is rich in fiber and omega-3 fats.

Canola oil cooking spray
2 cups pitted prunes
6 pieces thick-sliced, soft whole-grain bread (such as Rudi's "Honey Sweet Whole Wheat")
1 cup finely chopped walnuts
1 cup organic low-fat milk
4 omega-3-enriched eggs (such as Eggland's Best)
1 teaspoon pure vanilla extract
1 teaspoon cinnamon, plus more for "dusting"
3 ounces organic low-fat cream cheese
2 tablespoons sugar or Splenda "Brown Sugar Blend for Baking"

1. Preheat oven to 425 degrees. Spray the bottom and sides of a 9 x 13-inch baking dish with canola oil cooking spray.
2. Place the prunes in a small saucepan and add just enough water to cover; bring to a boil and cook prunes for 8–10 minutes. Remove prunes from the heat, drain and set aside to cool.
3. Tear bread into bite-sized pieces and loosely arrange in layers on the bottom of the prepared baking dish. Toss in the walnuts.
4. In a food processor or blender, add cooled prunes, milk, eggs, vanilla extract and cinnamon; process until smooth, about 1 minute. Pour the milk and egg mixture over the bread and walnuts, and toss lightly to coat. Transfer casserole to the oven and bake for 25 minutes.
5. Remove French toast pudding from the oven and allow it to cool on a wire rack before transferring it to the refrigerator; refrigerate until firm, at least two hours before frosting.
6. Meanwhile, make the frosting by mixing cream cheese and sugar (or Splenda) together in a small bowl until well blended.

7. Remove French toast pudding from the refrigerator a half-hour before serving; frost *lightly* with cream cheese mixture and then sprinkle with cinnamon. Cut the French toast pudding into rectangular serving pieces and arrange on a platter or individual plates. Serve at room temperature.

Nutrition Information: 220 calories, 2.5 g saturated fat, 16 g carbohydrate, 2 g dietary fiber, 10 g protein

Dressings, Dips, Soups and Salads

Creamy Tarragon Dressing

Serves: 4

Rich and smooth, Creamy Tarragon Dressing has a sweet, licorice flavor. The tarragon really pulls its own load here and gives the dressing a major flavor boost. Made from canola oil and flaxseed oil, this dressing is a great source of omega-3 essential fat. Serve this dressing on baby spinach leaves with chopped hard-boiled eggs (don't forget to use omega-3-enriched eggs.)

¼ cup low-fat plain yogurt
3 tablespoons canola-oil mayonnaise
½ cup loosely packed fresh tarragon leaves, coarsely chopped
1 teaspoon lemon juice
1 tablespoon flaxseed oil (we recommend Barlean's brand)
1 teaspoon brown sugar (or raw honey)

Toss all ingredients together into a blender or food processor and blend well for about 1 minute or until dressing is smooth and creamy. (*Note:* You can store this dressing in a covered container in the refrigerator for up to 2 days.)

Nutrition Information: 130 calories, 1 g saturated fat, 3 g carbohydrate, 0 g dietary fiber, 1 g protein

Roasted Red Pepper and Walnut Tapenade

Serves: 4

Traditionally, tapenade is made with capers, anchovies and olives, but since Ivy is not a big anchovy-flavor fan, our version offers a milder tasting and smoother condiment. It's also a healthful source of antioxidant vitamin C and omega-3 essential fats. For gourmet flair, serve Roasted Red Pepper and Walnut Tapenade with crudités, fish or meat. We're also crazy for this tapenade on all kinds of burgers (including turkey, beef and even ostrich).

1 jar (12-ounces) jar good-quality roasted red peppers (drained, rinsed and
   patted dry with paper towels)
½ cup walnuts
2 tablespoons extra-virgin olive oil
Juice from ½ lemon
⅛ teaspoon cayenne pepper
⅛ teaspoon salt

Combine all of the ingredients together in a food processor or blender and puree until a smooth paste is formed, about 1 minute. Store the tapenade in a covered container in the refrigerator until serving time. (*Note:* This recipe can be made 2–3 days in advance.)

Nutrition Information: 250 calories, 1.5 g saturated fat, 15 g carbohydrate, 1 g dietary fiber, 6 g protein

Caribbean Mango, Avocado and Black Bean Salad

Serves: 4

This invigorating dish is perfect for serving at your next "Beer-B-Q"—yes, even your good old beer-and-burger loving friends will appreciate this healthy recipe because it tastes so good! The vibrant tropical flavors in this refreshing salad blend sweet with tangy. Every mouthful offers a nutritional powerhouse of antioxidant vitamins C and E plus beta carotene, fiber, potassium and disease-fighting phytonutrients. For a complete meal, serve with grilled chicken.

1 mango, finely diced
1 red bell pepper, finely diced
¼ red onion, finely diced
1 teaspoon hot sauce (such as Tabasco)
1 teaspoon flaxseed oil (we recommend Barlean's brand)
½ cup chopped cilantro
1 avocado, finely diced
1 can (15.5 ounces) black beans, rinsed and drained
¼ teaspoon salt
1 tablespoon white vinegar

In a large glass or ceramic bowl, combine the diced mangoes, red pepper and red onion, and lightly toss. Add the hot sauce, oil and cilantro, and mix again. Fold in the avocado and beans. Add the salt and vinegar, and toss. Let stand 10–15 minutes before serving.

Nutrition Information: 150 calories, 1 g saturated fat, 19 g carbohydrate, 5 g dietary fiber, 4 g protein

Velvety Mushroom and Leek Soup

Serves: 6

Although we love to serve this soup for special holiday dinners, it's really a soup for all seasons. We gave this classic recipe a healthful makeover by ditching the butter and heavy cream; our version is low in saturated fat but still rich and creamy, plus it's a great source of calcium and antioxidants.

3 cups organic 2% low-fat milk
8 ounces (1 cup) silken tofu
1 cup organic chicken broth (such as Pacific Foods' "Organic Chicken Broth")
2 tablespoons extra-virgin olive oil, divided
2 bunches large leeks (4–6 stalks), washed and sliced into 1-inch rounds
½ pound button mushrooms, thinly sliced
¼ cup whole-wheat flour
½ teaspoon salt, plus more to taste
¼ teaspoon cayenne pepper, plus more to taste
1 tablespoon lemon juice
½ cup chardonnay (or other white wine)
Parsley, for garnish (optional)

1. In a blender puree milk, tofu and broth; set aside.
2. Heat 1 tablespoon olive oil in a large soup pot over medium-high heat; add leeks and sauté until tender but not brown. Remove the leeks from the pot and set aside.
3. Heat the remaining tablespoon of olive oil in the "dirty" soup pot over medium heat; add mushrooms and sauté until soft, about 5–8 minutes. Blend in flour and measured salt and cayenne pepper. Gradually whisk in the milk mixture. Cook, whisking constantly, until mixture thickens and comes to a boil.
4. Ladle a small amount (about ½ cup) of the broth into a small bowl and add the lemon juice and wine. Slowly add the lemon and wine mixture to the soup pot (go slowly so you don't curdle the broth). Add cooked leeks, and more salt and cayenne pepper to taste. Simmer for 10 minutes. Garnish with parsley and serve at once.

Nutrition Information: 230 calories, 2.5 g saturated fat, 25 g carbohydrate, 3 g dietary fiber, 10 g protein

Gazpacho

Serves: 8–10

Refreshing gazpacho is excellent served alongside grilled shrimp in the summertime. It's also great in Florida when the power goes out, and you have a bunch of perishable stuff in your refrigerator that's going to spoil if you don't do something with it in a go-go hurry! Ivy came up with this recipe with her mom during one of Florida's hurricanes. No need to wait for a hurricane to enjoy this delicious dish.

4 cloves garlic, crushed
¼ cup apple cider vinegar
⅓ cup extra-virgin olive oil
¼ teaspoon salt
1 teaspoon Worcestershire sauce
1 teaspoon Tabasco (or other hot sauce)
¼ teaspoon oregano
1 tablespoon brown sugar
2 cans (28 ounces each) diced tomatoes
1 yellow bell pepper, diced
1 cup fresh parsley, finely chopped
1½ cups minced onions
1 cup diced celery
2 small zucchini, diced
3 cups tomato juice

Garnish (optional):
Low-fat sour cream
Watercress sprigs

1. In a medium-sized bowl, add garlic, vinegar, oil, salt, Worcestershire sauce, Tabasco, oregano and brown sugar; whisk with a fork. Set dressing aside.
2. In a large sealable container, add the remaining ingredients. Then pour in the dressing and stir vegetables lightly. Transfer the gazpacho to the refrigerator and chill for at least 3 hours (or preferably overnight).
3. Serve in martini glasses or small bowls, and garnish with a dollop of low-fat sour cream and a sprig of watercress. Serve cold.

Nutrition Information: 180 calories, 2 g saturated fat, 22 g carbohydrate, 5 g dietary fiber, 4 g protein

Layered Chicken and Bean Trifle Salad

Serves: 8

This is chicken dressed to impress. Its elegant and "show-boaty" presentation is especially welcome on a buffet table. For a complete meal, serve with soup (such as tomato bisque) and fresh whole-grain bread. This visually appealing salad is rich in a wide spectrum of antioxidants, plus fiber, protein and heart-healthy monounsaturated fats.

Dressing:

½ cup freshly squeezed lime juice
1 tablespoon apple cider vinegar
1 tablespoon extra-virgin olive oil

1 crushed garlic clove
½ teaspoon ground cumin
Dash of salt

Salad:

1 tablespoon extra-virgin olive oil
2 chicken breasts, about 8 ounces total; cut into bite-sized cubes (preferably free-range, organic chicken)
1 teaspoon lemon pepper seasoning
2 cups torn mixed salad greens
1 can (15 ounces) black beans, rinsed and drained
1½ cups frozen corn (no need to thaw)
1 cup shredded-organic reduced-fat mozzarella cheese
1 cup mild white onion, chopped
2 cups multicolored bell peppers, (red, green and yellow)
2–4 scallions, chopped
½ cup prepared all-natural guacamole (or make your own with mashed avocados)
1 cup roughly broken blue corn tortilla chips (such as Garden of Eatin)

1. To make dressing, use a medium-sized bowl and add lime juice, vinegar, olive oil, garlic, cumin and salt; whisk with a fork. Set dressing aside.
2. For salad, heat extra-virgin olive oil in a large skillet over medium-high heat. Add chicken and lemon pepper; stir fry chicken until cooked through. When cooked, transfer chicken to a plate and set in freezer to cool for several minutes.

3. Using an 8-inch clear glass trifle bowl, layer salad ingredients in the following order: mixed greens, black beans, frozen corn, cheese, cooled chicken cubes, onion, bell pepper and scallions. Pour dressing on top of the salad; cover salad with clear plastic wrap and press down lightly with your hands. Refrigerate salad for a minimum of 2 hours, or overnight.

4. Just before serving, spread guacamole on top of the trifle and finish with the blue corn tortilla chips. Serve at once.

Nutrition Information: 300 calories, 3 g saturated fat, 32 g carbohydrate, 8 g dietary fiber, 23 g protein

Navy Bean and Leek Soup with Feta Cheese

Serves: 6

We call this hearty and fiber-rich soup our "Sunday dinner soup" because it's quick and easy to make (which is probably why Ivy makes it on Sundays, after we've been out and about all day). For a complete meal simply double the feta cheese and serve with a side salad and whole-grain rolls.

3 tablespoons extra-virgin olive oil
4 cloves garlic, minced
2 stalks leeks, washed and sliced into thin rounds
Salt, to taste
White pepper, to taste
2 cans (15.5 ounces each) navy beans, rinsed and drained
2 cups organic vegetable broth (such as Imagine "Organic Vegetable Broth")
2 cups water
½ cup crumbled low-fat feta cheese

1. Heat the olive oil in a Dutch oven or deep, heavy saucepan over medium-high heat. Add the garlic and leeks, and sauté for 3–4 minutes or until leeks are tender. Season to taste with salt and white pepper. Mix in the two cans of beans, vegetable broth and water.
2. Ladle half of the soup mixture into a blender and whirl until the beans are pureed; pour the pureed soup back into the pot. Season the soup with more salt and pepper to taste and heat over medium-high heat for 5 minutes.
3. Divide the soup among 6 bowls and top with feta cheese in the center of each bowl. Serve warm.

Nutrition Information: 470 calories, 3.5 g saturated fat, 62 g carbohydrate, 22 g dietary fiber, 24 g protein

Entrées

Glazed Jamaican BBQ Salmon

Serves: 4

Salmon is especially rich in omega-3 fats as well as protein and vitamins A, D, B_6 and B_{12}. For a complete meal, serve this grilled salmon with barbecued corn on the cob and grilled onions.

2 teaspoons white vinegar
2 teaspoons molasses
1 teaspoon tomato paste
1 tablespoon brown sugar
1 teaspoon allspice
1 teaspoon cinnamon
1 teaspoon salt
1 teaspoon ground ginger
½ teaspoon garlic powder
1 teaspoon cayenne pepper
1½ pounds salmon fillets
Extra-virgin olive oil cooking spray

1. In a small bowl, make the glaze by combining the vinegar, molasses and tomato paste; whisk to blend and set aside.
2. In a small sealable bag, combine the brown sugar, allspice, cinnamon, salt, ground ginger, garlic powder and cayenne pepper. Rub the spice mixture over both sides of the salmon.
3. Prepare a hot fire in a charcoal grill or preheat a gas grill or broiler to medium-high or 400 degrees. Away from the heat source, lightly coat the grill rack or broiler pan with cooking spray. Position the cooking rack 4–6 inches from the heat source.
4. Place the salmon on the grill rack or broiler pan. Grill or broil at medium-high heat for 3–4 minutes. Turn the fish over and baste with the glaze; continue cooking for another 4–5 minutes or until fish flakes easily with a fork. Transfer to a serving platter and serve immediately.

Nutrition Information: 270 calories, 1.5 g saturated fat, 8 g carbohydrate, <1 g dietary fiber, 34 g protein

Baked Halibut with Cilantro-Almond Pesto

Serves: 4

Go ahead and grab a glass of wine, then call and invite a few friends over for dinner. Then serve them this quick-fix dish. It looks impressive and tastes amazing. *Plus (in case any of your friends actually care) it provides a burst of nutrients, including omega-3 essential fats, antioxidant vitamin E, heart-healthy magnesium and phytonutrients (plant substances that help support a healthy immune system). Serve with sides of baked sweet potatoes and asparagus.*

½ cup loosely packed fresh cilantro
½ cup slivered almonds
2 tablespoons grated Parmesan cheese
1 teaspoon minced garlic
Juice from 1 lemon
⅛ teaspoon salt, plus more to taste
2 tablespoons extra-virgin olive oil, plus more to coat fish
1½ pounds halibut fillets (or any other firm white fish such as snapper or
    flounder)

1. Preheat oven to 450 degrees.
2. In a food processor, process the cilantro, almonds, Parmesan cheese, garlic, lemon juice, measured salt and extra-virgin olive oil for 15–20 seconds, or until well blended.
3. Brush the extra-virgin olive oil on both sides of the halibut and season lightly with salt. Place the halibut on a lightly oiled baking dish, and spread the pesto over the fillets. Bake for 10–15 minutes or until fish is cooked through. Serve at once.

Nutrition Information: 300 calories, 2 g saturated fat, 3 g carbohydrate, <1 g dietary fiber, 38 g protein

Sea Bass with Coconut Cream Sauce

Serves: 4

If you are as crazy about Thai food as we are, this recipe will be a hands-down winner! It's got such a unique combination of complementary flavors plus a rich, creamy and savory sauce. This recipe provides an excellent source of essential omega-3 fats, heart-healthy monounsaturated fats and protein. For a complete meal, serve the sea bass over brown rice with steamed snow peas (drizzle the coconut cream sauce on top of the veggies).

½ cup light coconut milk (such as Thai Kitchen "Light Coconut Milk")
¼ cup all-natural creamy peanut butter
Juice from ½ lime
2 teaspoons grated ginger
3 teaspoons soy sauce (such as Kikkoman)
⅛ teaspoon cayenne pepper, plus more to taste
Canola oil cooking spray
¼ cup chopped onion
Salt, to taste
1 pound Chilean sea bass fillets

1. In a food processor or blender, combine coconut milk, peanut butter, lime juice, ginger, soy sauce and cayenne pepper; process until smooth. Set sauce aside.
2. Spray a large nonstick skillet with canola oil cooking spray. Sauté onion for 3–4 minutes over medium heat until soft; season lightly with salt to taste. Clear onions to either side of the pan.
3. Season both sides of sea bass with salt and cayenne pepper. Place sea bass fillets in the center of the skillet and sear for 4–5 minutes each side. After searing the second side, add the sauce and bring to a boil. Flip the fish once and cook 1–2 more minutes. Serve immediately.

Nutrition Information: 240 calories, 3 g saturated fat, 6 g carbohydrate, 1 g dietary fiber, 25 g protein

Pan-Roasted Red Snapper
with Jalapeno-Pineapple Salsa

Serves: 4

This fish dish was inspired by a trip we took to Key West where we ate at a little shack of a restaurant that served outstanding food (wish we could remember the name of that place!). You'll get great anti-inflammatory benefits from the omega-3 fats in the fish as well as the bromelain in the pineapple. This recipe is also rich in protein, vitamin C and manganese. Serve this mouth-watering fish with a whole-grain side dish and green beans sautéed in garlic and extra-virgin olive oil.

Salsa:
2 cups coarsely chopped fresh pineapple
2 small jalapeno peppers, seeded and finely chopped
½ red onion, finely chopped
Juice from 1 lime
½ cup chopped fresh cilantro
1 teaspoon cumin
2 teaspoons honey
2 teaspoons hot sauce (such as Crystal "Louisiana Hot Sauce")
Fish:
2 pounds red snapper fillets
Extra-virgin olive oil
Salt, to taste
Cumin, to taste

1. In a nonreactive bowl, combine the pineapple, jalapeno peppers, onion, lime juice, cilantro, cumin, honey and hot sauce. Set salsa aside. (Can be made 3 hours ahead. Place in refrigerator and bring to room temperature before serving.)
2. Preheat oven to 400 degrees. Lightly coat a baking pan with extra-virgin olive oil, and then brush both sides of fish with the oil. Season fish on both sides with salt and cumin to taste.
3. Arrange fish skin-side up in baking pan. Bake 12–15 minutes or until fish is cooked through.
4. Serve fish immediately and top with salsa.

Nutrition Information: 290 calories, 0 g saturated fat, 20 g carbohydrate, 2 g dietary fiber, 52 g protein

Indian Lentil Dal

Serves: 4

Creamy and rich, this dish is delicious served over brown rice.

2 tablespoons extra-virgin olive oil
1 finely chopped mild onion
1 package (12 ounces) frozen butternut squash, thawed
¼ cup plus 2 tablespoons light coconut milk (such as Thai Kitchen "Light
    Coconut Milk"), divided
1 tablespoon plus 2 teaspoons fresh minced ginger, divided
3 cloves garlic, minced
1 cup lentils
2 teaspoons brown sugar
½ teaspoon salt
2 teaspoons ground cumin
2 teaspoons ground ginger
2 teaspoons turmeric
1 can (14 ounces) chopped tomatoes
2 cups water
1 cup organic 1% or 2% low-fat milk
¼ teaspoon cayenne pepper (or more to taste)
2 cups cooked brown rice

1. In a large saucepan over medium heat, heat oil and sauté onion until softened. Add butternut squash, ¼ cup coconut milk, 1 tablespoon minced ginger and garlic; stir and reduce heat to low.
2. Add the lentils, brown sugar, salt, cumin, ground ginger and turmeric to the pan. Stir until the lentils are well coated. Add tomatoes and 2 cups of water. Raise the heat to a boil, then reduce heat until mixture is at a fast simmer. Cook uncovered for 25 minutes, stirring frequently.
3. Add 1 additional cup of water plus remaining 2 tablespoons of coconut milk. Simmer for an additional 15 minutes. Add 1 more cup of water plus remaining 2 teaspoons of minced ginger and milk; simmer 10 more minutes.
4. Remove pan from heat, stir in the cayenne pepper (add more to taste), cover and let sit for 10 minutes. Serve warm over brown rice.

Nutrition Information: 480 calories, 3 g saturated fat, 80 g carbohydrate, 10 g dietary fiber, 20 g protein

Indonesian Baked Tofu with Peanut Sauce

Serves: 4

This full-bodied dish is absolutely bursting with flavor. The tofu provides an excellent source of vegetarian protein and also yields a good dose of iron, essential fats and phytoestrogens. Serve with simple sides like barley and roasted red peppers. (Note: you can reserve a little of the peanut sauce to flavor the peppers.)

¼ cup all-natural peanut butter
3 garlic cloves
1 tablespoon fresh minced ginger
1 tablespoon brown sugar
2 teaspoons soy sauce, plus more to taste
½ cup water
2 pounds extra-firm tofu, drained, pressed, patted dry and cut into about
    16 rectangles, 2 x 3 inches

1. Preheat the oven to 400 degrees, and line a baking sheet with aluminum foil.
2. In a blender, mix all ingredients except the tofu. Set peanut sauce aside.
3. Season each side of each piece of tofu with soy sauce, then rub the sauce into the tofu lightly with your hands.
4. Pour about half of the peanut sauce onto the baking sheet. Lay the tofu pieces on the sauce, then pour the rest of the sauce over the tofu. Bake tofu for 25 minutes, or until peanut sauce begins to harden and darken slightly. Serve at once.

Nutrition Information: 240 calories, 1.5 g saturated fat, 2 g carbohydrate, 1 g dietary fiber, 21 g protein

Pork Chops with Balsamic-Mango Chutney

Serves: 4

Pork, the "other white meat," is a healthy lean meat option, assuming you snip snap all visible fat. For this particular recipe, we paired the lean pork with chutney, which is a great way to spike your pork and give it a little life. Actually, Ivy's mom created the chutney for this recipe, which is just outrageous. Serve the pork with sides of baked sweet potatoes and a dollop of butter and chutney on top . . . yum's the word!

1 teaspoon organic butter
½ red onion, diced
1¼ cups chopped mango (you can also use frozen mangos, just chop and
    thaw)
½ cup yellow raisins
¼ cup balsamic vinegar
¼ cup brown sugar
¼ teaspoon salt
1 teaspoon extra virgin olive oil, plus more for rubbing on pork
4 pork chops (5–6 ounces each), trimmed of all visible fat
⅓ cup Chardonnay
Juice from 1 whole lemon
2 tablespoons water

1. Heat the butter in a small saucepan over medium-high heat; add the onion and sauté until the onion is soft, about 3 minutes. Add in the mango, raisins, vinegar, brown sugar and salt; bring mixture to a boil over medium-high and then reduce heat and simmer for 20 minutes, stirring occasionally. Remove chutney from heat and set aside. *(Note: the chutney can be made up to two days in advance; just keep in a sealed container in the refrigerator.)*
2. Dry the chops with a paper towel, rub extra virgin olive oil on both sides, then season with salt and white pepper to taste. Pour 1 teaspoon of the extra virgin olive into a large skillet, swirl to coat, and heat over moderately high heat; when the pan is very hot lay in the chops. Sauté to brown each lightly on both sides, about 3 minutes per side.
3. Pour the Chardonnay and lemon juice into the pan, cover the pan, and adjust heat to maintain a slow simmer. Cook pork slowly about 4 minutes, turn, and cook another 4 minutes on the other side.

Remove the chops to a side dish and add 2 tablespoons of the prepared chutney plus 2 tablespoons of water to the hot pan and heat briefly, until syrupy. Add the chops back to the pan and baste with the syrupy sauce as you simmer to re-warm. Serve at chops with 1 tablespoon of chutney on top.

Nutrition Information: 430 calories, 4 g saturated fat, 53 g carbohydrate, 2 g dietary fiber, 30 g protein

Spice-Rubbed Lamb Kabobs with Tahini Sauce

Serves: 4

We got the idea for this recipe after eating at Leila's, a cosmopolitan Middle-Eastern grille in downtown West Palm Beach. After Andy stopped admiring the belly dancers, and we started eating, we were hooked on the lamb kabobs! The combination of flavors is knock-out good, and the lamb is an excellent source of B-vitamins and minerals. And, if you choose lean cuts and meticulously snip off all visible fat, it's also low in saturated fat. The dipping sauce is a great source of essential fats. Serve lamb kabobs with whole-wheat couscous and grilled mixed vegetables.

1½ pounds completely trimmed lamb, preferably from the leg,
    cut into 2-inch chunks
½ cup good-quality red wine, such as Cabernet Sauvignon
2 teaspoons cinnamon
2 teaspoons chili powder
½ teaspoon cayenne pepper
½ teaspoon salt
½ cup tahini (sesame seed butter)
3 tablespoons lemon juice
2 teaspoons minced garlic cloves
⅓ cup low-fat yogurt or kefir
⅓ cup chopped parsley
Salt, to taste

1. Place lamb cubes in a gallon-size sealable plastic bag. Pour wine over meat and seal bag. Shake to coat, and let lamb marinate in the refrigerator for 4–8 hours.
2. Meanwhile, make the spice rub by adding cinnamon, chili powder, cayenne pepper and salt to a small sealable plastic bag. Shake to mix spices. Set aside.
3. To a food processor or blender add tahini, lemon juice, garlic, yogurt, parsley and salt to taste; puree until smooth and creamy. Refrigerate dipping sauce.
4. A half-hour before cooking, remove the dipping sauce and lamb from the refrigerator. Drain off wine from lamb and add spice rub to the gallon-size plastic bag previously used to marinate lamb; shake to coat lamb pieces.
5. Preheat the broiler and thread lamb chunks onto skewers.

6. Place lamb on an aluminum foil-lined baking sheet. Broil lamb 3–4 inches from the flame for a total of 10 minutes, turning to brown on all sides (the meat should be medium-rare). Remove lamb from broiler, and transfer to individual plates. Serve at once with individual small bowls of tahini dipping sauce.

Nutrition Information: 460 calories, 6 g saturated fat, 8 g carbohydrate, 2 g dietary fiber, 41 g protein

Tofu-Vegetable Lasagna Roll-Ups with Cheese Sauce

Serves: 4

We didn't realize some people would think the idea of eating tofu lasagna was unappetizing until just recently when we ran into an old friend, Gray Cooper. Ivy invited Gray and his wife over for dinner, which sounded like a great idea to him. Then Ivy said she would make tofu lasagna, and he burst out laughing (he thought it was a joke!). This reaction has taught us to refrain from telling unsuspecting dinner guests that tofu is involved in any recipe. All laughs aside, these lasagna roll-ups really are goooooood!

Salt, to taste
1 package (8 ounces) whole-wheat lasagna noodles
½ cup organic low-fat ricotta cheese
½ cup crumbled extra-firm tofu, drained and patted dry with paper towels
1 tablespoon extra-virgin olive oil
1 cup finely chopped onion
3 cloves garlic, minced
1 red bell pepper, diced
1 package (10 ounces) frozen chopped spinach, defrosted and squeezed dry
    with paper towels
½ teaspoon nutmeg
1 cup organic chicken broth
½ cup organic whole milk
3 wedges low-fat soft Swiss cheese (such as The Laughing Cow "Light Creamy
    Swiss Original")
¼ cup shredded Parmesan cheese

1. Preheat oven to 350 degrees.
2. Bring a large pot of water to a boil. When the water boils, add salt then the lasagna noodles. Cook the noodles until almost tender, or al dente (about 5–8 minutes). Drain the noodles, and set aside.
3. Combine the ricotta cheese and tofu together in a food processor, and puree until smooth.
4. Heat the oil in a medium skillet over medium-high heat. Add the onion, garlic and red bell pepper; sauté until vegetables are tender, about 4–5 minutes. Add chopped spinach to the skillet, and heat

through for 1 minute. Add the ricotta and tofu mixture to the veg-etables, and gently stir for 1 minute. Add nutmeg and season to taste with salt. Remove the skillet from the heat.

5. In a small pot, heat the chicken broth and milk over medium heat until small bubbles begin to form; add the soft Swiss cheese to the liquid, and return to a gentle bubble. Simmer sauce on low heat until cheese is melted, stirring frequently. Pour half of the cheese sauce into an 8 x 8-inch casserole.

6. Place the cooked lasagna noodles on a large cutting board or work surface. Spread each lasagna noodle with a layer of the vegetable mixture, and then roll them up and transfer to the casserole. Dot the bundles with spoonfuls of the cheese sauce. Sprinkle Parmesan cheese on top and transfer to the oven. Bake for 10 minutes. Remove from oven and serve at once.

Nutrition Information: 430 calories, 4.5 g saturated fat, 56 g carbohydrate, 10 g dietary fiber, 27 g protein

Mixed Mushroom and Rigatoni Bake with Gruyere

Serves: 4

This is fancy gourmet comfort food, perfect for hassle-free, spur-of-the-moment "impress-your-neighbors" entertaining. Our lightened version is rich in fiber and calcium. For a memorable meal serve this pasta bake with Creamy Roasted Red Pepper and Carrot Soup (see recipe in our Gold Coast Cure *book) and a simple side salad of mixed greens.*

1 tablespoon extra-virgin olive oil
2 sliced shallots
4 ounces shiitake mushroom caps, sliced
4 ounces oyster mushrooms, sliced
8 ounces button mushrooms, sliced
1 tablespoon chopped fresh sage
½ teaspoon salt
¼ teaspoon white pepper
3 cloves garlic, minced
2 tablespoons chardonnay (or other white wine)
1 cup frozen petite peas (such as Birds Eye)
¼ cup whole-wheat flour
2 cups organic 1% low-fat milk
½ cup low-fat organic mozzarella cheese
4 cups cooked whole-wheat rigatoni pasta
olive oil cooking spray
½ cup shredded Gruyère cheese
Fresh basil, for garnish

1. Preheat oven to 375 degrees.
2. Heat the oil in a large nonstick skillet over medium-high heat. Add the shallots; sauté 3 minutes. Add mushrooms, chopped sage, salt, pepper and garlic; sauté 5–8 minutes or until mushrooms are tender. Add chardonnay; cook 1 minute, stirring frequently. Mix in frozen peas; cook 1–2 more minutes. Remove from heat.
3. Place flour in a Dutch oven (or heavy soup pot) over medium-high heat; gradually add milk, stirring constantly with a whisk. Bring mixture to a boil; cook 1 minute or until slightly thick, stirring constantly with a whisk. Remove from heat; add the mozzarella cheese, stirring until melted. Add mushroom mixture and pasta to the cheese sauce, tossing well to combine. Spoon pasta mixture into an 8-inch square casserole lightly coated with cooking spray; sprinkle evenly with the

Gruyère cheese. Bake at 375 degrees for 30 minutes or until cheese melts and begins to brown. Garnish with fresh basil.

Nutrition Information: 470 calories, 5 g saturated fat, 63 g carbohydrate, 8 g dietary fiber, 27 g protein

Tofu Parmesan

Serves: 4

Even if you are wishy-washy about the thought of eating tofu, you're gonna love this. It's a healthy and simple remake of a traditional Italian favorite and a tasty way to get your tofu fix for the day.

Extra-virgin olive oil cooking spray
1 large Spanish onion, sliced
1 package (14 ounces) extra-firm tofu, drained and patted dry
Salt, to taste
2 teaspoons extra-virgin olive oil, divided
1 omega-3-enriched egg (such as Eggland's Best) beaten
¼ cup plus 2 tablespoons whole-wheat flour, divided
½ cup shredded Parmesan cheese
2 tablespoons wheat germ
1 small can (7 ounces) mushrooms, drained
1½ cups good-quality prepared marinara sauce (such as Rao's "Homemade Marinara")

1. Preheat oven to 350 degrees. Spray the bottom and sides of an 8 x 8-inch casserole with olive oil cooking spray.
2. Place onion slices in a microwave-safe bowl, cover and microwave on high for 2 minutes. Remove onions from microwave, drain water and set aside.
3. Slice tofu lengthwise into 4 thin rectangular blocks, and pat dry with paper towels. Season both sides of tofu blocks with salt to taste.
4. Pour 1 teaspoon extra-virgin olive oil into a large cast-iron skillet or nonstick skillet and spread oil lightly around the skillet with a paper towel. Begin heating the oil over low heat.
5. Meanwhile, in a medium-sized bowl beat the egg. Spread ¼ cup of the whole-wheat flour out on a clean, flat surface. Dredge both sides of the tofu blocks in the egg and then the flour.
6. Raise temperature on the stove top to medium-high, and place the tofu blocks on the hot skillet; sear for 2 minutes on each side, turning with a spatula, or until tofu is golden. Remove skillet from heat and set aside.
7. In a small bowl, mix together the remaining 2 tablespoons whole-wheat flour, Parmesan cheese and wheat germ. Mix in the remaining teaspoon of olive oil.

8. Arrange tofu blocks on the bottom of the prepared casserole. Spread cooked onions on top of the tofu, and then arrange the mushrooms on top of the onions. Pour the tomato sauce on top of the mushrooms, and sprinkle the Parmesan-wheat germ topping on top. Cover with aluminum foil and bake for 30 minutes.

9. Remove aluminum foil, and bake for an additional 15 minutes. Remove casserole from oven, and allow it to cool on a wire rack for 15 minutes before serving. Serve warm.

Nutrition Information: 200 calories, 1 g saturated fat, 21 g carbohydrate, 4 g dietary fiber, 13 g protein

---

Chicken Breasts Stuffed with Roasted Red Peppers and Goat Cheese

Serves: 4

This is not your everyday chicken dinner; it looks fancy and tastes "Oooooh la la"! If you don't like goat cheese you can use cream cheese instead. Whatever you choose, the recipe is still low in saturated fat and bundled with flavor. Serve with sides of a baked potato and grilled portobello mushrooms.

4 teaspoons extra-virgin olive oil, divided
3–4 cloves garlic, minced
1 jar (12 ounces) good-quality roasted red peppers, drained,
    patted dry with paper towels and finely chopped
2 tablespoons goat cheese (or cream cheese)
¼ cup fresh basil, chopped
2 whole boneless, skinless chicken breasts (about 1 pound total),
    cut in half and pounded thin
Salt, to taste
White pepper, to taste
½ cup white wine

1. Preheat the oven to 400 degrees.
2. In a large skillet add 2 teaspoons extra-virgin olive oil, and heat over medium-high heat. Add the garlic and peppers, and sauté for 2–3 minutes. Remove from heat, and stir in the cheese and basil; continue stirring until the cheese is melted through.
3. Season both sides of the chicken breasts with salt and white pepper to taste. Place ¼ of the roasted red pepper and goat cheese filling on one-half of each chicken breast; fold the chicken breasts over to form a "package." Press the sides of the chicken together with your fingertips to "seal" the package as best as you can.
4. Place the chicken in a glass baking dish and rub the remaining olive oil on the chicken; pour the wine on top. Cover with foil, and bake for 30 minutes. Remove chicken from the oven, and allow it to cool for 10 minutes before serving.

Nutrition Information: 350 calories, 3 g saturated fat, 12 g carbohydrate, 0 g dietary fiber, 39 g protein

Baked Mussels with Herbed Crumb Topping

Serves: 4

New Zealand Greenshell Mussels are especially rich in omega-3 essential fats. They are unlike the common black/blue mussels found elsewhere, and can be recognized by their distinctive green and gold shell coloring, superior meat yield and larger size. This larger-size mussel is grown quickly, resulting in a tender, succulent mussel. These delectable treats are easy to make and are perfect served over whole-grain pasta and bruschetta. Ta da! Dinner in a snap.

¼ cup wheat germ
¼ cup freshly grated Parmesan cheese
⅛ teaspoon salt
⅛ teaspoon cayenne pepper
¼ cup fresh basil leaves, minced
1 tablespoon extra-virgin olive oil
2 pounds frozen New Zealand Greenshell Mussels on the half shell

1. Preheat oven to 425 degrees. Line a large baking sheet with aluminum foil.
2. In a medium-sized bowl mix together the wheat germ, Parmesan, salt, cayenne pepper, basil and oil.
3. Arrange the frozen mussels on the baking sheet and sprinkle the herbed crumb topping evenly on top. Bake the mussels for 15 minutes. Serve at once.

Nutrition Information: 470 calories, 3.5 g saturated fat, 21 g carbohydrate, 1 g dietary fiber, 58 g protein

Tofu Enchiladas

Serves: 4

Enchiladas are practically a family staple—who doesn't love 'em? Gooey, cheesy and dripping with yummy. We, of course, have lightened up our version and snuck in some tofu. P.S. Definitely don't tell the kids about the tofu!

Extra-virgin olive oil cooking spray
1 package (14 ounces) extra-firm tofu, drained and patted dry
1 tablespoon extra-virgin olive oil
1½ cups diced onion
½ cup canned roasted red peppers, drained, patted dry and diced
1 teaspoon cumin
¼ teaspoon salt
1 cup frozen corn kernels
12 stone-ground corn tortillas (such as Tam-x-ico "Corn Tortillas")
1 cup tomato sauce (such as Hunts "Tomato Sauce")
1 can (4.5 ounces) chopped green chiles
¼ teaspoon cayenne pepper
¾ cup shredded organic low-fat Cheddar cheese

1. Preheat oven to 350 degrees, and spray a large rectangular baking pan with extra-virgin olive oil cooking spray.
2. Cut the tofu block in half, and then slice the tofu into 1-inch-long thin rectangular strips. Set the tofu on paper towels to drain excess water.
3. Heat the oil in a large sauté pan over medium-high heat; add the diced onion and roasted red peppers, and sauté until onion is soft, about 5 minutes.
4. Add the tofu to the pan and *gently* toss the tofu in with the onion and roasted red peppers. Season the tofu with the cumin and salt, and sauté the tofu until it browns lightly, about 5 minutes (be careful not to stir the tofu too much, or it will crumble). Gently toss the frozen corn kernels in with the tofu, and continue cooking for a few more minutes. Transfer the tofu and vegetables to a large bowl and allow to cool slightly.
5. Meanwhile, spray the "dirty" skillet with extra-virgin olive oil cooking spray and reheat. Working in batches of four, dip the tortillas in

a bowl of water and then transfer to the heated skillet and "fry" for about 1 minute each side.

6. To make the enchiladas, take a tortilla in your hand and place about 3 tablespoons of the tofu and vegetable filling in the center (be careful not to overfill the tortillas!). Carefully roll the tortilla in your hand, and place the seam side down in the prepared baking pan (you may need to overlap the enchiladas to make them fit in the baking pan).

7. In a small bowl, mix together the tomato sauce, chopped green chilis and cayenne pepper. Pour the tomato and green chile sauce over the top of the enchiladas, and sprinkle the cheese on top.

8. Bake for 30–35 minutes. Allow enchiladas to cool for 10 minutes before serving.

Nutrition Information: 310 calories, 1.5 g saturated fat, 49 g carbohydrate, 8 g dietary fiber, 17 g protein

On-the-Side Vegetables

Broiled Zucchini and Feta Boats

Serves: 6

We call this "visually impressive" cooking. These eye candy veggies are so simple to make and can quickly help dress up a rather humdrum looking dinner of grilled chicken or fish. And, of course, they are nutri-ent-rich and a good source of antiaging antioxidants vitamins C and A as well as folate.

1 tablespoon extra-virgin olive oil
1 tablespoon garlic, finely chopped
3 zucchini, halved lengthwise
Salt, to taste
Ground black pepper, to taste
½ cup low-fat feta cheese

1. Preheat broiler.
2. Heat olive oil in a large nonstick, oven-proof skillet (with ovenproof handle) set over medium-low heat. Add garlic, and sauté for 15 seconds or until lightly golden (be careful not to burn the garlic). Arrange zucchini halves cut-side down in skillet; season with salt and pepper to taste. Increase heat to medium, and cook zucchini for 5–6 minutes, or until just caramelized (again, be careful not to let the zucchini or garlic burn).
3. Turn the zucchini over and season lightly with salt and white pepper; cook an additional 1–2 minutes. Sprinkle feta cheese on the top of the zucchini and then transfer the zucchini to the broiler; broil for 2–3 minutes. Serve at once.

Nutrition Information: 60 calories, 1 g saturated fat, 4 g carbohydrate, 1 g dietary fiber, 3 g protein

Braised Carrots with Maple Syrup and Mint

Serves: 4

Even children will eat their carrots if you serve them this way! The natural sweetness of the carrots is enhanced with the maple syrup and mint. Carrots are rich in beta carotene, which is changed into vitamin A by your body. Vitamin A helps keep your eyes and skin healthy. Carrots also contain disease-fighting flavonoids and are a rich source of fiber.

2 pounds fresh carrots, peeled and sliced into thin rounds
1 teaspoon organic butter
1 teaspoon extra-virgin olive oil
1 tablespoon pure maple syrup
1 cup loosely packed fresh mint leaves, washed and dried with stems removed
Salt, to taste

1. Fill a large heavy soup pot half-full of water and bring to a boil; add the carrots and boil for 5 minutes. Drain the carrots and immediately rinse them with cold water.
2. Heat the butter and olive oil in the heavy soup pot over medium-high heat; add the carrots when the butter melts and sauté carrots for 3 minutes, stirring occasionally.
3. Add the maple syrup and mint leaves, then cook the carrots for another minute, or until the mint leaves just begin to wilt. Season to taste with salt, and serve at once.

Nutrition Information: 130 calories, 1 g saturated fat, 26 g carbohydrate, 7 g dietary fiber, 2 g protein

Roasted Summer Squash Combo

Serves: 4

Roasting really brings out the sweetness in vegetables and gives them a definitively richer flavor. This particular combination of mixed vegetables is easy to prepare and makes a tasty dish loaded with antioxidants. Serve these veggies as a side to grilled fish or beef.

2 tablespoons extra-virgin olive oil
1 tablespoon crushed garlic
1 teaspoon dried rosemary
2 medium zucchini, cut into ½ inch-thick slices
2 medium yellow summer squash, cut into ½ inch-thick slices
2 red onions, cut crosswise into ½ inch-thick slices
Salt, to taste
White pepper, to taste
¼ cup balsamic vinegar, or less to taste

1. Preheat the oven to 450 degrees.
2. In a small bowl, stir together the olive oil, crushed garlic and rosemary.
3. Line a large cookie sheet with aluminum foil and arrange vegetables evenly on the foil. Drizzle the oil mixture over the vegetables, and toss to coat. Season vegetables to taste with salt and white pepper. Transfer vegetables to the oven and roast for 20 minutes.
4. Remove vegetables from the oven and drizzle with balsamic vinegar to taste. Serve immediately or at room temperature.

Nutrition Information: 170 calories, 1 g saturated fat, 27 g carbohydrate, 5 g dietary fiber, 3 g protein

Ratatouille

Serves: 6

Ratatouille is a healthy and hearty southern French dish. There are many different variations; our version is a contemporary remake that relies on major shortcuts to save both time and pots. We've also added a snappy spicy twist with cayenne pepper. Ratatouille can be served hot, cold or warm and as a side dish to lamb, chicken, turkey or beef, or as a topping for whole-grain penne pasta, brown rice or whole-wheat couscous.

¼ cup extra-virgin olive oil, divided
3 cloves garlic, minced
1 large onion, sliced thinly
1 medium-sized eggplant, cut into ½ inch pieces
1 red bell pepper, chopped
2 zucchini, scrubbed, and cut into ½ inch-thick slices
1 can (14.5 ounces) diced tomatoes
½ teaspoon dried oregano
¼ teaspoon salt, or more to taste
¼ teaspoon cayenne pepper
½ cup shredded fresh basil leaves
½ cup grated Parmesan cheese

1. In a large Dutch oven or sauce pan, heat 2 tablespoons of the olive oil over medium heat. Add garlic and onion; cook until the onion is softened.
2. Add the remaining 2 tablespoons of olive oil and raise the temperature to medium-high. Add the eggplant and cook, stirring frequently, for 8 minutes, or until the eggplant is softened.
3. Add the pepper and zucchini and cook, stirring occasionally, until the vegetables are soft. Add the tomatoes, oregano, salt and cayenne pepper. Cover and simmer for 10 minutes. Add the fresh basil, and cook uncovered for 5–10 additional minutes.
4. The ratatouille may be made 1 day in advance, kept covered and refrigerated. Serve warm or cold with grated Parmesan cheese.

Nutrition Information: 160 calories, 2.5 g saturated fat, 12 g carbohydrate, 4 g dietary fiber, 5 g protein

Green Bean Casserole

Serves: 8

There are two types of people, those who love green bean casserole, and those who don't. Even if we only eat it once a year, we personally couldn't imagine a holiday meal without a really good green bean casserole. This lightened-up classic is healthy but still tasty enough to please all the die-hard green bean casserole lovers of the world.

1 tablespoon extra-virgin olive oil
1 medium onion, diced
1 red bell pepper, diced
½ pound button mushrooms, quartered
½ teaspoon salt, divided
½ teaspoon white pepper, divided
1½ pounds green beans, trimmed and cut into 2-inch pieces
1 tablespoon butter
6 tablespoons whole-wheat flour
2 cups organic 1% low-fat milk
Pinch of cayenne pepper
Pinch of nutmeg
Cooking spray (such as Crisco brand
    100% extra-virgin olive oil no-stick spray)
¼ cup grated Parmesan cheese
½ cup corn flakes, crushed

1. Heat the oil in a large skillet over medium heat. Add onion, and sauté until it begins to soften, about 2–4 minutes. Add bell pepper and mushrooms, and cook until softened and most of the liquid has evaporated, about 8 minutes. Season with ¼ teaspoon salt and ¼ teaspoon white pepper; set aside to cool.
2. Prepare an ice bath: Fill a large bowl with ice and water; set aside. Bring a medium-sized saucepan of water to a boil. Add beans, and cook until bright green and just tender, 4–5 minutes. Drain, and plunge into ice bath to stop cooking. When cooled, toss drained beans with mushroom mixture; set aside.
3. Melt the butter in a medium saucepan over medium-low heat. Alternate adding in flour and milk, whisk constantly until mixture has thickened, about 3 minutes. Stir in cayenne, nutmeg, and the remaining ¼ teaspoon salt and ¼ teaspoon white pepper. Remove

from heat, and let cool to room temperature, stirring occasionally. Pour over beans and mushroom mixture, and toss to coat.

4. Lightly oil a 9 x 13-inch glass or ceramic baking pan with cooking spray. Transfer the bean and mushroom mixture to the prepared baking dish. In a small bowl, mix the Parmesan cheese and corn flakes together; sprinkle Parmesan mixture over the top of the casserole. Cover casserole with aluminum foil.

5. Heat broiler, positioning rack about 8 inches from the heat. Cook casserole for 10 minutes. Uncover and cook until top is golden brown, about 30 seconds. Serve at once.

Nutrition Information: 130 calories, 2 g saturated fat, 17 g carbohydrate, 4 g dietary fiber, 6 g protein

Snow Peas with Ginger and Garlic

Serves: 4

This is a simple and classic Asian-inspired side dish. It's delicious served with buckwheat soba noodles and grilled shrimp or scallops. The snow peas are rich in antioxidants, vitamins C and A, iron and potassium, plus the ginger provides anti-inflammatory properties, and the garlic helps reduce your blood pressure.

1½ teaspoons organic butter
4 cups snow peas, trimmed (about 12 ounces)
1½ teaspoons minced peeled fresh ginger
1 teaspoon minced garlic
2 tablespoons soy sauce (such as Kikkoman)
1 teaspoon honey
Ground black pepper, to taste

1. Melt butter in a large nonstick skillet over medium-high heat. Add snow peas, ginger and garlic; sauté 4–5 minutes.
2. Remove snow peas from heat; stir in soy sauce and honey. Season snow peas to taste with black pepper, and serve at once.

Nutrition Information: 60 calories, 1 g saturated fat, 8 g carbohydrate, 2 g dietary fiber, 3 g protein

Spinach and Basil Stuffed Mushrooms

Serves: 4

Stuffed mushrooms are festive and fun. They make a great presentation and are perfect for serving as appetizers at a swanky soiree or as a side dish to beef, chicken or lamb. Unlike most stuffed mushrooms, our version is low in saturated fat and bursting with nutrients.

Extra-virgin olive oil cooking spray
1 package (10-ounces) frozen chopped spinach
12 large fresh white mushrooms (*Note:* Do not rinse mushrooms in water; brush off soil and other impurities using a soft brush or clean kitchen towel.)
1 tablespoon extra-virgin olive oil
2 cloves garlic, crushed
Salt, to taste
Cayenne pepper, to taste
2 tablespoons prepared hummus
2 tablespoons wheat germ
3 tablespoons shredded Parmesan cheese
⅓ cup chopped fresh basil

1. Preheat oven to 425 degrees. Spray a baking pan with olive oil cooking spray. Set baking pan aside.
2. Thaw the spinach, then drain well by squeezing excess liquid and patting as dry as possible with paper towels. Set aside.
3. Remove stems from mushrooms and set tops aside. Dice the mushroom stems.
4. Heat olive oil in a large nonstick skillet, and sauté mushroom stems and garlic for 2 minutes. Add thawed spinach, salt and cayenne pepper to taste. Cook over low heat for 1–2 minutes.
5. Stir hummus, wheat germ, Parmesan cheese and basil into the spinach mixture. Season with more salt and cayenne pepper to taste. Spoon mixture into mushroom tops (mushroom tops should be overstuffed).
6. Place stuffed mushrooms in the prepared baking pan. Bake for 10–12 minutes or until mushrooms are tender.

Nutrition Information: 80 calories, 1 g saturated fat, 6 g carbohydrate, 3 g dietary fiber, 5 g protein

Greek-Style Stuffed Tomatoes

Serves: 4

This A+ dish is one of the best recipes to serve at a luncheon or on a buffet. Even your non-tomato-loving guests will be so enamored with how pretty these stuffed tomatoes look they might even want to give them a try (or they will just admire looking at them and leave more for you!). Of course, they are healthy and brimming with nutrients and antioxidants, including that superstar lycopene.

5 medium-sized firm red tomatoes
Salt, to taste
Ground black pepper, to taste
¼ cup finely chopped black olives
¼ cup finely chopped parsley
¼ red onion, diced
1 tablespoon balsamic vinegar
2 teaspoons extra-virgin olive oil
¼ cup crumbled light feta cheese

1. Cut the tops off 4 tomatoes, and trim a thin slice off the bottoms so they sit upright easily. Hollow out the tomatoes with a spoon. Season the insides of the tomatoes with salt and pepper to taste.
2. Remove the stem from the remaining tomato then seed, peel and dice.
3. In a medium-sized bowl, combine the diced tomatoes, olives, parsley, onion, balsamic vinegar, olive oil and feta cheese; toss the mixture to combine. Fill the empty tomatoes with the stuffing and serve cold. (*Note:* you can refrigerate the tomatoes for up to 2 hours before serving.)

Nutrition Information: 80 calories, 1 g saturated fat, 8 g carbohydrate, 2 g dietary fiber, 3 g protein

Starches on the Side

Rosemary and Cheddar Rice Bake

Serves: 6

Ivy's mom gave us the idea for this superb dish, one that offers comfort food texture intertwined with gourmet flavor. This dish makes a great luncheon entrée served with roasted red pepper or tomato soup.

Extra-virgin olive oil cooking spray
1 box (10 ounces) frozen chopped spinach
2 omega-3-enriched eggs (such as Eggland's Best)
3 cups cooked short-grain brown rice
¾ cup shredded organic low-fat cheddar cheese
⅓ cup organic low-fat milk
1 teaspoon Worcestershire sauce
1 tablespoon chopped fresh rosemary
¼ teaspoon salt
⅛ teaspoon white pepper
2 tablespoons Parmesan cheese
¼ cup wheat germ

1. Preheat oven to 350 degrees. Spray the bottom and sides of an 8 x 8-inch casserole with extra-virgin olive oil cooking spray.
2. Thaw frozen spinach in microwave according to the directions.
3. Meanwhile, crack eggs into a large bowl and beat well.
4. Remove spinach from the microwave, drain water and pat dry with paper towels. Mix spinach in with the eggs. Stir in the rice, cheese, milk, sauce, rosemary, salt and pepper. Mix until well combined.
5. Transfer spinach and rice mixture to the prepared casserole. Bake for 25 minutes.
6. Meanwhile, mix together the Parmesan cheese and wheat germ in a small bowl. Remove casserole from oven after it has baked for 25 minutes, and top with the Parmesan and wheat germ mixture; return casserole to the oven and bake for an additional 10 minutes.
7. Remove casserole from the oven, and cool on a wire rack 10–15 minutes before cutting. Serve warm.

Nutrition Information: 200 calories, 2 g saturated fat, 29 g carbohydrate, 4 g dietary fiber, 12 g protein

Spring Quinoa Pilaf with
Macadamia Nuts and Fresh Dill

Serves: 6

Fresh and light, you'll love the simplicity of this tempting pilaf served with lamb. Quinoa is wheat- and gluten-free, rich in protein, and an excellent source of vital nutrients and fiber.

¼ cup macadamia nuts
1 tablespoon extra-virgin olive oil
¾ cup diced carrots
1¼ cups diced onions
⅛ teaspoon salt, plus more to taste
2 cups cooked quinoa
¼ cup chopped fresh dill

1. Place macadamia nuts in a zip-top plastic bag. Transfer the bag of nuts to a cutting board and pound with a mallet to make macadamia nut "crumbs." Set nuts aside.
2. Heat the oil in a large skillet over medium-high heat; add the carrots and onions, and sauté for several minutes until clear, yet crisp. Add salt. Stir in the quinoa, fresh dill and macadamia nuts, and sauté for an additional 1–2 minutes. If desired, season with a bit more salt.

Nutrition Information: 190 calories, 1 g saturated fat, 25 g carbohydrate, 3 g dietary fiber, 5 g protein

Jalapeno-Cheese Polenta Squares

Serves: 6

Quick! Run for the border, and don't look back. These Mexican-inspired jalapeno and cheese polenta squares make a great side dish to chicken, fish or meat. You can also serve them solo as an appetizer. Be sure to use a whole- grain cornmeal, which not only yields a richly flavored and textured polenta but also provides a good dose of fiber. Note: You may need to visit a natural foods store to find whole-grain cornmeal.

3 cups water
1 cup whole-grain cornmeal (we recommend Hodgson Mill or Arrowhead
   Mills brands)
¼ teaspoon salt
2–3 canned jalapeno peppers, minced (look for canned jalapeno peppers in
   the ethnic section of your supermarket)
¾ cup shredded low-fat organic Cheddar cheese
¼ cup whole-wheat flour
1 tablespoon extra-virgin olive oil

1. Bring water to a boil in a very heavy pot. Add cornmeal and salt; cook for about 5 minutes, stirring often. Mix in minced jalapeno peppers and cheese; stir until cheese melts.
2. Transfer cornmeal mixture to a square 8 x 8 inch casserole; spread mixture with the flat part of a spoon evenly in the dish. Refrigerate mixture for several hours or until very firm.
3. When cornmeal mixture is firm, cut into 12 square pieces. Dredge both sides of squares in whole-wheat flour.
4. Heat oil in a large nonstick skillet over medium-high heat; add polenta squares to hot oil, and cook 3–4 minutes per side (or until lightly browned). Remove skillet from heat, cover with a lid and let polenta sit for 5–6 minutes (or until warmed through). Serve immediately.

Nutrition Information: 150 calories, 1 g saturated fat, 22 g carbohydrate, 4 g dietary fiber, 6 g protein

Couscous with Gingered Raisins and Caramelized Onions

Serves: 6

The complexity of spices in this delicious pilaf is intoxicatingly scrumptious, especially served alongside lamb or grilled pork. Just be sure to use the whole-wheat couscous as opposed to the refined white stuff!

1 tablespoon organic butter
1 tablespoon extra virgin olive oil
1 red onion, finely chopped
Salt, to taste
1 tablespoon brown sugar
½ cup yellow raisins
1 tablespoon grated fresh ginger
1 teaspoon cinnamon
1¼ cups *whole-wheat* couscous
2 cups water
2 cups frozen corn kernels

1. Heat the butter and extra virgin olive oil in a large non-stick skillet over medium-high heat; when oil is hot add the onion and sauté until soft, about 5 minutes. Season onions to taste with salt. Lower the heat to medium-low and stir in the sugar, raisins, ginger and cinnamon and sauté for about 3 minutes, or until onions begin to caramelize.
2. Raise the heat back to medium-high and add the dry couscous into the skillet with the onions and raisins and toss to coat; pour the water into the skillet and cover with a large lid, stirring occasionally, for about 5 minutes, or until all the couscous has absorbed all of the liquid.
3. Remove the lid from the skillet and mix the frozen corn kernels in with the couscous. Cook, stirring occasionally, for an additional 5 minutes. Season couscous with salt to taste and serve at once.

Nutrition Information: 230 calories, 1.5 g saturated fat, 45 g carbohydrate, 5 g dietary fiber, 6 g protein

Twice-Baked Potatoes with Shallots

Serves: 4

Instead of using whipping cream in our twice-baked potatoes, we've substituted hummus, which adds flavor without sacrificing creaminess. Your thighs will thank you! You also get a wide variety of nutrients in each bite. These potatoes are very filling; each one is a meal itself (well, almost!).

2 Idaho baking potatoes (about 8 ounces each)
¼ cup prepared hummus (look for prepared hummus made with extra virgin
    olive oil in the deli section of your supermarket)
2 teaspoons dried tarragon
1 tablespoon shredded Parmesan cheese
Salt, to taste
White pepper, to taste
1 tablespoon extra virgin olive oil
3 shallots, thinly sliced

1. Preheat oven to 400 degrees. Use a fork to poke holes all over each potato; bake potatoes for 1 hour. Remove potatoes form the oven, but leave the oven on.
2. As soon as the potatoes are cool enough to handle, cut them in half length-wise and carefully scoop the insides of the potato out and transfer to a mixing bowl (taking care not to tear the potato shell). Mash the potatoes with a potato masher and mix in the hummus, tarragon, and shredded Parmesan cheese. Season potatoes with salt and white pepper to taste. Scoop the mashed potatoes back into the shells (shells should be somewhat over-stuffed) and place the over-stuffed potatoes on a baking sheet; bake potatoes in the 400 degree oven for 10–15 minutes.
3. Meanwhile, pour the extra virgin olive oil into a non-stick skillet and heat over medium-high heat; when oil is hot add the shallots and sauté until tender, about 2-3 minutes. Season shallots lightly with salt.
4. Remove the potatoes from the oven and pile the shallots on top of each potato. Serve at once.

Nutrition Information: 170 calories, 1 g saturated fat, 27 g carbohydrate, 3 g dietary fiber, 5 g protein

South of the Border Corn Fritters

Makes 6 Fritters

Our son calls these "special dinner pancakes," and they are the perfect healthy treat to serve alongside any chicken or fish dinner. When he's hungry, our little guy shouts out, "I'm starvin' Marvin!" To date, we have no idea who this Marvin guy is, but we sure bet Marvin would be impressed with how fast Blake's mommy can whip up these fritters!

1½ cups frozen corn kernels, thawed (will measure about 1 cup when thawed)
2 tablespoons canned chopped green chiles (can be found in ethnic section of supermarket)
2 omega-3 enriched eggs, beaten (such as Eggland's Best brand)
2 tablespoons plain yogurt
4 teaspoons extra virgin olive oil, divided
¾ cup stone-ground whole grain corn flour (available at natural foods stores)
½ teaspoon baking powder
¼ teaspoon salt, plus more to taste
1–2 pinches cayenne pepper, or more to taste

1. In a medium-sized bowl, toss together the corn kernels and canned chiles.
2. In another bowl, mix together the eggs, yogurt, and 2 teaspoons of the extra virgin olive oil. Stir the egg mixture into the bowl with the corn kernels. Mix in the whole grain corn flour, baking powder, salt and cayenne pepper and stir gently to combine all ingredients.
3. Pour 1 teaspoon of the extra virgin olive oil into a large non-stick skillet and swirl to coat; heat the oil over medium-high heat. When oil is hot, drop three large spoonfuls of the batter onto the hot skillet, cook for about 2-3 minutes per side, or until each corn fritter is lightly browned and insides are firm. Transfer the three cooked corn fritters from the skillet to a serving platter and set aside.
4. Repeat step three with the remaining teaspoon of extra virgin olive oil and remaining batter. When all fritters are done, serve at once.

Nutrition Information: 150 calories, 1 g saturated fat, 21 g carbohydrate, 3 g dietary fiber, 5 g protein

Baked Barley and Pecan Pilaf

Serves: 6

Enjoy the satisfying goodness of fiber-rich whole-grain barley in a delicious side dish. This simple pilaf is excellent with grilled chicken and sautéed spinach. Instead of cooking the barley stovetop, the baking process helps save you time, while infusing the barley with flavor. It tastes rich, but it's healthful and so delish!

2 tablespoons extra-virgin olive oil
½ cup finely chopped pecans
2 cups uncooked pearled barley
1 cup finely chopped scallions
1 cup finely chopped onions
½ teaspoon salt
¼ teaspoon white pepper
½ cup chopped parsley
2 cups organic free-range chicken broth (such as Imagine "Organic Free Range Chicken Broth")
¾ cup water

1. Preheat oven to 350 degrees.
2. In a large skillet, heat the olive oil over medium-high heat; toast the pecans for several minutes, taking care not to burn them. Remove the pecans from the skillet with a slotted spoon and set aside, keepinmg the pecan-infused oil in the skillet.
3. Add the barley, scallions and onions to the skillet, and sauté for several minutes, until barley is lightly toasted. Remove the skillet from the heat, and add the pecans back in. Season with salt, white pepper and parsley. Spoon the mixture into an 8 x 8-inch glass casserole.
4. Pour the chicken broth and water into a small saucepan and bring to a boil; pour the liquids over the barley mixture.
5. Bake the barley, uncovered, for 1 hour. Remove the casserole from the oven, and allow to cool on a wire rack for 15 minutes before serving.

Nutrition Information: 370 calories, 1.5 g saturated fat, 58 g carbohydrate, 12 g dietary fiber, 9 g protein

Tabbouleh with Mint and Cranberry

Serves: 4

Everyone in the family will love this mildly sweet whole-grain side dish, even picky kids! It's exceptionally rich in fiber and antioxidants. For a light and satisfying meal, serve tabbouleh with mixed greens and grilled shrimp.

2¼ cups plus ½ cup water, divided
1 cup bulgur wheat
¾ cup dried cranberries
¼ cup finely chopped pecans
1 small cucumber, seeds removed and diced
½ cup fresh mint, rinsed, patted dry, and chopped
1 teaspoon flaxseed oil (we recommend Barlean's brand)
Salt, to taste

1. Bring 2¼ cups water to a boil in a medium saucepan. Add the bulgur, and simmer for 10–12 minutes, or until all of the water is absorbed.
2. Meanwhile, place the cranberries and the remaining ½ cup water in a microwave-safe bowl, and microwave on high for 2 minutes; drain the water and blot the cranberries with paper towels to remove excess moisture.
3. When the bulgur is done, transfer the cooked grains to a large serving bowl, and stir in the cranberries, pecans, diced cucumber, mint, oil and salt to taste. Serve at once. (*Note:* If you want to make this recipe in advance, replace the flaxseed oil with extra-virgin olive oil and store in an air-tight container for up to 2 days.)

Nutrition Information: 260 calories, 0.5 g saturated fat, 48 g carbohydrate, 9 g dietary fiber, 5 g protein

Sweet Finale

Chocolate Blackberry Brownie Pudding

Serves: 6

This is somewhat of a cross between a bread pudding and a brownie. You can call it what you want, but it tastes outrageous! And it is so loaded with antioxidants, vitamins C and A, plus folate and even fiber, so you won't need to feel guilty for indulging.

Canola oil cooking spray
1 cup Nature's Path "Organic Millet Rice Oat Bran Flakes" (available in the natural foods section of your supermarket)
1 cup frozen blackberries
¼ cup mini dark chocolate chips (such as Ghirardelli "Double-Chocolate Chips")
¼ cup unsweetened cocoa powder (such as Ghirardelli brand)
3 omega-3-enriched eggs (such as Eggland's Best)
¼ cup plus 2 tablespoons brown sugar
¼ cup low-fat plain yogurt or kefir
½ cup organic whipping cream

1. Preheat oven to 350 degrees, and spray the bottom of an 8 x 8 casserole with canola oil cooking spray.
2. Spread the cereal, blackberries and chocolate chips evenly on the bottom of the casserole.
3. In a medium-sized bowl, whip the eggs; beat in the sugar and yogurt or kefir. Add the egg mixture to the casserole, and gently toss all ingredients together until well combined. Bake for 40–45 minutes or until the pudding is firm when pierced with a toothpick. Meanwhile, pour the whipping cream into a medium-sized stainless steel bowl; whip with a handheld mixer until firm (about 2–3 minutes).
4. Remove the pudding from the oven, and let cool on a rack for 10 minutes. Serve in small bowls with 1 small dollop of whipped cream per serving.

Nutrition Information: 210 calories, 5 g saturated fat, 30 g carbohydrate, 4 g dietary fiber, 4 g protein

Tart Persian Lime Custard

Serves: 4

Gail, Ivy's mom, specially created this sinfully rich custard for Andy, whose absolute favorite dessert is key lime pie (he loves key lime pie so much, we even had to serve it at our wedding!). This custard dessert has all of the rich, creamy and tart delight of traditional key lime pie minus the excess amounts of sugar and saturated fat. It totally quenches Andy's key lime pie craving and saves Ivy from having to hear Andy complain about why she never makes key lime pie. Thanks mom!

½ cup organic whole milk
¼ cup plus 2 teaspoons sugar, divided
1 omega-3-enriched egg plus 1 egg yolk
3 tablespoons freshly squeezed Persian lime juice
2 tablespoons reduced-fat sour cream
Pinch of salt
¼ cup organic whipping cream
Mini lime slices, for garnish

1. Preheat oven to 350 degrees.
2. Beat milk and ¼ cup sugar with an electric mixer until well blended. Add egg and egg yolk to mixture, and beat on high for 30 seconds. Add lime juice and beat for another 20 seconds.
3. Pour mixture into four ramekins. Pour water ½ inch deep into a pan and carefully place the four ramekins in the water; place the pan in the center of the oven, and bake for 25 minutes.
4. Meanwhile, in a small bowl mix together sour cream and the remaining 2 teaspoons sugar and salt. Remove ramekins from the oven, and add the sour cream mixture on top of the custards.
5. Transfer the custards back to the oven, increase oven temperature to 425 degrees, and bake for another 5 minutes. Remove custards from the oven, and chill in the refrigerator several hours.
6. Pour the whipping cream into a medium-sized stainless steel bowl; whip with a handheld mixer until firm (about 2–3 minutes.) Garnish custards with a dollop of fresh whipping cream and mini slices of lime.

Nutrition Information: 170 calories, 5 g saturated fat, 20 g carbohydrate, 0 g dietary fiber, 3 g protein

Molasses Spice Cookies

Makes 20 Cookies (Serving size = 1 cookie)

Our son, Blake, works very hard every year helping his mommy make Santa's favorite cookies (Dad is not much help!). Since Santa needs to stay trim enough to fit down all of those narrow chimneys, we've reduced the total fat and saturated fat in this recipe by using Land O' Lakes "Soft Baking Butter with Canola Oil." We've also increased the fiber by using whole wheat pastry flour and decreased the empty sugar calories by half. Best of all, Santa doesn't even know the healthy changes have been made!

½ cup Splenda "Brown Sugar Blend for Baking"
½ cup Land O' Lakes "Soft Baking Butter with Canola Oil"
½ cup molasses
1 omega-3-enriched egg (such as Eggland's Best)
2¼ cups whole-wheat pastry flour
2 teaspoons baking soda
1 teaspoon ground cinnamon
½ teaspoon ground cloves
½ teaspoon ground ginger
¼ teaspoon salt
1/2 cup water
¼ cup brown sugar

1. Combine Splenda and soft baking butter in a large bowl; beat with a mixer at medium speed until light and fluffy. Add molasses and egg; beat well.
2. In a separate bowl, combine flour, baking soda, cinnamon, cloves, ginger and salt, stirring with a whisk. Add flour mixture to sugar mixture; beat at low speed just until blended. Cover and freeze 1 hour.
3. Preheat oven to 375 degrees.
4. Place water in a small bowl, and place brown sugar in another bowl. Shape dough into 2-inch balls, and then flatten slightly into the shape of a cookie. Dip one side of each unbaked cookie in water; dip wet side in sugar.
5. Place the dough, sugar side up, 1 inch apart on baking sheets coated with cooking spray.
6. Bake at 375 degrees for 12–15 minutes, or until cookies just begin

to brown. Remove cookies from pans, and cool on a wire rack. Use a spatula to transfer cookies to a serving platter. Refrigerate cookies for 10–15 minutes before serving.

Nutrition Information: 160 calories, 2 g saturated fat, 25 g carbohydrate, 2 g dietary fiber, 2 g protein

Pumpkin Pudding

Serves: 8

Love pumpkin pie? Then our healthy alternative is a must try! Our Pumpkin Pudding has the taste and texture of real-deal pumpkin pie without the crust and a lot less sugar, too!

4 omega-3-enriched whole eggs (such as Eggland's Best)
1 can (12 ounces) 2% low-fat evaporated milk
1 can (12 ounces) organic whole milk (use the evaporated milk can to measure)
1 cup canned pumpkin
¼ cup plus 2 tablespoons brown sugar
1 teaspoon cinnamon
½ teaspoon salt
½ teaspoon allspice
1 teaspoon vanilla extract
½ cup organic heavy whipping cream
1 tablespoon sugar (or Splenda)

1. Preheat oven to 375 degrees.
2. In a large bowl, beat the eggs together with an electric mixer. Add the two cans of milk and pumpkin; mix well. Blend in the brown sugar, cinnamon, salt, allspice and vanilla extract.
3. Pour the pumpkin mixture into an 8 x 8–inch casserole, and place the casserole in a larger baking pan; add water to the large baking pan until the water is about 1½ inches deep. Carefully transfer the pan to the oven, and bake for 1 hour, or until a knife inserted in the middle comes out clean. Remove the pudding from the oven, transfer to the refrigerator, and refrigerate for 2 hours.
4. Meanwhile, pour the whipping cream and 1 tablespoon sugar (or Splenda) into a small stainless steel bowl; whip with a handheld mixer until firm (about 2–3 minutes). "Frost" the top of the pudding with *half* of the whipped cream (store the remaining half of the whipped cream in a covered container in the refrigerator for another use). Sprinkle cinnamon lightly on top of the whipped cream, and serve at once.

Nutrition Information: 220 calories, 6 g saturated fat, 23 g carbohydrate, 1 g dietary fiber, 9 g protein

Palm Beach Pineapple-Walnut Bread Cake

Serves: 8

Palm Beach fashion sensation Lilly Pulitzer would love this South Florida–inspired vitamin-C-rich pineapple treat. It's the perfect way to satisfy your sweet tooth.

Canola oil cooking spray
3 tablespoons Land O' Lakes "Soft Baking Butter with Canola Oil"
¼ cup plus 1 tablespoon Splenda "Brown Sugar Blend for Baking," divided
1 teaspoon plus 1/4 teaspoon pure lemon extract, divided
5 omega-3-enriched eggs (such as Eggland's Best)
½ cup 2% low-fat organic milk
1 can (20 ounces) crushed pineapple with no added sugar, drained
6 pieces toasted whole-grain sprouted bread (such as Food for Life "Ezekiel 4:9
    Sprouted Grain Bread"), broken into bite-sized pieces
½ cup chopped walnuts
¼ cup low-fat sour cream

1. Preheat oven to 350 degrees. Spray canola oil cooking spray on the bottom and sides of an 8 x 8-inch casserole.
2. In a large bowl, with a mixer on medium speed, beat butter, ¼ cup Splenda "brown sugar" and 1 teaspoon lemon extract for about 1 minute, scraping the bowl frequently. Add eggs; beat on high for 2 minutes, or until light and fluffy. Add milk, and beat for 1 minute. Fold in the pineapple, and hand mix until well combined.
3. Place the toasted bread pieces and walnuts in the prepared casserole, and toss gently. Pour the pineapple mixture over the bread and walnuts, and toss lightly to coat. Bake for 40–45 minutes.
4. Meanwhile, in a small bowl, make the glaze by whisking together the sour cream, remaining tablespoon of Splenda "brown sugar" and remaining ¼ teaspoon lemon extract. Set glaze aside.
5. Remove cake from the oven, and top with the glaze. Return to the oven, and bake for another 5 minutes. Transfer cake to a wire rack and cool for 15–20 minutes before serving.

Nutrition Information: 300 calories, 3.5 g saturated fat, 31 g carbohydrate, 4 g dietary fiber, 11 g protein

Pear Crisp with Almond-Crumble Topping

Serves: 6

This is a universal crowd-pleasing treat; it is light while being rich at the same time (you just have to taste it to see what we mean). By using whole-wheat flour, Splenda "Brown Sugar Blend for Baking" and a canola oil-butter blend, we've created a dessert so healthy it almost isn't fair to even call it dessert.

Canola oil cooking spray
5 firm pears, thinly sliced
2 tablespoons Splenda "Brown Sugar Blend for Baking"
1 teaspoon pure almond extract
1 tablespoon cornstarch

Almond-Crumble Topping:
½ cup whole-wheat flour
1 tablespoon Splenda "Brown Sugar Blend for Baking"
½ cup slivered almonds
2 tablespoons Land O' Lakes "Soft Baking Butter with Canola Oil"

1. Preheat oven to 400 degrees and spray a 10-inch pie dish with canola oil cooking spray.
2. Add the sliced pears, Splenda "Brown Sugar Blend for Baking," almond extract and cornstarch to the pie dish; toss with your hands to coat the pears, and set aside.
3. Prepare the almond-crumble topping: Put flour, Splenda "Brown Sugar Blend for Baking," and slivered almonds in a food processor. Pulse five or six times to chop the nuts. Scatter Land O' Lakes "Soft Baking Butter with Canola Oil" over dry ingredients. Pulse again until butter is combined. Empty the mixture into a bowl, and gently rub it between your fingers.
4. Divide the almond-crumble topping evenly over the pears, patting down gently. Bake for 35 minutes.
5. Remove the pear crisp from the oven and transfer to a wire rack. Cool for at least 15 minutes before cutting and serving.

Nutrition Information: 250 calories, 2 g saturated fat, 38 g carbohydrate, 6 g dietary fiber, 4 g protein

Cherry Upside-Down Cake

Serves: 12

Self-decorating upside-down cakes are quick and easy, just mix, bake and voilà! This is the ideal dessert for serving to guests you want to impress. For a special treat, serve with a dollop of fresh whipped cream.

Canola oil cooking spray
¾ cup brown sugar
¼ cup plus 2 tablespoons Land O' Lakes "Soft Baking Butter with Canola Oil," divided
2½ cups (12 ounces) frozen pitted cherries, thawed
1½ cups whole-wheat flour
2 teaspoons baking powder
¼ teaspoon salt
½ cup Splenda "Brown Sugar Blend for Baking"
2 omega-3-enriched eggs yolks, and whites separated
½ cup organic 2% low-fat milk
1 teaspoon pure lemon extract
¼ teaspoon cream of tartar

1. Preheat oven to 350 degrees.
2. Spray a 9-inch round metal cake pan with canola oil cooking spray, and add brown sugar and 2 tablespoons Land O' Lakes "Soft Baking Butter with Canola Oil"; heat over medium heat, and stir until butter melts. Spread the sugar-butter mixture evenly over the bottom of the pan, and arrange the thawed cherries on top. Lightly mash the cherries with a paper towel. Set cake pan aside.
3. In a medium-sized bowl, mix together the flour, baking powder and salt.
4. In a large bowl, combine the remaining ¼ cup Land O' Lakes "Soft Baking Butter with Canola Oil" and Splenda "Brown Sugar Blend for Baking"; beat with an electric mixer at high speed until ingredients are well combined. Add egg yolks, one at a time, beating well after each addition.
5. Add flour mixture and milk alternately to butter mixture, beginning and ending with the flour mixture; mix after each addition. Beat in lemon extract.

6. In a small bowl, beat egg whites and cream of tartar with a mixer at medium speed until stiff peaks form. Fold egg whites into batter; pour batter over cherries in prepared pan. Bake at 350 degrees for 35 minutes or until a wooden toothpick inserted in the center comes out clean. Cool in pan for 15 minutes; run a knife around outside edge. Place a plate upside down on top of cake pan; invert cake onto plate. Serve at room temperature.

Nutrition Information: 240 calories, 3 g saturated fat, 38 g carbohydrate, 2 g dietary fiber, 4 g protein

Blueberry Cobbler

Serves: 6

What's better than blueberry cobbler? Lots of blueberry cobbler! Our version is so healthy you don't even need to feel guilty about indulging. This good old-fashioned dessert is a snap to make, too. For a special occasion serve Blueberry Cobbler with a small scoop of all-natural vanilla ice cream. Yummy!

Canola oil cooking spray
3½ cups fresh blueberries (or use frozen blueberries and thaw at room
    temperature for 3 hours)
1 teaspoon pure lemon extract
2 teaspoons cornstarch
½ cup Splenda "Brown Sugar Blend for Baking," divided
1 cup whole-wheat flour
1 teaspoon baking powder
1 omega-3-enriched egg (such as Eggland's Best)
1 tablespoon Land O' Lakes "Soft Baking Butter with Canola Oil," melted

1. Preheat the oven to 350 degrees and spray an 8 x 8-inch glass casserole with canola oil cooking spray.
2. Place the blueberries in the prepared casserole and toss lightly with the lemon extract, cornstarch and ½ cup Splenda.
3. In a medium-sized bowl, combine the flour, remaining Splenda and baking powder. Add the egg, and crumble ingredients together with your hands (the mixture will be dry). Crumble the topping evenly over the blueberries. Drizzle melted butter on top.
4. Bake uncovered for 40 minutes. Cool at room temperature before serving.

Nutrition Information: 250 calories, 1 g saturated fat, 47 g carbohydrate, 4 g dietary fiber, 4 g protein

Apple-Cranberry Torte

Serves: 6

This is a revised and lightened-up French recipe for what has become one of our family's favorite desserts. It only takes about 20 minutes of preparation, and it's worth every decadent bite!

Canola oil cooking spray
⅓ cup whole-wheat flour
1 tablespoon baking powder
⅛ teaspoon salt
3 omega-3-enriched eggs (such as Eggland's Best), divided
½ cup brown sugar, divided
⅓ cup organic 2% low-fat milk
2 tablespoons high-oleic canola oil
1 tablespoon pure almond extract
3 large Granny Smith apples, cored, peeled and sliced into thin rounds
½ cup dried cranberries
2 tablespoons Land O' Lakes "Soft Baking Butter with Canola Oil," melted

1. Heat the oven to 400 degrees. Spray a 9-inch springform pan with canola oil cooking spray.
2. Mix together the flour, baking powder and salt in a medium bowl.
3. In large bowl, beat together 2 eggs and ¼ cup of brown sugar until thick. Beat in the milk, oil and almond extract. Whisk the dry ingredients into the egg mixture, and stir gently to blend. Fold in the apples and dried cranberries.
4. Pour the batter into the springform pan, and place in the middle of the oven. Bake for 35 minutes.
5. Meanwhile, make the glaze in a small bowl by beating together the remaining 1 egg, remaining ¼ cup brown sugar and the melted Land O' Lakes "Soft Baking Butter with Canola Oil."
6. Remove the torte from the oven and pour the glaze evenly over the top. Return the torte to the oven, and bake an additional 12–15 minutes, or until torte is firm but not brown. Remove the torte from the oven, and allow to cool in the pan for at least 10 minutes. Run a knife around the edge of the pan and unmold, but keep the torte on the bottom of the pan. Cut and serve.

Nutrition Information: 280 calories, 2 g saturated fat, 42 g carbohydrate, 3 g dietary fiber, 5 g protein

10 Two Weeks of 30-Minute "Nearly Homemade" Gourmet and Family-Friendly Meals

This chapter has been created specifically for the time-crunched. We're going to help you make fabulous meals quickly and easily. We'll show you how to put a sensational whole-foods meal on the table in less than thirty minutes flat.

The first part of the chapter is comprised of "Nearly Homemade Gourmet Dinners," where we'll show you how to take advantage of shortcut cooking techniques. What's our secret? With so many great-tasting, healthful convenience foods so readily available, why waste time with unnecessary work? Instead, we'll show you how to use readily available, healthful prepared foods as a base, then mix in fresh ingredients to yield amazing meals that take a fraction of the time it would take to prepare from scratch. We call it "convenience cuisine."

We'll also show you how to use our shortcut cooking technique to make no-fuss "Family-Friendly Meals." Even if your children and teenage kids are not particularly enamored with eating healthfully, we've got fit and fabulous kid-friendly dinners they can't help but love. You don't even need to tell anyone these meals are healthy; they taste so good no one will suspect they are actually good for you. Our no-fuss meals are guaranteed to make everyone in the family happy.

Plan Ahead

Organization and preplanning are essential for fast and easy meal prep. Plus, meals tend to be healthful when planned. Before you begin to prepare one of our "Nearly Homemade" meals, it's helpful to do the following:

- Check your pantry and your freezer. Do you need to shop for ingredients?
- Plan your weekly menu in advance. This ten-minute investment pays big dividends in stress relief later in the week. Scan recipes you intend to make, then make up your shopping list for the week. Divide your grocery shopping list into the eight categories:

  1. Frozen
  2. Produce
  3. Breads, Grains, Flour
  4. Canned and jarred foods
  5. Dairy
  6. Meats, Fish, Chicken
  7. Condiments, Spices
  8. Other

  (*Note:* Since some of the foods we recommend may not be available in your local supermarket it's helpful to have a second list of foods ready for your visit to the natural foods store.)
- Decide first thing in the morning what you will make for dinner. Thaw frozen items such as meat and fish in the refrigerator.
- Scan any unfamiliar recipe. Be familiar with the prep steps before you begin cooking.

Part I: Gourmet Meals

Pasta with Clam Sauce
Broccoli with Balsamic Vinaigrette

Serves: 4

1 teaspoon plus 1 tablespoon extra-virgin olive oil, divided
4 cloves garlic, chopped
1 Spanish onion, chopped
Salt, to taste
White pepper, to taste
8 ounces dry whole-wheat fettuccine (we like Hodgson Mill "Fettuccine with Flaxseeds")
2 cups fresh chopped sea clams, drained
2 cups Rao's "Marinara Sauce"
6 cups broccoli florets (to save time, buy bagged, precut broccoli florets)
3–4 tablespoons Balsamic vinegar
½ cup shredded Parmesan cheese

1. Bring a large pot of water to a boil. Meanwhile, heat a large non-stick skillet over medium heat. Add 1 teaspoon of the olive oil. When the oil is hot, add the garlic and onion, and cook, stirring occasionally, until the onion is golden, about 5 minutes. Season the onion with a dash of salt and white pepper.
2. Add pasta to the boiling water. Add the clams to the skillet with the onion; season with salt and pepper, then add the marinara sauce, and cook uncovered for 5 minutes, stirring occasionally.
3. After the pasta has been cooking for 5–6 minutes, carefully drop the broccoli into the water with the pasta, and cook for an additional 3 minutes, or until the broccoli is tender. Drain the pasta and broccoli into a colander, rinse with cool water and separate the broccoli, transferring the broccoli to a medium-sized bowl.
4. Toss the broccoli with the remaining tablespoon of oil and balsamic vinegar plus salt and white pepper to taste.
5. On individual plates, serve pasta topped with sauce and Parmesan cheese. Serve broccoli on the side.

Nutrition Information: 510 calories, 3 g saturated fat, 70 g carbohydrate, 12 g dietary fiber, 33 g protein

Parmesan Fish Bake
Lemony Corn Chowder
Tomato Salad

Serves: 4

⅓ cup Hellmann's "Canola Oil Mayonnaise"
⅓ cup Parmesan cheese
1 teaspoon Dijon mustard
2 tablespoons chopped fresh dill
4 tilapia fillets (about 6 ounces each)
1 tablespoon plus 2 tablespoons extra-virgin olive oil, divided
½ cup minced onion
1½ cups frozen corn kernels
1 package (16 ounces) Imagine "Organic Creamy Corn Soup"
⅓ cup water
Juice from ½ lemon
2 teaspoons Tabasco (or other hot sauce)
4 tomatoes, sliced
1 tablespoon balsamic vinegar
Salt, to taste
Black pepper, to taste

1. Heat oven to 450 degrees. Line a baking sheet with aluminum foil.
2. Mix mayonnaise, Parmesan cheese and mustard together in a small bowl; gently stir in dill. Place fish on lined baking sheet, and spread mayonnaise mixture evenly on top of each fillet.
3. Bake fish for 11–12 minutes, or until topping turns golden and fish is cooked through.
4. Meanwhile, heat 1 tablespoon of the extra-virgin olive oil in a large soup pot over medium-high heat; add the onion, and sauté for 3–4 minutes or until onion is soft. Add corn kernels, soup, water, lemon juice and Tabasco. Reduce heat to low, and simmer for 3–4 minutes.
5. Arrange sliced tomatoes on a platter, and drizzle with remaining 2 tablespoons of extra-virgin olive oil and balsamic vinegar; season to taste with salt and black pepper. Serve meal at once.

Nutrition Information: 650 calories, 7 g saturated fat, 36 g carbohydrate, 5 g dietary fiber, 42 g protein

Pasta à la Vodka
Seared Chicken
Mixed-Greens Salad with Italian Dressing

Serves: 4

1 packet Good Seasons "Italian Salad Dressing"
¼ cup plus 2 tablespoons water
¼ cup flaxseed oil (we recommend Barlean's brand)
2 tablespoons balsamic vinegar
2 tablespoons lemon juice
Salt, to taste
¾ pound uncooked Gia Russa "Whole Wheat Roman Rigatoni"
2 teaspoons extra-virgin olive oil, divided
2 shallots, chopped
2 cups prepared marinara sauce (such as Rao's "Homemade Marinara" or
    Alessi "All Natural Marinara Pasta Sauce")
½ cup prepared hummus (such as Hannah "Hommus" in deli section of grocery)
1 can (14.5 ounces) Hunt's "Diced Tomatoes with Sweet Onion"
¼ cup finely chopped fresh basil
2 shots vodka
1 tablespoon organic heavy whipping cream
1 pound boneless, skinless chicken breasts, cut into strips
Paprika, to taste
8 cups prewashed, ready-to-eat mixed greens

1. Bring a large pot of water to a boil.
2. Meanwhile, in a clean salad dressing bottle, add the packet of Good
   Seasons "Italian Salad Dressing," water, flaxseed oil, balsamic vinegar and lemon juice; shake well until ingredients are well blended.
   Refrigerate until serving time.
3. Add salt and rigatoni to the boiling water, and cook for 10 minutes.
4. Meanwhile, heat 1 teaspoon extra-virgin olive oil in a large skillet
   over medium-high heat; add shallots, and cook for 2 minutes. Whisk
   in marinara sauce and hummus; continue stirring until hummus is
   well blended. Stir in canned tomatoes. Add basil, and simmer for
   2–3 minutes. Add vodka and heavy cream, and simmer another 2
   minutes. Pour sauce into a covered dish, and set aside.
5. Drain the rigatoni, and place on individual serving plates.
6. Heat remaining 1 teaspoon of extra-virgin olive oil in the "dirty" skillet. Meanwhile, season chicken with a generous amount of paprika
   to cover all sides, plus salt to taste. Stir-fry chicken in the olive oil for

4–5 minutes, stirring constantly, until chicken is cooked through.

7. Top rigatoni with vodka sauce and chicken strips. Serve with a side of salad drizzled with Italian dressing (1 tablespoon dressing per person).

Nutrition Information: 820 calories, 4 g saturated fat, 94 g carbohydrate, 15 g dietary fiber, 41 g protein

Salmon Burgers with Creamy Dill Sauce on Toasted Buns
Roasted Red Pepper and Tomato Soup

Serves: 4

1 teaspoon plus 1 tablespoons extra-virgin olive oil, divided
1 large Spanish onion, chopped
1 soft-can (16 ounces) Pacific Foods "Roasted Red Pepper and Tomato Soup"
2 tablespoons orange juice concentrate
1 can (12 ounces) good-quality roasted red peppers, drained and diced
½ cup water
2 tablespoons low-fat sour cream
½ cup fresh chopped dill
Juice from ½ lemon
2 tablespoons prepared hummus
1 teaspoon Dijon mustard
1 can (16 ounces) Alaskan salmon, drained and flaked
1 omega-3 enriched egg, lightly beaten
⅓ cup wheat germ
¼ cup grated Parmesan cheese
½ cup finely chopped parsley
2 garlic cloves, crushed
⅛ teaspoon cayenne pepper
4 whole-wheat grain burger buns (such as Alvarado Street Bakery "Sprouted Burger Buns")
Extra-virgin olive oil cooking spray

1. Preheat oven to 400 degrees.
2. In a medium-sized stock pot, add 1 tablespoon extra-virgin olive oil. Over medium heat, sauté the onions until soft and translucent. Add the Pacific Foods "Roasted Red Pepper and Tomato Soup," orange juice concentrate and diced red peppers. Working in batches, puree the soup in a blender. Pour soup back into the pot, and add ½ cup water; simmer over low heat for 5 minutes.
3. Meanwhile, make the dill sauce by whisking the sour cream, chopped dill, lemon juice, hummus and mustard together in a small bowl. Set sauce aside.
4. In a medium bowl, combine flaked canned salmon, egg, wheat germ, Parmesan cheese, parsley, garlic and cayenne pepper. Divide into 4 equal parts, and form ½-inch thick patties.
5. Open the buns and spray the inside of each bun with extra-virgin olive oil, and place buns, face-side down, on the oven rack, and toast for 5-6 minutes.

6. Meanwhile, pour remaining 1 tablespoon of extra-virgin olive oil, in a large, flat griddle or skillet, spread the oil around the pan gently with a paper towel, and heat on medium-high heat. Cook patties 4–5 minutes each side, shaping and patting down continuously with a spatula, until lightly browned.
7. Serve salmon burgers on buns drizzled with dill sauce and a cup of soup on the side.

Nutrition Information: 590 calories, 5 g saturated fat, 57 g carbohydrate, 7 g dietary fiber, 40 g protein

Chicken Pesto Pizza
Tomato Salad with Red Onions and Plums

Serves: 4

1 12-inch (10-ounce) Boboli "Whole Wheat Italian Bread Shell"
3 tablespoons prepared pesto, divided
4 cups fresh baby spinach leaves (to save time buy prewashed)
1 cup shredded, low-fat organic mozzarella cheese
½ cup canned Valley Fresh "Premium Chunk White Chicken in Water,"
    drained and patted dry (*Note:* Canned chicken is in the supermarket near
    the canned tuna.)
Salt, to taste
3 firm plums, seeds removed and diced
2 red, firm tomatoes (such as Red Diamond), chopped
2 small cucumbers, seeds removed and diced
1 red onion, diced
½ teaspoon salt
2 tablespoons flaxseed oil (we recommend Barlean's brand)
2 teaspoons honey
2 teaspoons crushed garlic
1 tablespoon plus 1 teaspoon balsamic vinegar

1. Preheat oven to 400 degrees, and line a cookie sheet with aluminum foil.
2. Place the Boboli shell on the aluminum foil-lined cookie sheet, and spread 2 tablespoons of the prepared pesto on top of the bread shell. Layer the spinach leaves and mozzarella on top.
3. In a small bowl, mix together the canned chicken with the remaining tablespoon of the prepared pesto. Spread the chicken on top of the spinach and mozzarella cheese. Season with salt to taste. Bake for 15 minutes.
4. Meanwhile, in a medium-sized bowl, add the plums, tomatoes, cucumbers, red onion, salt, flaxseed oil, honey, garlic and balsamic vinegar. Mix the salad ingredients together lightly, and set aside.
5. Remove the pizza from the oven. Cut the pizza with a pizza cutter, and serve with a side of the tomato salad.

Nutrition Information: 510 calories, 6 g saturated fat, 58 g carbohydrate, 5 g dietary fiber, 24 g protein

Seared Thai-Style Peanut-Crusted Ahi Tuna
Roasted Red Potatoes with Vegetables

Serves: 4

7 medium red-skinned potatoes, washed and cut into one-eighths
3 red bell peppers, chopped into bite-sized pieces
2½ cups baby carrots
1 large red onion, chopped into bite-sized pieces
6–8 cloves garlic, coarsely chopped
2 tablespoons extra-virgin olive oil
Salt, to taste
Coarse black pepper, to taste
1½ pounds center-cut Ahi tuna or 4 (4–6-ounce) 1-inch thick sushi-quality tuna
   steaks
3 tablespoons all-natural peanut butter
1 packet, A Taste of Thai "Spicy Thai Peanut Bake" seasoning (www.atasteofthai.com)
Canola oil cooking spray

1. Preheat oven to 450 degrees, and line two cookie sheets with aluminum foil.
2. Divide the potatoes, peppers, carrots, red onions and garlic on top of the cookie sheets; toss potatoes and vegetables with the olive oil until all of the potatoes and vegetables are well coated. Season with salt and pepper to taste. Roast for 25 minutes.
3. *Note:* If using the center-cut Ahi tuna, trim and cut the tuna into 1-inch steaks. Rub the peanut butter onto both sides of the tuna steaks, pressing the peanut butter firmly onto the tuna. Evenly coat both sides of the tuna steaks with a generous amount of the "Spicy Thai Peanut Bake."
4. Spray a large nonstick heavy skillet with canola oil cooking spray, and heat over medium-high heat. When the skillet is hot, add the tuna steaks, cover with a lid, and sear for 1–2 minutes. Flip the tuna steaks with a spatula, reduce the heat to medium, and sear the tuna for another 1–2 minutes (tuna should be medium-rare when done). Transfer the tuna to individual serving plates.
5. Remove the roasted potatoes and vegetables from the oven, and serve alongside the tuna steaks. Serve at once.

Nutrition Information: 510 calories, 2.5 g saturated fat, 40 g carbohydrate, 7 g dietary fiber, 48 g protein

Sirloin Steak Salad on Mixed Greens with Corn, Gorgonzola Cheese, and Smoked Tomato Vinaigrette

Serves: 4

4 omega-3-enriched eggs
4 cups frozen corn kernels
1 pound extra-lean top sirloin steak (look for organic and grass-fed beef, if
    possible), trimmed of all visible fat, and cut into strips
Salt, to taste
Coarse black pepper, to taste
1 teaspoon plus 1 tablespoon extra-virgin olive oil, divided
¼ cup Drew's All-Natural Dressing and Marinade "Smoked Tomato"
1 tablespoon balsamic vinegar
6 cups mixed greens (prewashed)
½ large red onion, diced
½ cup crumbled Gorgonzola cheese

1. Place eggs in a large pot of water; bring the water to a boil, and boil the eggs for 10 minutes.
2. Place corn in a microwave-safe container, and thaw in the microwave for 3 minutes, or until just barely warm.
3. Season both sides of the sirloin strips with salt and coarse black pepper.
4. Pour 1 teaspoon extra-virgin olive oil onto a large nonstick skillet, and gently rub the oil over the skillet using a paper towel; heat the oil over medium-high heat. When the oil is hot, add the sirloin strips, and sauté for 3–4 minutes, or until sirloin is medium-rare. Remove the sirloin from the heat, and set aside to cool.
5. Meanwhile, remove the eggs from the water and run under cool water; when the eggs are cool enough to handle, remove the shells. Finely chop the eggs, and set aside.
6. Pour the prepared dressing and marinade in a small bowl; whisk in the remaining olive oil and vinegar.
7. Divide the salad greens onto four plates. Layer the corn, sirloin, egg, red onion and Gorgonzola on top of each plate of mixed greens. Drizzle with dressing, and serve at once.

Nutrition Information: 500 calories, 8 g saturated fat, 43 g carbohydrate, 6 g dietary fiber, 38 g protein

Part II: Family-Friendly Meals

Turkey and Black Bean Pita Pizza
Green Beans

Serves: 4

4 (6-inch) whole-wheat or oat-bran pitas (such as Toufayan brand)
2 teaspoons plus 1 tablespoon extra-virgin olive oil, divided
1 pound extra-lean ground turkey
1 cup diced onions
1 can (15 ounces) black beans, rinsed and drained
¼ cup tomato puree
1 teaspoon cumin
1 teaspoon chili powder
1 teaspoon brown sugar
1 teaspoon paprika
Salt, to taste
1 cup organic low-fat shredded Cheddar cheese
Tabasco or other hot sauce, to taste (optional)
2 packages (9 ounces each) frozen cut green beans (such as Birds Eye "Cut
    Green Beans")
Juice from ½ lemon

1. Preheat oven to 400 degrees.
2. Toast pitas on cookie sheets for 2–3 minutes. Remove pitas from oven, and set aside, but keep the oven on.
3. Heat 2 teaspoons extra-virgin olive oil in a large skillet over medium-high heat; add the ground turkey, and sauté for several minutes. Stir in the onions, and sauté until turkey is cooked through and onions are soft. Mix in the black beans, tomato puree, cumin, chili powder, brown sugar, paprika and salt to taste. Cook for an additional 2–3 minutes.
4. Divide turkey and bean mixture evenly on top of each pita, then top with equal amounts of cheese. If desired, drizzle Tabasco or other hot sauce on top of the cheese. Place pita pizzas on a cookie sheet, and bake for 10 minutes.

5. Meanwhile, remove the outer wrapping from the frozen green beans, and place the green beans in a microwave-safe bowl. Microwave on high for 3–4 minutes or until green beans are warm. Toss green beans with remaining 1 tablespoon of extra-virgin olive oil and lemon juice. Season with salt to taste.

6. Remove the pita pizzas from the oven, and serve with green beans.

Nutrition Information: 580 calories, 2.5 g saturated fat, 72 g carbohydrate, 16 g dietary fiber, 51 g protein

---

Baja Fish Tacos
Roasted Red Peppers

Serves: 4

6 red peppers, sliced into thin strips
2 tablespoons extra-virgin olive oil, divided
Salt, to taste
¼ cup prepared hummus (such as Hannah brand)
¼ cup canola oil mayonnaise
½ cup chopped fresh cilantro
2 tablespoons low-fat plain yogurt or kefir
1 package (1.25 ounces) Ortega "Taco Seasoning Mix" (use only 3 tablespoons)
1½ pounds cod, or other white fish fillets, cut into 1-inch pieces
2 tablespoons lime juice
8 all-natural taco shells (such as Garden of Eatin' "Yellow Corn Taco Shells")

Toppings:
2 avocados, chopped
3 cups prepared pico de gallo (look for this in the deli section of your
    supermarket—Hannah brand is good)
3 cups frozen corn kernels, thawed

1. Preheat oven to 400 degrees.
2. Line a large cookie sheet with aluminum foil, and arrange red pepper slices on the foil. Drizzle 1 tablespoon olive oil on the red peppers, and toss to coat with your hands. Season to taste with salt.
3. Roast red peppers in the oven for 25 minutes, or until soft.
4. In a food processor or mini cuisinart, puree hummus, mayonnaise, cilantro, yogurt and 1 tablespoon Ortega seasoning mix. Set taco sauce aside.
5. In a medium-sized bowl, toss cod with 1 tablespoon extra-virgin olive oil, lime juice and 1 tablespoon Ortega seasoning mix.
6. Transfer seasoned fish into a large skillet and cook, stirring constantly, over medium-high heat for 3–4 minutes, or until fish flakes easily when tested with a fork. Season fish with 1 more tablespoon of Ortega seasoning mix.
7. Transfer taco shells to the oven, and warm for 2–3 minutes.

8. Remove taco shells from the oven, and scoop fish filling evenly into the shells. Add the avocado, pico de gallo and corn kernel toppings at the table. Serve with taco sauce and a side of roasted red peppers.

Time-Crunch Note: If you are really pressed for time, you can substitute 24 ounces of canned Alaskan salmon for the fresh cod and skip preparation step numbers 5 and 6. Instead, just sprinkle canned salmon with 2 tablespoons or more of Ortega seasoning mix and continue with step number 7.

Nutrition Information: 810 calories, 5 g saturated fat, 77 g carbohydrate, 15 g dietary fiber, 44 g protein

Classic Tuna Casserole
Broccoli Florets with Thyme

Serves: 4

Olive oil cooking spray
1 package (9 ounces) frozen Amy's "Macaroni and Cheese"
1 tablespoon extra-virgin olive oil
1 cup chopped onion
1 red bell pepper, finely chopped
2 tablespoons whole-wheat flour
⅛ teaspoon salt
⅛ teaspoon white pepper
1 cup organic 1% low-fat milk
2 cans (6 ounces each) chunk white albacore tuna, drained
1 cup frozen petite peas
1 cup frozen yellow corn kernels
¼ cup wheat germ
¼ cup shredded Parmesan cheese
½ cup corn flakes
2 packages (8.5 ounces each) frozen Birds Eye "Baby Broccoli Florets with Thyme"

1. Preheat oven to 375 degrees. Spray an 8 x 8-inch casserole dish with olive oil cooking spray.
2. Remove wrapper from frozen Amy's meal, and place macaroni and cheese in the microwave; cook on high for 4 minutes.
3. Meanwhile, heat oil in a large saucepan over medium heat; add onion and red bell pepper, and sauté until vegetables are tender (about 3 minutes). Stir in flour, salt and white pepper. Reduce heat to medium, and slowly add milk; stir for 2–3 minutes, or until mixture thickens.
4. Mix in Amy's Macaroni and Cheese, canned tuna, frozen peas and frozen corn; stir for 1–2 minutes, or until peas and corn are just thawed. Transfer tuna and macaroni mixture to the prepared casserole.
5. In a medium-sized bowl, crumble together the wheat germ, Parmesan and corn flakes; divide wheat germ and Parmesan mixture evenly on top of the casserole. Spray the top of the casserole lightly with olive oil cooking spray, and then transfer the casserole to the oven. Bake for 12–15 minutes, or until the top is just browned.

6. While casserole is cooking, place frozen broccoli in a microwave-safe dish. Cover, and microwave on high for 5 minutes (stir halfway through cooking). Drain broccoli, and mix in contents of herb pouch.
7. Cut casserole when done, and serve with broccoli.

Nutrition Information: 400 calories, 3 g saturated fat, 47 g carbohydrate, 10 g dietary fiber, 34 g protein

Chicken and Cheddar Quesadillas with Apple-Cranberry Relish
Creamy Butternut Squash Soup

Serves: 4

3 teaspoons high-oleic canola oil, divided
½ cup dried cranberries
2 Granny Smith apples, diced
¼ teaspoon cinnamon
⅛ teaspoon allspice
2 teaspoons brown sugar, divided
1 box (12 ounces) Birds Eye "Frozen Cooked Winter Squash"
½ onion, minced
1 box (16 ounces) Pacific Foods "Creamy Butternut Squash Soup"
1 cup organic 2% low-fat milk
¼ teaspoon nutmeg
Salt, to taste
Extra-virgin olive oil cooking spray
1 pound cooked rotisserie chicken breast pieces with skin removed (you'll find rotisserie chicken in the deli section of your supermarket)
1 cup shredded low-fat organic Cheddar cheese
4 whole-grain tortilla wraps (such as Tamxico's "100% Whole Wheat Tortilla Wrap-itz")

1. Place 1 teaspoon canola oil, cranberries, apples, cinnamon, all-spice and 1 teaspoon brown sugar in a small saucepan; cover and cook, stirring occasionally, until apples are soft, about 5 minutes. Set apple-cranberry relish aside.
2. Meanwhile, place frozen squash in a microwave-safe dish; cover, and microwave on high for 3–4 minutes.
3. Heat the remaining 2 teaspoons of canola oil in a saucepan over medium-high heat; add onions, and sauté until tender, 2–3 minutes; stir in thawed squash, Pacific Foods "Creamy Butternut Squash Soup," milk, nutmeg, remaining 1 teaspoon of brown sugar and salt to taste. Bring soup to a simmer. Remove from heat and cover to keep warm.
4. Spray a flat griddle or large nonstick skillet with nonstick cooking spray, and heat over medium-high heat. Place two of the tortillas on the pan. After heating tortillas for about a minute, place one-quarter of the apple-cranberry relish, chicken and cheese on one side of each tortilla. Turn heat down to medium, and fold tortillas in half,

covering filling, and press down lightly with your fingertips. Heat for 2 minutes, and turn over for another 2 minutes, or until cheese melts. Remove quesadillas from the pan, and repeat the process with the remaining ingredients.
5. Serve warm quesadillas with butternut squash soup.

Nutrition Information: 540 calories, 3.5 g saturated fat, 67 g carbohydrate, 8 g dietary fiber, 49 g protein

Mexican Lasagna

Serves: 4

Extra-virgin olive oil cooking spray
1 tablespoon extra-virgin olive oil
½ pound extra-lean ground turkey
1 cup finely chopped onion
1 green bell pepper, finely chopped
7 ounces (½ of a 14 ounce package) extra-firm tofu, drained, patted dry with
    paper towels and crumbled
1 package (1.25 ounces) McCormick "Taco Seasoning Mix
1 can (14.5 ounces) diced tomatoes, drained
1 can (15 ounces) pinto beans, drained
1 cup frozen corn kernels, thawed
1 cup shredded organic low-fat Cheddar cheese, divided (or as a low-saturated
    fat alternative, use shredded rice cheese, such as Galaxy Nutritional Foods
    "Cheddar Rice Shreds")
1 omega-3-enriched egg, beaten
½ cup organic low-fat cottage cheese
8 stone-ground corn tortillas (such as Tamxico's "Corn Tortilla")
1 cup thinly sliced scallions

1. Preheat oven to 375 degrees. Spray the bottom and sides of an 8 x 8-inch casserole with cooking spray.
2. Heat oil in a large skillet over medium-high heat; brown turkey with onions and green peppers. Mix in crumbled tofu, taco seasoning and canned tomatoes; cook for 3 minutes.
3. Meanwhile, lightly mash beans in a bowl with potato masher or back of a large spoon. Stir beans into turkey and tofu mixture. Mix in the thawed corn kernels. Cook for 1–2 minutes.
4. In a medium-sized bowl, combine ½ cup of the shredded cheese (or rice shreds), egg and cottage cheese.
5. Spread half of the turkey and tofu mixture into the prepared casserole. Pour half of the cheese and egg mixture on top. Top with 4 tortillas, overlapping if necessary. Repeat layers. Cover with aluminum foil, and bake 35 minutes. Uncover, and top with remaining ½ cup of shredded cheese (or rice shreds), and cook an additional 5 minutes. Top with scallions. Let casserole cool for 15 minutes before cutting and serving.

Nutrition Information: 570 calories, 3 g saturated fat, 75 g carbohydrate, 15 g dietary fiber, 42 g protein

Pork Chops with Apple-Sauerkraut
Roasted Sweet Potato Fries

Serves: 4

Extra-virgin olive oil cooking spray
3 tablespoons extra-virgin olive oil, divided
Coarse salt, to taste
Coarse black pepper, to taste
1½ pounds sweet potatoes, scrubbed, left unpeeled, and cut into thin fries
4 boneless, center-cut pork chops (about 1¼ pounds), trimmed of all fat
White pepper, to taste
Cardamom, to taste
3 tablespoons whole-wheat flour
1 large red onion, chopped
2 Granny Smith apples, chopped
1 jar (28 ounces) sauerkraut, rinsed with water, drained and patted dry
2 tablespoons brown sugar
1 tablespoon Land O' Lakes "Soft Baking Butter with Canola Oil"

1. Preheat the oven to 450 degrees, and spray a cookie sheet with cooking spray.
2. In a small bowl, whisk together 2 tablespoons of the extra-virgin olive oil with salt and pepper to taste. Transfer the sweet potatoes to the oiled cookie sheet, and toss with the seasoned oil mixture. Arrange the sweet potatoes in rows, not touching, and roast in the upper one-third of the preheated oven, for 20–25 minutes, turning once with a spatula.
3. Meanwhile, place the pork chops in a zip-top bag, and pound thin with a kitchen mallet. Season the pork with salt, white pepper and cardamom to taste. Dust both sides of pork chops with whole-wheat flour.
4. Pour the remaining 1 tablespoon of extra-virgin olive oil into a large skillet, and lightly spread the oil around the skillet with your fingertips. Heat the oil over medium-high heat; add the pork chops, and brown on both sides, cooking each side 3–4 minutes.
5. Add the chopped red onions to the skillet with the pork, and cook for 2 minutes, stirring the onions constantly. Stir in the apples, and cook for 2–3 minutes, or until apples begin to soften. Remove the pork chops from the skillet, and set aside on a clean plate. Stir in the

sauerkraut, brown sugar, more cardamom and white pepper to taste, and the Land O' Lakes "Soft Baking Butter with Canola Oil"; continue stirring and cooking the sauerkraut for 3–4 minutes.

6. Remove the sweet potato fries from the oven (they should be golden and crisp) and sprinkle with coarse salt and pepper to taste. Divide sauerkraut onto 4 individual plates, and serve with pork chops on top and roasted sweet potato fries on the side. Serve at once.

Nutrition Information: 540 calories, 4 g saturated fat, 67 g carbohydrate, 12 g dietary fiber, 30 g protein

Li'l BBQ Turkey and Cheese Loaves
Black Bean Corn Salsa
Green Beans

Serves: 4

Extra-virgin olive oil cooking spray
3 packages (9 ounces) frozen Birds Eye "Italian Green Beans"
1 pound extra-lean ground turkey
⅓ cup wheat germ
1½ cups diced onion
1 omega-3-enriched egg, beaten
½ teaspoon salt, plus more to taste
2 teaspoons cumin, divided
½ cup shredded low-fat organic Cheddar cheese
¼ cup all-natural barbecue sauce
3 cups frozen corn kernels
1 can (15.5 ounces) black beans, rinsed and drained
2–3 crushed garlic cloves
1 cup prepared pico de gallo (look for this in the deli section of your
     supermarket; buy fresh if possible)
1 tablespoon lime juice
1 tablespoon plus 2 teaspoons extra-virgin olive oil, divided
¼ cup chopped fresh cilantro, rinsed and patted dry
White pepper, to taste

1. Preheat the oven to 400 degrees. Spray 12 muffin tins with extra-virgin olive oil cooking spray.
2. Open the 3 packages of frozen green beans, and transfer to a large microwave-safe bowl; microwave on high for 5 minutes. Set aside.
3. In a large mixing bowl, add the ground turkey, wheat germ and diced onions; mix thoroughly with your hands to combine all ingredients. Stir in the egg, measured salt, 1 teaspoon of the cumin and shredded Cheddar cheese. Divide the turkey mixture evenly among the 12 prepared muffin tins, pressing down lightly with your fingertips; spread the barbecue sauce over the tops. Bake turkey loaves at 400 degrees for 20 minutes, or until turkey is no longer pink.
4. Meanwhile, place the frozen corn kernels in a medium-sized microwave-safe bowl, and heat in the microwave, for 2 minutes. Remove the corn from the microwave, and add to the bowl the black beans, garlic, pico de gallo, lime juice, 2 teaspoons of the

extra-virgin olive oil, 1 teaspoon cumin, cilantro and salt to taste. Stir all ingredients until well blended and set aside.

5. Toss the green beans with the remaining 1 tablespoon of extra-virgin olive oil, salt and white pepper to taste.
6. Remove the barbecued turkey and cheese loaves from the oven, and allow the loaves to cool for several minutes before removing them from the muffin tins. Serve with sides of green beans and black bean corn salsa.

Nutrition Information: 640 calories, 2.5 g saturated fat, 90 g carbohydrate, 21 g dietary fiber, 52 g protein

Daily Vitamin Planner and Supplement Shopping Guide

11

In doing research for our first book, *The Gold Coast Cure,* we investigated a multitude of nutritional supplementation options. As you know, Ivy's diagnosis with MS was what sparked our interest into lifestyle modification in the first place. Fortunately, Andy's medical background was a major help when it came to researching the benefits of nutritional supplements. After weighing many factors, including cost, scientific evidence supporting health benefits, safety, side effects and convenience, we determined most adults could greatly benefit from a properly designed supplement regimen. Plenty of scientific evidence supports our recommendations, including guidelines published in esteemed medical journals such as the *New England Journal of Medicine* and the *Journal of the American Medical Association.* Our supplement regimen works on many levels to combat the inflammation, insulin resistance and malnutrition that contribute to obesity, accelerated aging and many chronic diseases.

The benefits gained from nutritional supplements occur after long-term commitment and long-term use. Significant evidence shows the risk of developing conditions such as osteoporosis, cancer, heart disease and even multiple sclerosis can be reduced by supplementing with a select group of vitamins, minerals and essential fats. Research leads us to believe supplements can help you look younger, too.

In addition to protecting against disease and improving health, you may notice it's easier to lose weight with the help of supplements than without. The nutrients we recommend assist your body in regulating appetite, burning fat for energy and keeping food cravings under control. The essential fats will help decrease insulin resistance and make it easier for you to lose weight. Over time, you should also notice an improvement in the appearance of your skin, hair and nails. Those of you who suffer from an inflammation-mediated condition, such as arthritis, fibromyalgia or even asthma, will likely notice an improvement of your symptoms, an increased feeling of well-being and increased energy. If you have high cholesterol or even high blood pressure you may see objective improvement. You may even notice an improvement in your memory and your mood. While these results won't occur overnight, they will occur if you are diligent about following our entire *Fitter, Firmer, Faster* program. Consistency is crucial.

It's important to understand scientists have yet to discover any "magic bullet" antioxidant, vitamin, mineral, supplemental nutrient or even food that in and of itself promotes lasting good health. In fact, we doubt such a cure-all nutrient or food will ever be identified. It's impossible for researchers to isolate exactly which antioxidants, minerals, phytonutrients and vitamins found in the whole foods we recommend are responsible for helping to protect against disease and fight the aging process. The most likely, most widely accepted, explanation is the nutrients in whole foods work synergistically, not in isolation.

Natural Team Players

In nature, each whole food offers a unique set of nutrients, and each nutrient offers a unique set of biological properties. For example, strawberries are not only rich in the antioxidant vitamin C, they also contain vitamin E and folic acid as well as various nonvitamin phytonutrients—all of these substances work together to enhance your health and fight the aging process. The nutrients in whole foods work synergistically as part of an elaborate network. Some nutrients work specifically to enhance the health benefits of others. For example, vitamins E and C when taken along with selenium in supplement form, enhance the benefits of beta-carotene. Together, these antioxidants work in synergy and have the potential to protect cells, delay the aging process and prevent degenerative diseases.

We ask you to put this same logic to work in designing your supplementation regimen. Avoid à la carte nutritional supplementation. Avoid mega-dosing. Avoid changing your regimen every time you read something new in the paper. A properly structured supplementation regimen should contain a wide spectrum of vitamins, minerals and antioxidants in balanced amounts and dosages shown to protect against disease. The safety and efficacy of the supplements we recommend, when taken together in reasonable doses, has stood the test of time.

The Daily Vitamin Planner

It's important certain vitamins and supplements be taken together and others taken separately for maximal absorption. You should take your supplements *with* food during the three main meals you eat each day. Be sure to follow the serving size suggestions provided on the back of the supplement label because each brand varies slightly. For example, with some multivitamin brands you need to take two or three capsules every day to get the dosages on the label, and with some brands all the nutrients you need are found in just one pill. Some supplements, such as calcium and vitamin C, *must* be split into multiple doses, as it is not possible to absorb all you need all at once. Try to follow our daily vitamin planner as closely as possible.

Note: If you are familiar with our earlier *Gold Coast Cure* book, you'll notice our daily vitamin planner has not changed, although we have broadened the acceptable ranges for some of the recommended vitamins and essential fats.

Recommended Supplements and Doses
1. Multivitamin/multimineral supplement
2. Calcium with magnesium and vitamin D: 1000 mg calcium + 400 mg magnesium + 400–800 IUs vitamin D

3. Natural vitamin E with seleniuml: 100–400 IUs Natural Vitamin E + 100–200 mcg selenium
4. Vitamin C with bioflavonoids: 1000 mg vitamin C + 200–500 mg bioflavonoids
5. GLA (gamma linoleic acid): 1300 to 2600 mg
6. Fish oil (containing EPA and DHA): 1000–2000 mg combined EPA and DHA (dosage can be as high as 4000 mg)

Take at Breakfast

- Take your entire multivitamin, multi-mineral supplement.
- Take half your daily dose of vitamin C with bioflavonoids. Half your daily dose contains about 500 milligrams of vitamin C and about 100–250 milligrams of bioflavonoids.
- Take half your daily dose of calcium with magnesium and vitamin D. Half your daily dose contains about 500 milligrams of calcium, 200 milligrams of magnesium, and 200–400 IUs of vitamin D.

Take at Lunch

- Take the other half of your daily dose of vitamin C with bioflavonoids.
- Take the other half of your daily dose of calcium with magnesium and vitamin D.

Take at Dinner

- Take your entire daily dose of natural vitamin E with selenium. The daily dose contains between 100 to 400 IUs of vitamin E and between 100 to 200 micrograms of selenium.
- Take your entire daily dose of GLA. The daily dose is 1300–2600 milligrams of evening primrose oil.
- Take your entire daily dose of fish oil containing both DHA (docosahexanoic acid) and EPA (eicosahexaenoic acid). This daily dose should contain between 1000 and 2000 milligrams of combined EPA and DHA and may be as high as 4000 milligrams of combined DHA and EPA.

The Supplement Shopping Guide

All of the following supplements meet our standards for quality. All contain the vitamins and minerals your body needs in optimal doses. If you choose to take different brands, perhaps to save money, it's crucial you choose products of the highest quality that contain approximately the same dosages in approximately the same combination we have recommended in the text of this chapter. Doses don't need to be exactly the same, but they should be very close. Read labels carefully to determine how many pills or how many teaspoons are needed to make one serving.

Note: Many of the supplements we recommend can be purchased at a discount through The Vitamin Shoppe online at *www.vitaminshoppe.com.* You can also call 1-800-223-1216 for referral to a store near you. Swanson Health Products also sells a number of the products we recommend at a discount online at *www.swansonvitamins.com.* You can also order by catalog. To request a catalog call 1-800-437-4148.

Multivitamin, Multimineral Supplement

1. Product made by: *Wyeth*
   Product name: "Centrum Silver"
   We recommend: one tablet per day
   Where to purchase: just about any pharmacy, grocery store, or vitamin store
   Note: This product is actually better for adults of all ages than the standard "Centrum" product, so don't worry if you are less than 50 years old. There are no "mega-doses" of any vitamins or minerals in this product.

2. Product made by: *GNC*
   Product name: "Liquid Ultra Mega"
   We recommend: one tablet per day
   Where to purchase: online at *www.GNC.com* or any GNC store

3. Product made by: *Swanson Health Products*
   Product name: "High Potency Soft Multiple without Iron"
   We recommend: two softgels, once per day
   Where to purchase: online at *www.swansonvitamins.com*

4. Product made by: *Twin Lab*
   Product name: "Daily One Caps without Iron"

We recommend: one tablet per day
Where to purchase: many retail stores, The Vitamin Shoppe, and through Swanson Health Products by catalog (call 1-800-437-4148) or online at *www.swansonvitamins.com*

5. Product made by: *Dr. Weil Nutritional Supplements*
Product name: "Weil Daily Mulitvitamin for Optimum Health"
We recommend: one tablet per day
Where to purchase: The Vitamin Shoppe or online at *www.drweil.com*

6. Product made by: *Olay*
Product name: "Complete Woman's Multivitamin 50+"
We recommend: one tablet per day
Where to purchase: supermarkets and drugstores nationwide
Note: This product is appropriate for adult men and women alike.

Calcium with Magnesium and Vitamin D

1. Product made by: *Carlson Laboratories*
Product name: "Liquid Cal-Mag"
We recommend: a total of four tablets per day, divided into two doses
Where to purchase: Available at most major vitamin stores, or call Carlson direct at 1-888-234-5656, or online at *www.carlsonlabs.com*
Note: This product also contains vitamin D even though this fact is not clear from the name.

2. Product made by: *Solaray*
Product name: "Cal-Mag Citrate with Vitamin D"
We recommend: a total of six tablets per day, divided into two doses
Where to purchase: The Vitamin Shoppe

3. Product made by: *Schiff*
Product name: "Super Calcium-Magnesium with Vitamin D and Boron"
We recommend: a total of three tablets per day, divided into three doses
Where to purchase: The Vitamin Shoppe, online at *www.schiffvitamins.com*, or through Swanson Health Products by catalog (call 1-800-437-4148) or online at *www.swansonvitamins.com*

4. Product made by: *Twin Lab*
Product name: "Calcium 500 Tabs"
We recommend: a total of two tablets, divided into two doses
Where to purchase: The Vitamin Shoppe, online at *www.twinlab.com*, or Swanson catalog (call 1-800-437-4148) or order online at *www.swansonvitamins.com*

5. Product made by: *Nature's Way*

Product name: "Calcium, Magnesium and Vitamin D"
We recommend: a total of two tablets, divided into two doses
Where to purchase: The Vitamin Shoppe, online at *www.naturesway.com*, or Swanson catalog (call 1-800-437-4148) or order online at *www.swansonvitamins.com*

6. Product made by: *Solgar*
Product name: "Calcium, Magnesium with Vitamin D"
We recommend: a total of five tablets, divided into three doses (take one tablet at breakfast plus two tablets at lunch and dinner)
Where to purchase: The Vitamin Shoppe or online at *www.solgar.com*

Natural Vitamin E with Selenium (Mixed Tochopherols Only)

1. Product made by: *Solaray*
Product name: "Bio E Gamma Plex with Selenium"
We recommend: two tablets per day
Where to purchase: The Vitamin Shoppe

2. Product made by: *The Vitamin Shoppe*
Product name: "E-400 IU Plus Selenium"
We recommend: one tablet per day
Where to purchase: The Vitamin Shoppe

Vitamin C with Bioflavonoids

1. Product made by: *Solgar*
Product name: "HY BIO"
We recommend: a total of two tablets per day, divided into two doses
Where to purchase: online at *www.solgar.com* or locate a retailer near you by calling 1-877-SOLGAR-4
Note: This product contains 500 milligrams vitamin C plus 500 milligrams bioflavonoids per tablet.

2. Product made by: *The Vitamin Shoppe*
Product name: "Ester-C 500 Complex"
We recommend: a total of two tablets per day, divided into two doses
Where to purchase: The Vitamin Shoppe
Note: This product contains 500 milligrams vitamin C plus 200 milligrams bioflavonoids per tablet.

3. Product made by: *Solaray*
Product name: "Super Bio-Plex Vit C & Bioflavonoids"
We recommend: a total of two pills per day, divided into two doses
Where to purchase: The Vitamin Shoppe

Note: This product contains 250 milligrams vitamin C plus 250 milligrams bioflavonoids per tablet.

4. Product made by: *Carlson Laboratories*
   Product name: "Super-C-Complex"
   We recommend: a total of two pills per day, divided into two doses
   Where to purchase: Available at most major vitamin stores, or call Carlson direct at 1-888-234-5656 or online at www.carlsonlabs.com
   Note: This product contains 500 milligram vitamin C plus 500 milligram bioflavonoids per pill.

5. Product made by: *Source Naturals*
   Product name: "Ester C 500"
   We recommend: a total of two pills per day, divided into two doses
   Where to purchase: Available at most major vitamin stores or online at *www.sourcenaturals.com*
   Note: This product contains 500 milligrams vitamin C plus 130 milligrams bioflavonoids per pill.

6. Product made by: *Swanson Health Products*
   Product name: "Buffered C with Bioflavonoid Capsules"
   We recommend: a total of two pills per day, divided into two doses
   Where to purchase: Swanson catalog (call 1-800-437-4148) or online at *www.swansonvitamins.com*
   Note: This product contains 500 milligrams vitamin C plus 200 milligrams bioflavonoids per pill.

GLA (from Evening Primrose Oil)

1. Product made by: *Barlean's Organic Oils*
   Product name: "Organic Evening Primrose Oil"
   We recommend: two soft gels per day will provide 1,300 milligrams of evening primrose oil.
   Where to purchase: online at *www.barleans.com* or try your local natural foods store
   Note: It's vital to buy only the highest quality essential fat supplements in order to insure freshness. We've come to rely exclusively on Barlean's "Evening Primrose Oil" for producing a consistently high-quality, fresh product.

Fish Oil (Containing EPA and DHA)

Note: It's imperative to buy only the highest quality, freshest pharmaceutical-grade fish oil to ensure product integrity and biological efficacy. Both Barlean's and Nordic Naturals produce an exceptionally fresh product with absolutely no fishy aftertaste, time and time again. The fish oils manufactured by these companies undergo rigid quality control procedures, including molecular distillation, and they surpass all national and international standards for environmental pollutants, including dioxins, PCBs, pesticides and heavy metals.

1. Product made by: *Barlean's*
   Product name: "Fresh Catch Fish Oil"
   We recommend: one teaspoon every day
   Where to purchase: many health food and vitamin stores or online at *www.barleans.com* or call 1-800-445-3529

2. Product made by: *Barlean's*
   Product name: "Healthy Adult" or "EPA-DHA" (both products contain the same amount of EPA and DHA)
   We recommend: two soft gels every day
   Where to purchase: many health food and vitamin stores or online at *www.barleans.com* or call 1-800-445-3529

3. Product made by: *Nordic Naturals*
   Product name: "Ultimate Omega"
   We recommend: two soft gels every day
   Where to purchase: many health food and vitamin stores or online at *www.nordicnaturals.com* or call 1-800-662-2544

The Daily Vitamin Planner for Children

Children twelve and under do benefit from taking a daily multivitamin and a daily essential fat supplement, and should take their supplements with food. They don't need to take all of the higher-dose supplements we recommend to adults. Teenagers can follow our recommendations for adults.

- **Take at Breakfast:** Multivitamin, multi-mineral supplement
- **Take at Dinner:** Essential fat supplement

Supplement Shopping Guide for Children

It's most important your children take their vitamins to ensure adequate nutrition. Because of the high demand for energy and essential nutrients, children are at particular risk of undernutrition, which can affect their growth, overall health, behavior and even mental abilities.

To compound the problem, many children are picky eaters and will only eat a limited variety of nutrient-rich foods. A good multivitamin, multimineral supplement can fill important gaps in your child's diet with nutrients that play a vital role in proper brain, immune and nervous system function. Because children's bodies cannot store all of the essential vitamins and minerals they need, these substances must be supplied on a regular basis. A good nutritional supplement can help make up for the days your children don't eat as well as they should.

Multivitamin, Multi-Mineral Supplement

1. Product made by: *Northwest Natural Products*
   Product name: "L'il Critters Gummy Vites"
   We recommend: Children ages two through twelve should take two gummy bear vitamins per day.
   Where to purchase: *www.gummybearvitamins.com* or at popular drugstores, discount stores and grocery stores nationwide

2. Product made by: *Wyeth*
   Product name: "Centrum Kids Rugrats Extra Calcium"
   We recommend: Children between two and four years old should take one-half tablet daily. Children ages four through twelve years old should take one tablet daily.
   Where to purchase: most major drugstores, grocery stores or vitamin stores nationwide
   Note: The higher calcium dose in this product makes it a good choice if your children avoid dairy products.

3. Product made by: *Schiff*
   Product name: "Children's Chewable Vitamins with Minerals"
   We recommend: Children between two and four years old should chew one tablet once a day. Children ages four through twelve years old should chew two tablets daily.
   Where to purchase: The Vitamin Shoppe or online at *www. schiffvitamins.com,* or Swanson catalog (call 1-800-437-4148) or online at *www.swansonvitamins.com*

4. Product made by: *Bayer Health Care*
   Product name: "Flintstones Plus Calcium"
   We recommend: Children between two and four years old should chew one-half tablet once a day. Children ages four through twelve years old should chew one tablet daily.
   Where to purchase: drugstores and supermarkets nationwide
   Note: Again, this is a good product if your children avoid dairy products.

5. Product made by: *Country Life*
   Product name: "Tall Tree Children Chewable Multiple"
   We recommend: Children between two and four years old should chew one-half wafer once a day. Children ages four through twelve should chew one wafer once a day.
   Where to purchase: The Vitamin Shoppe or online at *www.vitaminlife.com* or call 1-866-998-8855

6. Product made by: *Kirkland*
   Product name: "Children's Chewable"
   We recommend: Children between two and four years old should chew one-half tablet once a day. Children ages four through twelve should chew one tablet once a day.
   Where to purchase: Costco

Essential Fat Supplement (Containing EPA, DHA, and GLA)

We also highly recommend children take an essential fat supplement for optimal health and growth. Essential fats, especially the omega-3 essential fats found in fish oil, have been shown to play a significant role in visual and brain development in children. The omega-3 fats are "smart fats" that researchers have linked to an improvement in children's attention, concentration, learning ability and behavior. Children suffering from inflammation-mediated conditions such as asthma and allergies also benefit from fish oil supplementation. Don't worry about your kids not liking the taste of fish or fish oil; we unconditionally guarantee the high-quality fish oil supplement brands we recommend have absolutely no fishy taste; they actually taste good (honest!).

1. Product made by: *Barlean's*
   Product name: "Fresh Catch Fish Oil" (good for children who can't swallow pills)
   We recommend: one-half teaspoon every day
   Where to purchase: many health food and vitamin stores or online at *www.barleans.com* or call 1-800-445-3529

2. Product made by: *Nordic Naturals*
   Product name: "ProEFA Liquid" (good for children who can't swallow pills)
   We recommend: Children under the age of four should take one-quarter teaspoon daily. Children ages four through twelve should take one-half teaspoon daily.

Where to purchase: many health food and vitamin stores, online at *www.nordicnaturals.com* or call 1-800-662-2544

3. Product made by: *Nordic Naturals*
Product name: "Omega 3-6-9 Junior"
We recommend: Children under the age of four should take two soft gels daily. Children ages four through twelve can take three or four soft gels daily.
Where to purchase: many health food and vitamin stores, or online at *www.nordicnaturals.com* or call 1-800-662-2544

Appendix A

Brand-Name "Fit Foods" Shopping Guide

Healthful prepared and convenience foods play an essential role in allowing us to maintain our sanity in today's hectic lifestyles. We wouldn't dare ask you to give up convenience for the sake of health. Nor will we insist you read every single label searching for nutritious alternatives to your favorite "ready-made" foods. In this section we've done the work for you! We've read the nutrition labels and the ingredients lists on hundreds of packaged food products available at the supermarket and the natural foods store. We've taste-tested these products and have compiled a listing of some of the best-tasting "whole foods" convenience items on the market. For bona fide junk food lovers, we've included a special list for you with more healthful alternatives to some of your favorite "not-so-healthful" foods. Take our three convenience foods shopping lists with you the next time you're out food shopping. You'll be delighted to learn how wide the variety of healthful convenience foods available truly is.

List #1: Supermarket Shopping List

The vast majority of larger metropolitan supermarkets carry the majority of the items on this list. Some of these items can be found in the "natural foods" or "health foods" section of your local supermarket. If you live in a smaller city you may need to visit your local natural foods store to obtain the widest possible selection. In addition, why not cut, paste and copy the items in these lists so they correspond with the organization of the aisles in your own supermarket?

OMEGA-3-ENRICHED EGGS

Eggland's Best
Egg Innovations "Cage Free
  Omega-3 Eggs"

Organic Valley "Omega-3 Brown
  Eggs"

CHEESE

Wholesome Valley "Organic
  Cheddar 33% Less Fat"
Wholesome Valley "Organic
  Mozzarella 15% Less Fat"
Organic Valley "Monterey Jack
  Reduced Fat"
Organic Valley "Shredded
  Mozzarella Cheese"
Organic Valley "Parmesan"
Organic Valley "Blue Cheese
  Crumbles"
Horizon Organic "Shredded
  Reduced Fat Cheese"

Horizon Organic "Shredded Part
  Skim Mozzarella Cheese"
Horizon Organic "Part Skim String
  Cheese"
The Laughing Cow "Light Gourmet
  Cheeses"
Cracker Barrel "2% Milk Reduced
  Fat Sharp White Cheddar"
Laura Chenel's Chevre "Goat's
  Milk Cheese"
Boursin "Light Cheese"

CHEESE ALTERNATIVES

These melt very well and contain zero grams saturated fat.

Galaxy Nutritional Foods "Rice
  Shreds Mozzarella Flavor"

Galaxy Nutritional Foods "Rice
  Shreds Cheddar Flavor"
Lisanatti "Almond Cheese"

CANOLA OIL BUTTER BLEND

Land O' Lakes "Soft Baking Butter with Canola Oil"
(contains 30% less saturated fat than regular butter)

PLAIN SOY MILK

Unsweetened versions are also available in many natural foods stores.

Silk "Unsweetened Soymilk" (the best choice because it has no added sugars)

Sun Soy "Creamy Original"
Silk "Plain Soymilk"
Organic Valley Soy Milk "Original"

CHOCOLATE SOY MILK

To reduce the sugar content, try diluting the chocolate flavors listed here with plain soy milk. Use ½ cup plain soy milk mixed with ½ cup chocolate soy milk.

Sun Soy "Chocolate"
Silk "Chocolate Soymilk"

Organic Valley Soy Milk "Chocolate"

BUTTER ALTERNATIVE SPREADS

Made without trans fats these products are best for "no-heat" use such as for spreading on toast.

Smart Balance "67% Buttery Spread"
Smart Balance "Omega Plus with Flax Spread"

Earth Balance "Organic Whipped Buttery Spread"
Earth Balance "Natural Margarine"

YOGURT

Stonyfield Farm "Low Fat Plain Yogurt"
Stonyfield Farm "No Fat Plain Yogurt"
Dannon "Low Fat Plain Yogurt"

Dannon "No Fat Plain Yogurt"
Fage Authentic Greek Yogurt "Total 2%"
Fage Authentic Greek Yogurt "Total 0%"

KEFIR

Lifeway "Low Fat Plain Kefir"

Helios "2% Reduced Fat Plain Kefir"

TOMATO SAUCE

Rao's "Homemade Marinara
Sauce"

Rao's "Homemade Puttanesca
Sauce"

Rao's "Tomato Basil Sauce"

Gia Russa "Marinara Sauce"

Gia Russa "Hot Sicilian Sauce"

Victoria "All Natural Marinara
Sauce" (also available organic)

Victoria "All Natural Hot and Spicy
Vodka Sauce"

Victoria "All Natural Mushroom
Sauce"

Victoria "All Natural Eggplant
Sauce"

Victoria "All Natural Artichoke
Sauce"

Victoria "All Natural Tomato Basil
Sauce" (also available organic)

Victoria "All Natural Roasted
Garlic Sauce" (also available
organic)

Joey Pots and Pans "Marinara
Sauce"

Emeril's "Roasted Gaaahlic Pasta
Sauce"

Emeril's "Roasted Red Pepper Pasta
Sauce"

Amy's "Wild Mushroom Pasta
Sauce"

Amy's "Puttanesca Pasta Sauce"

Amy's "Garlic Mushroom Pasta
Sauce"

Amy's "Tomato and Basil Pasta
Sauce"

Alessi "All Natural Marinara Pasta
Sauce" (smooth and chunky
varieties are available)

PREPARED DELI FOODS

Many supermarket delicatessens offer the following healthful pre-pared foods manufactured by Hannah (*www.hannahfoods.net*).

Hannah "Taboule"

Hannah "Olive Spread"

Hannah "Pico de Gallo"

Hannah "Hommus"

ALL-NATURAL PEANUT BUTTER

Smucker's "Natural Peanut Butter" (Chunky or Smooth)
Smart Balance "Omega Peanut Butter"

ALL-NATURAL "PEANUT-FREE" SUNFLOWER SEED BUTTER

These products are especially good for people allergic to peanuts. To learn more about SunGold products visit *www.sunbutter.com*.

SunGold "Sunbutter Natural"

SunGold "Sunbutter Honey
Crunch"

SunGold "Sunbutter Creamy"

SunGold "Sunbutter Natural
Crunch"

ALL-NATURAL SESAME SEED BUTTER (TAHINI)

Arrowhead Mills "Sesame Tahini"

RICE PILAF MIXES

For a truly homemade-tasting pilaf try sautéing garlic and shallots in extra-virgin olive oil. Add the cooked pilaf and thawed frozen corn kernels then heat through.

Near East Whole Grain Blends "Chicken and Herbs with Brown Rice, Barley, and Grains"

Near East Whole Grain Blends "Brown Rice Pilaf"

Near East Whole Grain Blends "Roasted Garlic with Bulgar, Brown Rice, and Grains"

Near East "Rice Pilaf with Lentil"

Near East "Rice Pilaf Toasted Almond"

Near East "Brown Rice Pilaf Mix"

Near East "Rice Pilaf Mix with Wheat"

Near East "Roasted Garlic with Brown Rice"

Near East "Chicken and Herbs with Brown Rice, Barley, and Pearled Wheat"

Rice-A-Roni "Savory Whole Grains Chicken and Herb Classico"

TABBOULEH

Try mixing a prepared tabbouleh from your local deli with fresh lemon juice, diced tomato, flaxseed oil and one of the following mixes:

Near East "Tabbouleh Wheat Salad Mix"

Fantastic Foods "Tabouli"

PITA BREAD

The Baker "Whole Wheat Pita"
Toufayan "Whole Wheat Pita"

Toufayan "Oat Bran Pita"

WHOLE-GRAIN BREAD

Many of these breads are kept in the frozen foods section. You may need to visit a natural foods store for the best variety. The sprouted breads marked with an asterisk (*) are flour-free.

Mestemacher "Pumpernickel"

Mestemacher "Whole Rye Bread

Mestemacher "Organic Linseed Bread"

Mestemacher "3 Grain Bread"

Mestemacher "Fitness Bread"

The Baker "9-Grain Whole Wheat"

The Baker "Low-Carb Flax Bread"

Nature's Own Healthline Sugar Free "100% Whole Grain Wheat"

Rudi's Organic Bakery "Honey Sweet Whole Wheat Bread"

Pepperidge Farm "100% Whole Wheat Hearty Texture"

Alvarado Street Bakery "California Style Complete Protein Bread"*

Alvarado Street Bakery "Sprouted Soy Crunch Bread"*

Alvarado Street Bakery "Ultimate Kids Bread"

Alvarado Street Bakery "Sprouted Wheat Bread"*

Alvarado Street Bakery "Sprouted Sourdough"*

Alvarado Street Bakery "Sprouted Rye Seed Bread"*

Alvarado Street Bakery "Sprouted Wheat Cinnamon Raisin Bread"*

Food for Life "Ezekiel 4:9 Sprouted Grain Bread"*

Food for Life "Ezekiel 4:9 Cinnamon Raisin Bread"*

Food for Life "7 Sprouted Grains"*

Food for Life "Genesis 1:29"*

Food for Life "Ezekiel 4:9 Sesame"*

Food for Life "Sesame Spelt"

WHOLE-GRAIN PIZZA SHELLS

Boboli "Whole Wheat Italian Bread Shell"

WHOLE-GRAIN HAMBURGER AND HOT DOG BUNS

Alvarado Street Bakery "Sprouted Wheat Hot Dog Buns"

Alvarado Street Bakery "Sprouted Wheat Burger Buns"

Food for Life "Ezekiel 4:9 Sesame Sprouted Grain Burger Buns"

Food for Life "Sprouted Wheat Hot Dog Buns"

ENGLISH MUFFINS

Thomas' English Muffins Hearty Grains "100% Whole Wheat"

CEREAL

Post Healthy Classics "Shredded
Wheat & Bran"

Post Healthy Classics "Shredded
Wheat Spoon Size"

Kellogg's "Raisin Bran"

Kashi "The Breakfast Pilaf, Seven
Whole Grains and Sesame"

Kashi "Heart to Heart"

Kashi "Go Lean"

Kashi "Seven in the Morning"

Kashi "Good Friends"

Kashi "Vive" Cereal

Kashi "Mighty Bites Cinnamon"
Cereal (for Kids)

Kashi Mighty Bites "Honey
Crunch" Cereal (for Kids)

Nature's Path "Organic Flax Plus
Multigrain Cereal"

Nature's Path "8 Grain Synergy"

Nature's Path "Millet Rice Oat
Bran Flakes"

Nature's Path "Multigrain Oatbran"

Nature's Path "Optimal Slim"

Nature's Path "Heritage Bites"

Kretschmer "Original Toasted
Wheat Germ"

Uncle Sam Cereal "Original"

Uncle Sam Cereal "With Real
Mixed Berries"

Alpen "No Sugar Added—Muesli"

Familia "Swiss Muesli—No Sugar
Added"

Krusteaz "Zoom Quick Hot Cereal"

PASTA, SPAGHETTI AND
LASAGNA NOODLES

Gia Russa "Whole Wheat Penne
Regate"

Gia Russa "Rotini"

Gia Russa "Roman Rigatoni"

Gia Russa "Whole Wheat Angel
Hair Pasta"

Gia Russa "Whole Wheat Thin
Spaghetti"

Gia Russa "Whole Wheat
Linguine"

Gia Russa "Whole Wheat Lasagna"

Barilla Plus "Penne"

Barilla Plus "Spaghetti"

De Cecco "Whole Wheat Fusilli"

De Cecco "Enriched Whole Wheat
Linguine"

Annie's Organic "Whole Wheat
Spaghetti"

Hodgson Mill Organic "Fettuccini
with Milled Flaxseed"

Hodgson Mill Organic "Spirals
with Milled Flaxseed"

Hodgson Mill Organic "Penne with
Milled Flaxseed"

Hodgson Mill "Angel Hair"

Hodgson Mill "Whole Wheat
Spaghetti"

Hodgson Mill "Whole Wheat
Penne"

Hodgson Mill "Whole Wheat Bow
Tie"

ALL-FRUIT JELLY

Jelly is a calorie-rich condiment intended to be used in moderation.

St. Dalfour Preserves "Black Cherry"

St. Dalfour Preserves "Blackberry"

St. Dalfour Preserves "Blackcurrant"

St. Dalfour Preserves "Raspberry"

St. Dalfour Preserves "Strawberry"

St. Dalfour Preserves "Wild Blueberry"

Smucker's Simply Fruit "Black Cherry"

Smucker's Simply Fruit "Blueberry"

Smucker's Simply Fruit "Concord Grape"

Smucker's Simply Fruit "Strawberry"

Smucker's Simply Fruit "Red Raspberry"

ALL-NATURAL PUDDINGS

These puddings are good low-saturated fat options for your daily sweet treat.

Kozy Shack "Crème Caramel Flan"

Kozy Shack "Original Rice Pudding"

Kozy Shack "Old Fashioned Tapioca"

Kozy Shack "Real Chocolate Pudding"

Kozy Shack "Natural Vanilla Pudding"

Kozy Shack "Dulce de Leche"

Kozy Shack "Cinnamon Raisin Rice"

Kozy Shack "Creamy Banana"

SALAD DRESSINGS

Purchase only dressings made from extra-virgin olive oil, expeller-pressed canola oil or expeller-pressed walnut oil.

Annie's Naturals "Balsamic Vinaigrette"

Annie's Naturals "Organic Buttermilk Dressing"

Annie's Naturals "Caesar Dressing"

Annie's Naturals "Cilantro & Lime Vinaigrette"

Annie's Naturals "Cowgirl Ranch Dressing"

Annie's Naturals "French Dressing"

Annie's Naturals "Roasted Red Pepper Vinaigrette"

Annie's Naturals "Organic Thousand Island Dressing"

Annie's Naturals "Tuscany Italian Dressing"

Annie's Naturals "Gardenstyle Dressing"

Briana's Homestyle "Poppyseed Dressing"

Briana's Homestyle "Real French Vinaigrette"

Briana's Homestyle "Blush Wine Vinaigrette"

Drew's All Natural Dressing and Marinade "Kalamata Olive and Caper"

Drew's All Natural Dressing and Marinade "Romano and Caesar"

Drew's All Natural Dressing and Marinade "Rosemary Balsamic"

Drew's All Natural Dressing and Marinade "Soy Ginger"

Drew's All Natural Dressing and Marinade "Garlic Italian"

Drew's All Natural Dressing and Marinade "Roasted Garlic"

WHOLE-GRAIN CRACKERS

Wasa "Multi-Grain Crisp Bread"

Wasa "Hearty Rye"

Wasa "Golden Sourdough"

Wasa "Crispbread Light Rye"

Wasa "Crispbread"

Wasa "Crispbread Cinnamon Toast"

Wasa "Crispbread Toasted Wheat"

Ryvita "Tasty Light Rye"

Ryvita "Flavorful Fiber"

Ryvita "Toasted Sesame Rye"

Ryvita "Tasty Dark Rye"

Ryvita "Tasty Light Rye"

Triscuit "Reduced Fat"

CANNED SOUPS

Amy's "Lentil Soup"
Amy's "Split Pea Soup"
Amy's "Lentil Vegetable Soup"
Amy's "Chunky Tomato Bisque"
Health Valley Organic "Black Bean Soup"
Health Valley Organic "Lentil"
Health Valley Organic "Potato Leek"
Health Valley Organic "Tomato"

Health Valley Organic "Mushroom Barley"
Health Valley Organic "Split Pea"
Wolfgang Puck "Organic Split Pea"
Wolfgang Puck "Thick and Hearty Lentil and Vegetable"
Wolfgang Puck "Organic Spicy Bean"
Wolfgang Puck "Organic Tortilla"

DRIED SOUPS AND CHILI

We sometimes add shredded cheese to these soups for extra protein and calcium.

Fantastic Foods "Jumpin' Black Bean"
Fantastic Foods "Country Lentil"
Fantastic Foods "Split Pea"

Fantastic Foods "Cha Cha Chili"
Fantastic Foods "Five Bean Soup"
Fantastic Foods "Vegetable Barley"

GOURMET CREAMY VEGETABLE SOUPS

Pacific Foods "Creamy Tomato Soup"
Pacific Foods "Roasted Red Pepper and Tomato Soup"
Pacific Foods "Creamy Butternut Squash Soup"
Pacific Foods "Creamy Roasted Carrot Soup"
Imagine "Organic Creamy Tomato Soup"

Imagine "Organic Sweet Potato Soup"
Imagine "Organic Creamy Tomato Basil Soup"
Imagine "Organic Sweet Corn Soup"
Imagine "Creamy Portobello Mushroom Soup"

ALL-NATURAL CHICKEN BROTHS AND GRAVIES

Pacific Foods "Free Range Chicken Broth" (organic version)

Pacific Foods "Organic Vegetable Broth"

Pacific Foods "Organic Mushroom Broth"

Pacific Foods "Beef Broth"

Pacific Foods "Mushroom Gravy"

Pacific Foods "Natural Beef Gravy"

Pacific Foods "Natural Turkey Gravy"

Pacific Foods "Natural Chicken Gravy"

Imagine "Vegetable Broth"

Imagine "Beef Broth"

Imagine "Free Range Chicken Broth"

MARINATED TUNA IN A FLAVOR-FRESH POUCH

Use on salads, with whole-grain pasta or brown rice. You can also mix them with a little canola oil mayonnaise or eat them straight up.

StarKist Tuna Creations "Hickory Smoked"

StarKist Tuna Creations "Zesty Lemon Pepper"

StarKist Tuna Creations "Herb & Garlic"

StarKist Tuna Creations "Sweet & Spicy"

MAYONNAISE

Hellmann's "Canola Oil Mayonnaise"

Smart Balance "Omega Plus Light Mayonnaise"

Spectrum Naturals "Canola Oil Mayonnaise"

CANNED "NO-SUGAR ADDED" FRUITS

Del Monte "Pineapple Tidbits in 100% Juice" (packaged in plastic cups)

Del Monte "Diced Peaches in 100% Juice" (packaged in pull-top cans)

Mott's Healthy Harvest Apple Sauce with no sugar added "Country Berry"

Mott's Healthy Harvest Apple Sauce with no sugar added "Summer Strawberry"

Mott's Healthy Harvest Apple Sauce with no sugar added "Peach Medley"

FROZEN ENTREES

Kashi all-natural "Lemon Rosemary
Chicken"
Kashi all-natural "Black Bean and
Mango"
Kashi all-natural "Southwest Style
Chicken"

Kashi all-natural "Chicken Pasta
Pomodoro"
Kashi all-natural "Lime Cilantro
Shrimp"

FROZEN SEASONED VEGETABLE SIDE DISHES

Birds Eye "Herb Garden Collection:
Baby Broccoli & Cauliflower
Florets with Chives"
Birds Eye "Herb Garden Collection:
Petite Peas & Mushrooms with
Chives"

Birds Eye "Green Beans with
Thyme"
Birds Eye "Baby Broccoli with
Thyme"
Tabatchnick "Creamed Spinach"

FROZEN VEGGIE BURGERS

Avoid veggie burgers made with hydrogenated oil or with the relatively unhealthful omega-6 vegetable oils such as corn oil or soybean oil.

Amy's "California Veggie Burger"
Amy's "Texas Veggie Burger"
Amy's "Chicago Veggie Burger"
Amy's "All American Veggie
Burger"

Boca Burger "Roasted Onion"
Boca Burger "Vegan"
Boca Burger "Garden Vegetable"
Boca Burger "Grilled Vegetable"

List #2: Natural Foods Store Shopping List

You should be able to find almost all of the following foods at any well-stocked natural foods store. Many health-oriented supermarkets also carry a variety of items on this list.

MUSTARDS

We often mix gourmet mustards with a small amount of canola-oil mayonnaise, then brush the paste on top of raw fish and bake for a simple, delicious dinner entrée.

Annie's Natural Organic "Horseradish Mustard"

Annie's Natural Organic "Honey Mustard"

Annie's Natural Organic "German Mustard"

Annie's Natural Organic "Asian Mustard"

FLAXSEED OIL

(Buy high-quality refrigerated flax oil.)

Barlean's "Flax Oil"

GROUND FLAXSEEDS

Barlean's "Forti-Flax"

Bob's Red Mill "Golden Flaxseed Meal"

ORGANIC TOMATO SAUCES

Amy's Premium Organic Pasta Sauce "Family Marinara"

Amy's Premium Organic Pasta Sauce "Tomato Basil"

Amy's Premium Organic Pasta Sauce "Garlic Mushroom"

Amy's Premium Organic Pasta Sauce "Roasted Garlic"

Amy's Premium Organic Pasta Sauce "Puttanesca"

Muir Glen Organic "Sun Dried Tomato"

Muir Glen Organic "Italian Herb"

Muir Glen Organic "Balsamic Roasted Onion"

Muir Glen Organic "Fire Roasted Tomato"

Muir Glen Organic "Portobello Mushroom"

Muir Glen Organic "Garden Vegetable"

Muir Glen Organic "Spicy Tomato"

Muir Glen Organic "Tomato Basil"

Muir Glen Organic "Four Cheese"

Muir Glen Organic "Mushroom Marinara"

PASTA, SPAGHETTI, AND LASAGNA NOODLES

Sprouted whole-grain pastas are the gold-standard for health and weight loss.

Vita Spelt "Whole Grain Spelt Pasta"
Eden Organic Pasta Company's "100 Percent Whole Grain Kamut Spirals"
Food for Life "Ezekiel 4:9 Organic Sprouted Penne Pasta"
Food for Life "Ezekiel 4:9 Organic Sprouted Linguine Pasta"
Food for Life "Ezekiel 4:9 Organic Sprouted Fettuccine Pasta"
Food for Life "Ezekiel 4:9 Organic Sprouted Spaghetti Pasta"
Westbrae Natural "Organic Whole Wheat Lasanga"
Ancient Quinoa Harvest "Supergrain Spaghetti"

CANNED CHILI

Amy's "Medium Chili"
Amy's "Medium Black Bean Chili"
Shelton's Chicken Chili with Black Beans (Spicy or Mild)
Shelton's Turkey Chili with Beans (Spicy or Mild)
Health Valley "Spicy Black Bean Chili"

CRACKERS

Hain Pure Foods "Reduced Fat Wheatettes"
Dr. Kracker "Klassic 3 Seed"
Dr. Kracker "Pumpkin Seed Cheese"
Dr. Kracker "Seeded Spelt"
Dr. Kracker "Sunflower Cheese"
Dr. Kracker "Muesli"
Dr. Kracker "Graham"
Dr. Kracker "Seedlander"

WHOLE-GRAIN BREADS

French Meadow Bakery "Healthy Hemp Sprouted Bread"
French Meadow Bakery "Men's Bread for Vitality and Energy"
French Meadow Bakery "Woman's Bread"
Shiloh Farms "Sprouted Five Grain Bread"

WHOLE-GRAIN PILAF

Seeds of Change "Zesty Cilantro
  Quinoa Blend"
Seeds of Change "Tomato Basil
  Quinoa Blend"

Seeds of Change "French Herb
  Quinoa Blend"

COUSCOUS

Always choose whole-wheat couscous over the white refined stuff.

Fantastic Foods "Whole Wheat
  Couscous"
Hodgson Mill "Whole Wheat
  Couscous"
Hodgson Mill "Whole Wheat
  Couscous with Milled Flaxseed
  and Soy"

Hodgson Mill "Whole Wheat
  Couscous Garlic and Basil with
  Milled Flaxseed and Soy"
Hodgson Mill "Whole-Wheat
  Parmesan Cheese Couscous
  with Milled Flaxseed and Soy"

HOT CEREAL

Bob's Red Mill "Creamy
  Buckwheat Hot Cereal"
Bob's Red Mill "10 Grain Hot
  Cereal"
Bob's Red Mill "5 Grain Rolled Hot
  Cereal"
Bob's Red Mill "7 Grain Hot
  Cereal"
Bob's Red Mill "8 Grain Wheatless
  Hot Cereal"
Bob's Red Mill "Apple, Cinnamon,
  & Grains Hot Cereal"
Bob's Red Mill "Grains & Nuts Hot
  Cereal"
Bob's Red Mill "Spice N' Nice Hot
  Cereal"
Hodgson Mill "Cracked Wheat All
  Natural Hot Cereal"
Hodgson Mill "Bulgur Wheat with
  Soy Hot Cereal"

Hodgson Mill "Multi Grain Hot
  Cereal with Milled Flaxseed and
  Soy"
Arrowhead Mills "Four Grain Plus
  Flax Hot Cereal"
Arrowhead Mills "Seven Grain Hot
  Cereal"
Arrowhead Mills "Wheat Free
  Seven Grain Hot Cereal"
McCann's "Steel Cut Irish
  Oatmeal"
Erewhon "Oatbran with Toasted
  Wheat Germ"
Erewhon "Organic Instant Oatmeal
  with Added Oat Bran"
Erewhon "Organic Instant Oatmeal
  Apple Cinnamon"
Erewhon "Organic Instant Oatmeal
  with Raisins, Dates and
  Walnuts"

COLD CEREAL

Food for Life "Ezekiel 4:9 Sprouted
Grain Cereal: Golden Flax"
Barbara's "Grain Shop"
Food for Life "Ezekiel 4:9 Sprouted
Grain Cereal: Cinnamon Raisin"
Barbara's Bakery "Multigrain
Shredded Spoonfuls"
Bob's Red Mill "Old Country Style
Muesli"
Arrowhead Mills "Spelt Flakes"
Arrowhead Mills "Kamut Flakes"
Arrowhead Mills "Amaranth
Flakes"
Arrowhead Mills "Oat-bran Flakes"
Arrowhead Mills "Maple
Buckwheat Flakes"
Erewhon "Whole Grain Wheat
Flakes"
Erewhon "Fruit-n-Wheat"
Erewhon "Kamut Flakes"
Erewhon "Raisin Bran"

DRIED BEAN SOUP MIXES

Bob's Red Mill "13 Bean Soup Mix"

FROZEN WHOLE-GRAIN DINNER ROLLS

Alexia Whole Grain "Hearty Whole Wheat Rolls with Flaxseeds"

CHICKEN SAUSAGE

Han's brand (*www.hansallnatural.com*) chicken sausages are much lower in saturated fat than regular sausages, contain no artificial growth stimulants or hormones, no antibiotics and no nitrates.

Han's All Natural Gourmet Sausage
"Sun-dried Tomato and Basil
Organic"
Han's All Natural Gourmet Sausage
"Chicken"
Han's All Natural Gourmet Sausage
"Apple-Spokane Chicken"
Han's All Natural Gourmet Sausage
"Artichoke and Calamata Olive
Chicken"
Han's All Natural Gourmet Sausage
"Italian Mild Chicken"
Han's All Natural Gourmet Sausage
"Italian Spicy Chicken"
Han's All Natural Gourmet Sausage
"Roasted Red Pepper and Garlic
Chicken"
Han's All Natural Gourmet Sausage
"Spinach and Feta Chicken"
Applegate Farms Certified Organic
"Andouille Chicken and Turkey
Sausage"
Applegate Farms Certified Organic
"Fire Roasted Red Pepper
Sausage"
Applegate Farms Certified Organic
"Chicken and Apple Sausage"
Applegate Farms Certified Organic
"Sweet Italian Sausage"

ALL-NATURAL HOT DOGS

Han's All Natural Uncured Skinless
   Hotdog "California Brand,
   Chicken"
Han's All Natural Uncured Skinless
   Hotdog "Chicago Brand, Pork"

Applegate Farms "Organic
   Uncured Chicken Hot Dogs"
Applegate Farms "Organic
   Uncured Turkey Hot Dogs"

ALL-NATURAL BOLOGNA

Shelton's "Uncured Turkey
   Bologna"

Applegate Farms "Sliced Turkey
   Bologna"

NATURAL CHICKEN BURGERS

Bell & Evans "Chicken Burgers"

ORGANIC TURKEY BURGERS

Applegate Farms "Organic Turkey Burgers"

NUTTY SNACK BITES
AND PARTY FOODS

Find them at Whole Foods, Target and Sam's Club. You can also go
online at *www.mrsmays.com*.

Mrs. May's "Almond Crunch"
Mrs. May's "Pecan Crunch"
Mrs. May's "Peanut Crunch"
Mrs. May's "Cashew Crunch"
Mrs. May's "Pinenut Crunch"
Mrs. May's "Sunflower Crunch"

Mrs. May's "Sesame Crunch"
Mrs. May's "Black Sesame"
Mrs. May's "Pumpkin Crunch"
Mrs. May's "Blueberry and Peanut"
Mrs. May's "Banana and Peanut"

List #3: The Junk-Food Lovers' Shopping List

In this list we provide more healthful all-natural alternatives to some of your favorite junk foods. We have found there is a healthier way to satisfy almost any craving. If you are lucky enough to have a health-oriented supermarket in your town, you'll have no problem finding the foods we mention in this section. For example, supermarkets specializing in natural and organic foods such as Whole Foods Market (*www.wholefoods.com*) are becoming more and more popular as consumer demand increases. These stores carry a huge variety of brand-name natural food products. Many "traditional" supermarkets also feature a wide variety of health-oriented food products, as well. If you can't find the brand names we mention below in your local supermarket give any well-stocked natural foods store a try.

CHIPS

All-natural chips made with good oils do the least damage. Watch your portion size if you are a chip eater. No more than one serving per day. Read the label to see what a "serving" is . . . usually no more than fifteen to twenty chips, not half the bag!

Kettle "Blue Corn"
Kettle "Sesame Rye with Caraway"
Kettle "Sweet Brown Rice & Black Bean"
Kettle "Five Grain Yellow Corn"
Kettle "Little Dippers"
Kettle "Sesame Blue Moons"
Kettle "Lightly Salted Low Fat Kettle Krisps"

Kettle "Hickory Barbecue Low Fat Kettle Krisps"
Kettle "French Onion Low Fat Kettle Krisps"
Garden of Eatin' "Black Bean Chips"
Garden of Eatin' "White Rounds"
Garden of Eatin' "Red Chips"
Garden of Eatin' "Sesame Blues"

NONDAIRY CREAMERS

These products have no trans fats.

Silk "Plain Creamer"
Silk "Hazelnut Creamer"

Silk "French Vanilla Creamer"

TACO SHELLS
Garden of Eatin' "Yellow Corn Taco Shells"

WHOLE-GRAIN TORTILLA WRAPS
Food for Life "Ezekiel 4:9 Sprouted
   Grain Tortillas"

Tamxico's "100% Whole Wheat
   Tortilla Wrap-itz"

STONE-GROUND CORN TORTILLAS
Tamxico's "Corn Tortillas"

BAKED AND REFRIED BEANS
Amy's "Vegetarian Baked Beans"
Amy's "Organic Refried Beans with
   Green Chiles"

Amy's "Refried Black Beans"

MICROWAVE POPCORN
Farmer Steve's "100% Organic
   Popcorn"
Newman's Own Organics "Light
   Butter Flavored Pop's Corn"
Smart Balance "Smart 'N Healthy
   Popcorn"

Newman's Own Organics "No
   Butter/No Salt 94% Fat Free
   Pop's Corn"
Garden of Eatin' "Organic
   Microwave Popcorn—No Oil
   Added"

WHOLE-GRAIN PANCAKES
AND WAFFLE MIXES
Bob's Red Mill "10 Grain Pancake
   and Waffle Mix"
Bob's Red Mill "Buckwheat
   Pancake and Waffle Mix"
Hodgson Mill "Multi Grain
   Buttermilk Pancake Mix with
   Milled Flaxseed & Soy"

Hodgson Mill "Buckwheat Pancake
   Mix"
Hodgson Mill "Whole Wheat
   Buttermilk Pancake Mix"
Hodgson Mill "Whole Wheat
   Insta-Bake Mix"

FROZEN WHOLE-GRAIN GOURMET WAFFLES

Van's "Wheat Free"

Van's "Wheat Free Flax"

Van's "Wheat Free Apple
Cinnamon"

Van's "Wheat Free Blueberry"

Van's "Belgian 7 Grain Waffles"

Van's "Buckwheat Waffles with
Blueberries and Raspberries"

SNACK BARS

Save the Forest Organic Trail Mix
Bars "Cranberry Crunch"

Save the Forest Organic Trail Mix
Bars "Banana Chocolate Nut"

Zoe Foods "Chocolate Flax and
Soy Bar"

Zoe Foods "Apple Crisp Flax and
Soy Bar"

Zoe Foods "Peanut Butter Flax and
Soy Bar"

Zoe Foods "Lemon Flax and Soy
Bar"

CEREAL BARS

Nature's Choice "Multigrain Cherry
Cereal Bars"

Nature's Choice "Multigrain Triple
Berry Cereal Bars"

Nature's Choice "Multigrain
Strawberry Cereal Bars"

Nature's Choice "Multigrain
Raspberry Cereal Bars"

Nature's Choice "Multigrain
Blueberry Cereal Bars"

Nature's Choice "Multigrain Apple-
Cinnamon Cereal Bars"

Kashi TLC "Honey Almond Flax"
Chewy Granola Bars

Kashi TLC "Trail Mix" Chewy
Granola Bars

Kashi TLC "Peanut Peanut Butter"
Chewy Granola Bars

Kashi Crunchy Granola Bars

BOXED DESSERT MIXES

Arrowhead Mills "Chocolate Chip
Cookie Mix"

Arrowhead Mills "Oatmeal Raisin
Cookie Mix"

Arrowhead Mills "Peanut Butter
Cookie Mix"

Arrowhead Mills "Brownie Mix"

Dr. Oetker Simple Organics
"Lemon Cake Mix"

Dr. Oetker Simple Organics
"Marble Cake Mix"

Dr. Oetker Simple Organics
"Vanilla Cake Mix"

Dr. Oetker Simple Organics
"Chocolate Cake Mix"

HEALTHIER BOXED DESSERT MIXES

Made with whole-wheat flour, fit and fabulous homemade frosting is easy to make and tastes delicious. Whisk together 1 cup (8 ounces) whipped cream cheese with 3–4 tablespoons powdered sugar, 2 teaspoons vanilla extract, a gentle squeeze of lemon juice, and 2–3 tablespoons light sour cream. If you prefer chocolate frosting, just add unsweetened cocoa. Add granulated sugar to taste.

Nature's Path "Organic Chocolate Chip Cookie Mix"

Nature's Path "Hemp Plus Brownie Mix"

Nature's Path "Double Fudge Brownie Mix"

Hodgson Mill "Brownie Mix with Whole Wheat Flour and Milled Flaxseed"

Hodgson Mill "Whole Wheat Wild Blueberry Muffin Mix"

Hodgson Mill "Whole Wheat Gingerbread Mix"

Fearn "Carrot Cake Mix"

Fearn "Banana Cake Mix"

Fearn "Spice Cake Mix"

CAKE-LIKE BREAD

These sweet breads contain no sugar and are rich in fiber and nutrients.

Sunnyvale Organic Bakery "Fruit, Date, and Pecan"

Sunnyvale Organic Bakery "Stem Ginger"

Sunnyvale Organic Bakery "Cherry, Fig, & Orange"

Sunnyvale Organic Bakery "Rich Fruit"

Sunnyvale Organic Bakery "Carrot & Raisin with Almond"

Nature's Path "Whole Rye Manna Bread"

Nature's Path "Carrot Raisin Manna Bread"

Nature's Path "Multi Grain Manna Bread"

Nature's Path "Fruit & Nut Manna Bread"

Nature's Path "Whole Wheat Manna Bread"

PREPARED COOKIES

Barbara's Bakery "Old Fashioned Oatmeal Crisp Cookies"

Barbara's Bakery "Chocolate Chip Cookies"

Country Choice "Oatmeal Raisin Cookies"

Country Choice "Double Fudge Brownie Cookies"

Country Choice "Oatmeal Chocolate Chip Cookies"

Country Choice "Chocolate Chip Walnut Cookies"

Country Choice "Ginger Cookies"

Country Choice "Old Fashioned Oatmeal Cookies"

Country Choice "Peanut Butter Cookies"

BOXED WHOLE-GRAIN BREAD MIXES

An easy way to add fiber and omega-3 essential fats to your diet is to add ground flaxseed to your homemade breads and muffins.

Bob's Red Mill "100% Whole Wheat Bread Mix"

Bob's Red Mill "Cornbread and Cornmeal Muffin Mix"

ALL-NATURAL JELLY ALTERNATIVE

Medford Farms "Apple Butter Spread—No Sugar Added"

Medford Farms "Pear Butter Spread—No Sugar Added"

ALL-NATURAL SHORTENING

Organic palm oil is trans-fat free and contains less saturated fat than butter.

Spectrum Naturals "Organic Shortening"

GRANOLA

Zoe Foods "Cranberries Currants Flax and Soy Granola Cereal"

Zoe Foods "Honey Almond Flax and Soy Granola Cereal"

Zoe Foods "Apple Cinnamon Flax and Soy Granola Cereal"

Nature's Path "Organic Pumpkin Flax Plus Granola"

MEATLESS "SAUSAGE" AND "BEEF"

Lightlife "Gimme Lean! Sausage Style"

Lightlife "Gimme Lean! Ground Beef Style"

VEGETARIAN ENTRÉE AND MEAL HELPERS

Fantastic Foods "Nature's Burger"
Fantastic Foods "Sloppy Joe Mix"
Fantastic Foods "Taco Filling"

Fantastic Foods "Tofu Scrambler"
Fantastic Foods "Vegetarian Chili"

INTERNATIONAL FOODS

Fantastic Foods "Falafel" (Near East
brand also makes a falafel mix)
Fantastic Foods "Instant Black
Beans"

Fantastic Foods "Instant Refried
Beans"
Fantastic Foods "Spinach Parmesan
Hummus"

ICE CREAM

Watch your portion size. No more than one small scoop!

Breyers "Natural Vanilla"
Breyers "Chocolate"
Breyers "Maple Walnut"
Breyers "French Vanilla"
Breyers "Neapolitan"

Breyers "Strawberry"
Breyers "French Vanilla"
Breyers "Butter Pecan"
Breyers "Coffee"
Breyers "Butter Almond"

CREAMY FRUIT POPSICLES

Visit *www.fruitfull.com* to learn more.

FruitFull "Strawberry Cream"
FruitFull "Mango Cream"
FruitFull "Peaches 'n' Cream"

FruitFull "Rasberry 'n Cream"
FruitFull "Banana"
FruitFull "Piña Colada"

FROZEN SOUPS

Tabatchnick "Vegetable Soup"
Tabatchnick "Split Pea Soup"
Tabatchnick "Vegetable Barley
Soup"
Tabatchnick "Lentil with Carrots
Soup"
Tabatchnick "Be My Baby Chili"
Tabatchnick "Santa Fe Black Bean"
Tabatchnick "Golden Cream of
Mushroom Soup"

Tabatchnick "Cream of Broccoli"
Tabatchnick "Thick and Creamy
Corn Chowder"
Tabatchnick "New England Potato
Soup"
Tabatchnick "Barley and
Mushroom Soup"
Tabatchncik "Vegetable Soup"
Tabatchnick "Minestrone Soup"

FROZEN ALL-NATURAL POTATO FRIES

Alexia "Sweet Potato Julienne Fries with Sea Salt"

Alexia "Oven Fries with Olive Oil, Rosemary and Garlic"

Alexia "Rissole Potatoes with Garden Herbs"

Alexia "Oven Reds with Olive Oil"

Alexia "Parmesan and Roasted Garlic"

Alexia "Julienne Fries with Sea Salt"

Alexia "Oven Reds with Olive Oil, Sun-Dried Tomatoes and Pesto"

FROZEN SAUSAGE PATTIES

Wellshire Farms All-Natural "Turkey-Maple Sausage Patties"

FROZEN MEATLESS "MEATBALLS

Nate's "Classic Flavor Meatless Meatballs"

Nate's "Savory Mushroom Meatless Meatballs"

Nate's "Zesty Italian Meatless Meatballs"

FROZEN VEGETARIAN "CHICKEN" NUGGETS

Nate's "Chicken Style Nuggets"

FROZEN MEATLESS "SAUSAGE"

Boca Burger Meatless Sausage "Bratwurst" (contains zero grams saturated fat)

FROZEN MEATLESS "GROUND BURGER"

Boca Burger Meatless "Ground Burger" (contains zero grams saturated fat and 3 grams of fiber; add to sloppy joes, tacos, chili, and so on.)

FROZEN BURRITOS

Amy's "Bean and Rice Burrito— Non Dairy"

Amy's "Bean and Cheese Burrito"

Amy's "Breakfast Burrito"

Amy's "Black Bean and Vegetable Burrito"

Amy's "Southwestern Burrito"

FROZEN MACARONI AND CHEESE

Amy's "Macaroni & Cheese"

Amy's "Macaroni & Soy Cheese"

FROZEN LASAGNA ENTREES

Amy's "Vegetable Lasagna"   Amy's "Garden Vegetable Lasanga"
Amy's "Tofu Vegetable Lasagna"

FROZEN MEXICAN FOOD

Amy's "Black Bean and Vegetable   Nate's "Black Bean and Soy
   Enchilada"   Cheese Taquitos"
Amy's "Santa Fe Enchilada"   Nate's "Chicken Style Taquitos"
Amy's "Mexican Tamale Pie"   Nate's "Beef Style Taquitos"
Amy's "Chili and Cornbread"

FROZEN INDIAN ENTREES

Amy's "Indian Samosa Wraps"   Amy's "Indian Mattar Paneer"
Amy's "Indian Palak Paneer"

FROZEN VEGETARIAN ENTREES

Amy's "Country Dinner"   Amy's "Veggie Loaf with Gravy"
Amy's "Brown Rice and   Amy's "Tofu Scramble with Brown
   Vegetables"   Rice and Vegetables"
Amy's "Brown Rice, Black Eyed
   Peas and Vegetables"

ALL-NATURAL FROZEN PIZZA

These brands are made primarily from whole-wheat flour. To boost
the fiber and nutritional content add your own fresh vegetables to
these delicious frozen pizzas.

A.C. LaRocco "Cheese and Garlic   A.C. LaRocco "Polynesian Pizza"
   Pizza"   A.C. LaRocco "Tomato Feta Pizza"
A.C. LaRocco "Greek Sesame   A.C. LaRocco "Shitake Mushroom
   Pizza"   Pizza"
A.C. LaRocco "Garden Vegetarian   Amy's "Spinach Pizza"
   Pizza"   Amy's "Cheese Pizza"
A.C. LaRocco "Quattro Formaggio   Amy's "Mushroom and Olive
   Pizza"   Pizza"
A.C. LaRocco "Spinach and   Amy's "Rice Crust Cheese Pizza"
   Artichoke Pizza"

FROZEN READY-MADE PIZZA CRUST

French Meadow Bakery "Spelt Organic Pizza Crust"

READY-MADE PIE

These brands are trans-fat-free.

Natural Feast "Apple Gourmet Streusel Pie"

Natural Feast "Blueberry Gourmet Streusel Pie"

Natural Feast "Chocolate Mousse Pie"

Wholly Healthy "Truly Natural Apple Pie"

Wholly Healthy "Truly Natural Cherry Pie"

Wholly Healthy "Truly Natural Pumpkin Pie"

Wholly Healthy "Truly Natural Blueberry Pie"

READY-MADE COOKIE DOUGH

Wholly Healthy "Truly Natural Peanut Butter Cookie Dough"

Wholly Healthy "Truly Natural Chocolate Chip Cookie Dough"

Wholly Healthy "Truly Natural Oatmeal Raisin Cookie Dough"

FROZEN RAVIOLI

Soy Boy "Roasted Red Pepper and Tofu Filling" (not whole wheat, but low in saturated fat and high in fiber)

Appendix B

Selected References

Chapter 1: Ditch Dieting and Go for Whole Foods

Festa A, et al. "Chronic subclinical inflammation as part of the insulin resistance syndrome: the Insulin Resistance Atherosclerosis Study (IRAS)." *Circulation.* 2000 Jul 4; 102(1):42–7.

Ford ES. "Does exercise reduce inflammation? Physical activity and C-reactive protein among US adults." *Epidemiology.* 2002 Sep; 13(5):561–8.

Hotamisligil GS, et al. "Increased adipose tissue expression of tumor necrosis factor-alpha in human obesity and insulin resistance." *J Clin Invest.* 1995 May; 95(5):2409–15.

Papanicolaou DA, et al. "The pathophysiologic roles of interleukin-6 in human disease." *Ann Intern Med.* 1998 Jan 15; 128(2):127–37.

Xu, H, et al. "Chronic inflammation in fat plays a crucial role in the development of obesity-related insulin resistance." *J Clin Invest.* 2003 Dec; 112(12):1821–30.

Yudkin JS, et al. "Inflammation, obesity, stress and coronary heart disease: is interleukin-6 the link?" *Atherosclerosis.* 2000 Feb; 148(2):209–14.

Chapter 2: Choose "Fit Foods"

Ajani UA, et al. "Dietary fiber and C-reactive protein: findings from national health and nutrition examination survey data." *J Nutr.* 2004 May; 134(5):1181–5.

Anderson JW, et al. "Meta-analysis of the effects of soy protein intake on serum lipids." *N Engl J Med.* 1995 Aug 3; 333(5):276–82.

Feskanich D, et al. "Milk, dietary calcium, and bone fractures in women: a 12-year prospective study." *Am J Public Health.* 1997 Jun; 87(6):992–7.

Hibbeln JR. "Fish Consumption and major depression." *Lancet.* 1998 Apr 18; 351(9110):1213.

Mamalakis G, et al. "Depression and adipose essential polyunsaturated fatty acids." *Prostaglandins Leukot Essent Fatty Acids.* 2002 Nov; 67(5):311–8.

Owusu W, et al. "Calcium intake and the incidence of forearm and hip fractures among men." *J Nutr.* 1997 Sep; 127(9):1782–7.

Studer M, et al. "Effect of different antilipidemic agents and diets on mortality: A systematic review." *Arch Intern Med.* 2005 Apr 11; 165(7):725–30.

Yoshizawa K, et al. "Mercury and the risk of coronary heart disease in men." *N Engl J Med.* 2002 Nov 28; 347(22):1755–60.

Zemel MB, et al. "Calcium and dairy acceleration of weight and fat loss during energy restriction in obese adults." *Obes Res.* 2004 Apr; 12(4):582–90.

Zhang J, et al. "Fish consumption and mortality from all causes, ischemic heart disease, and stroke: an ecological study." *Prev Med.* 1999 May; 28(5):520–9.

Chapter 3: Avoid Fake and Fattening Foods

James MJ, et al. "Dietary polyunsaturated fatty acids and inflammatory mediator production." *Am J Clin Nutr.* 2000 Jan; 71(1 Suppl):343S–8S.

Keys A, et al. "The diet and 15-year death rate in the seven countries study." *Am J Epidemiol.* 1986 Dec; 124(6):903–15.

Willett WC, et al. "Intake of trans fatty acids and risk of coronary heart disease among women." *Lancet.* 1993 Mar 6; 341(8845):581–5.

Chapter 4: Plan You Day's Meals with the "Fit-Body Plate"

Cordain L, et al. "Influence of moderate daily wine consumption on body weight regulation and metabolism in healthy free-living males." *J Am Coll Nutr.* 1997 Apr; 16(2):134–9.

Facchini F, et al. "Light-to-moderate alcohol intake is associated with enhanced insulin sensitivity." *Diabetes Care.* 1994 Feb; 17(2):115–9.

Friedman LA and Kimball AW. "Coronary heart disease mortality and alcohol consumption in Frammingham." *Am J Epidemiol.* 1986 Sep; 124(3):481–9.

Greenfield JR, et al. "Moderate alcohol consumption, dietary fat composition, and abdominal obesity in women: evidence for gene-environment interaction." *J Clin Endocrinol Metab.* 2003 Nov; 88(11):5381–6.

Gronbaek M, et al. "Mortality associated with moderate intakes of wine, beer, or spirits." *BMJ.* 1995 May 6; 310(6988):1165–9.

Iwai N, et al. "Relationship between coffee and green tea consumption and all-cause mortality in a cohort of a rural Japanese population." *J Epidemiol.* 2002 May; 12(3):191–8.

Kahn HS, et al. "Stable behaviors associated with adults' 10-year change in body mass index and likelihood of gain at the waist." *Am J Public Health.* 1997 May; 87(5):747–54.

Kiechl S, et al. "Insulin sensitivity and regular alcohol consumption: large, prospective, cross sectional population study (Bruneck study)." *BMJ*. 1996 Oct 26; 313(7064):1040–4.

Liu S, et al.. "A prospective study of alcohol intake and change in body weight among US adults." *Am J Epidemiol*. 1994 Nov 15; 140(10):912–20.

Ross GW, et al. "Association of coffee and caffeine intake with the risk of Parkinson disease." *JAMA*. 2000 May 24–31; 283(20):2674–9.

Salazar-Martinez E, et al. "Coffee consumption and risk for type 2 diabetes mellitus." *Ann Intern Med*. 2004 Jan 6; 140(1):1–8.

Chapter 7: Resistance Circuit Training: The Secret to Getting Fitter, Firmer, Faster

Blair SN, et al. "Physical fitness and all-cause mortality. A prospective study of healthy men and women." *JAMA*. 1989 Nov 3; 262(17):2395–401.

Braun WA, et al. "Acute EPOC response in women to circuit training and treadmill exercise of matched oxygen consumption." *Eur J Appl Physiol*. 2005 Aug; 94(5–6):500–4.

Burleson MA Jr, et al. "Effect of weight training exercise and treadmill exercise on post-exercise oxygen consumption." *Med Sci Sports Exerc*. 1998 Apr; 30(4):518–22.

Paffenbarger RS Jr, et al. "Physical activity, all-cause mortality, and longevity of college alumni." *N Engl J Med*. 1986 Mar 6; 314(10):605–13.

Smith JK, et al. "Long-term exercise and atherogenic activity of blood mononuclear cells in persons at risk of developing ischemic heart disease." *JAMA*. 1999 May 12; 281(18):1722–7.

Tabata I, et al. "Effects of moderate-intensity endurance and high-intensity intermittent training on anaerobic capacity and VO2max." *Med Sci Sports Exerc*. 1996 Oct; 28(10):1327–30.

Tremblay A, et al. "Impact of exercise intensity on body fatness and skeletal muscle metabolism." *Metabolism*. 1994 Jul; 43(7):814–8.

Westcott WL, et al. "Effects of regular and slow speed resistance training on muscle strength." *J Sports Med Phys Fitness*. 2001 Jun; 41(2):154–8

Chapter 11: Daily Vitamin Planner and Supplement Shopping Guide

Anderson RA. "Chromium, glucose intolerance and diabetes" *J Am Coll Nutr*. 1998 Dec; 17(6):548–55.

Bates D, et al. "A double-blind controlled trial of long-chain n-3 polyunsaturated fatty acids in the treatment of multiple sclerosis." *J Neruol Neurosurger Psychiatry.* 1989 Jan; 52(1):18–22.

Church TS, et al. "Reduction of C-reactive protein levels through use of a multivitamin." *Am J Med.* 2003 Dec 15; 115(9):702–7.

Dawson-Hughes B, et al. "A controlled trial of the effect of calcium supplementation on bone density in postmenopausal women." *N Engl J Med.* 1990 Sep 27; 323(13):878–83.

Enstrom JE, et al. "Vitamin C intake and mortality among a sample of the United States population." *Epidemiology.* 1992 May; 3(3):194–202.

Fletcher RH and Fairfield KM. "Vitamins for chronic disease prevention in adults: clinical applications" *JAMA.* 2002 Jun 19; 287(23):3127–9.

Geleijnse JM, et al. "Blood pressure response to fish oil supplementation: metaregression analysis of randomized trials." *J Hypertens.* 2002 Aug; 20(8):1493–9.

Geusens P, et al. "Long-term effect of omega-3 fatty acid supplementation in active rheumatoid arthritis. A 12-month, double-blind, controlled study." *Arthritis Rheum.* 1994 Jun; 37(6):824–9.

He K, et al. "Fish consumption and risk of stroke in men." *JAMA.* 2002 Dec 25; 288(24):3130–6.

Ishikawa T, et al. "Effects of gammalinolenic acid on plasma lipoproteins and apolipoproteins." *Atherosclerosis.* 1989 Feb; 75(2–3):95–104.

Kawano Y, et. al. "Effects of magnesium supplementation in hypertensive patients: assessment by office, home, and ambulatory blood pressures" *Hypertension.* 1998 Aug; 32(2):260–5.

Knekt P, et al. "Serum selenium and subsequent risk of cancer among Finnish men and women." *J Natl Canc Inst.* 1990 May 16; 82(10):864–8.

Lieberman DA, et al. "Risk factors for advanced colonic neoplasia and hyperplastic polyps in asymptomatic individuals." *JAMA.* 2003 Dec 10; 290(22):2959–67.

Munger KL, et al. "Vitamin D intake and incidence of multiple sclerosis" *Neurology.* 2004 Jan 13; 62(1):60–5.

Reid IR, et al. "Effects of calcium supplementation on serum lipid concentrations in normal older women: a randomized controlled trial." *Am J Med.* 2002 Apr 1; 112(5):343–7.

Rimm E.B. "Folate and vitamin B6 from diet and supplements in relation to risk of coronary heart disease among women." *Bibl Nutr Dieta.* 2001; (55):42–5.

Salonen RM, et al. "Six-year effect of combined vitamin C and E supplementation on atherosclerotic progression: the Antioxidant Supplementation in Atherosclerosis Prevention (ASAP) Study." *Circulation.* 2003 Feb 25; 107(7):947–53.

Schnyder G, et al. "Effect of homocysteine-lowering therapy with folic acid, vita-
    min B12, and vitamin B6 on clinical outcome after percutaneous coronary
    intervention: the Swiss Heart Study: a randomized controlled trial." *JAMA.*
    2002 Aug 28; 288(8):973–9.

Shapses SA, et al. "Effect of calcium supplementation on weight and fat loss in
    women" *J Clin Endocrinol Metab.* 2004 Feb; 89(2):632–7.

Stephens NG, et al. "Randomised controlled trial of vitamin E in patients with
    coronary disease: Cambridge Heart Antioxidant Study (CHAOS)." *Lancet.*
    1996 Mar 23; 347(9004):781–6.

Utiger RD. "The need for more vitamin D." *N Engl J Med.* 1998 Mar 19;
    338(12):828–9.

Zandi PP, et al. "Reduced risk of Alzeheimer disease in users of antioxidant vita-
    min supplements: the Cache County study." *Arch Neurol.* 2004 Jan;
    61(1):82–4.

Appendix C

Converting to Metrics

Volume Measurement Conversions

U.S.	METRIC
1/4 teaspoon	1.25 ml
1/2 teaspoon	2.5 ml
3/4 teaspoon	3.75 ml
1 teaspoon	5 ml
1 tablespoon	15 ml
1/4 cup	62.5 ml
1/2 cup	125 ml
3/4 cup	187.5 ml
1 cup	250 ml

Weight Conversion Measurements

U.S.	METRIC
1 ounce	28.4 g
8 ounces	227.5 g
16 ounces (1 pound)	455 g

Cooking Temperature Conversions

Celsius/Centigrade	0°C and 100°C are arbitrarily placed at the melting and boiling points of water and standard to the metric system
Fahrenheit	Fahrenheit established 0°F as the stabilized temperature when equal amounts of ice, water, and salt are mixed.

To convert temperatures in Fahrenheit to Celsius, use this formula:

$$C = (F-32) \times 0.5555$$

So, for example, if you are baking at 350°F and want to know that temperature in Celsius, use this calculation:

$$C = (350-32) \times 0.5555 = 176.66°C$$

Index

About the Authors

Andrew Larson, M.D., FACS, is a board certified general surgeon with special interests in surgical nutrition, advanced laparoscopic surgery and bariatric surgery. He earned his medical degree from the University of Pennsylvania and has published multiple peer-reviewed journal articles and presented research at national conferences. Dr. Larson is a member of multiple medical societies including the American Society for Bariatric Surgery, the Society of American Gastrointestinal and Endoscopic Surgeons, the American Medical Association and the International Federation for the Surgery of Obesity. Dr. Larson is the coauthor of *Chicken Soup for the Soul Healthy Living: Weight Loss* (HCI, 2005). He holds a fellowship in the American College of Surgeons and is a board member of the Palm Beach County Medical Society. Dr. Larson is the medical director for JFK Medical Center's Bariatric Wellness and Surgical Institute. His private surgical practice is based at JFK Medical Center just outside of West Palm Beach, Florida.

Ivy Larson, B.S., ACSM, is a certified American College of Sports Medicine Health Fitness Instructor. She holds additional professional certifications as a fitness instructor and fitness-testing specialist through the Fitness Institute International. Currently, Ivy works as an independent contractor teaching group nutrition and cooking classes, developing exercise programs, and counseling patients on diet and healthy living strategies. Ivy takes advantage of her love for cooking to create the healthy whole foods recipes in her books.

Together, the Larsons previously authored *The Gold Coast Cure: The 5-Week Health and Body Makeover* (HCI, 2005), offering the latest research regarding diet, exercise and disease prevention in an easy-to-follow lifestyle plan. The couple has appeared on the *Montel Willians Show*, CNN, the internationally syndicated *Harvest Show*, and over seventy television news shows and radio talk shows across the country. *The Gold Coast Cure* has been featured on ediets.com, the country's leading interactive online dieting site, in leading magazines including *Woman's Day*, the *National Examiner*, *Fit Magazine*, *Women's Health and Fitness*, *Get Active*, *Great Life* and *Chicken Soup for the Soul Magazine*, and in numerous newspapers around the country. Andrew and Ivy and their son, Blake, reside on Florida's Gold Coast.

www.goldcoastcure.com
www.goldcoastsurgery.com

Andrew Larson, M.D.
Ivy Ingram Larson

The GOLD
COAST
CURE

The 5-Week
Health & Body Makeover

A Lifestyle Plan to Shed Pounds, Gain Health
and Reverse 10 Diseases

Code #2351 • Hardcover • $21.95
Code #5636 • Paperback • $15.95

Finally, the diet that slims and tones also heals the
immune system and prevents degenerative diseases.

To order direct: Telephone (800) 441-5569 • www.hcibooks.com
Prices do not include shipping and handling. Your response code is BKS.

The Ethics of the Ordinary in Healthcare

Concepts and Cases

John Abbott Worthley

Health Administration Press
Chicago, IL

READING

The following article is distinctive in two major respects: first, it is among the most insightful illuminations of the microethics of healthcare in print; and second, it originally appeared in a most unlikely journal and, consequently, has been little noticed. George Luthringer convincingly maintains that the quiet struggles in the routine day of the ordinary healthcare professional are at the core of ethical professionalism. Although he addresses his reflection to the subspecialty of nutrition sup-
rt, his discourse is rigorously relevant to all of healthcare.

Early on he sets the tone of his perception, the same tone that inspires
book: "It is the ethical dilemmas of ordinary practitioners in ordinary
es during ordinary times that are both the most difficult to resolve
the most significant for patient well-being." Anticipating chapter 4,
esses the professional duty to manage competing values. Germane
pter 3, he argues that it is what we do—our conduct—not who we
ur character—that is key to the pursuit of microethics. Through-
examples of seven routine dilemmas is a practical emphasis on
dignity and a determination to seek balance and reconciliation in
gles of everyday professional life. In perhaps his most brilliant
ary, Luthringer offers some salient tenets for our consideration:

nsible moral behavior inevitably entails risks to self-esteem
ofessional relationships.
tle manipulation and quiet deception so common in
re degrade the very people they are meant to serve.
annot be singular when reality is plural.
es are both necessary and treacherous.

• The peril of acknowledging a rightful place for self-interest must be countered by a demand for objective limits on self-service.

What you are about to read is as good as it gets in the literature of healthcare ethics. Enjoy it!

THE ETHICS OF ORDINARY TIME

George F. Luthringer

There is, it seems, a good chance that Nancy Cruzan's long journey to death will be more than a tale "full of sound and fury, signifying nothing." Certainly, the social and political contexts surrounding the provision of nutritional support to patients with no prospects for meaningful life have shifted. More sensitive and rational decisions look possible, still within a framework which affirms and protects the sacredness of life.

Only those, however, who live in ignorance of the personal and professional realities faced in enteral and parenteral feeding will assume that the central moral issues of this practice are now resolved. The high drama of intense public conflict notwithstanding, it is the ethical dilemmas of ordinary practitioners in ordinary places during ordinary times that are both the most difficult to resolve and the most significant for patient well-being.

Like chronic illness, they are almost always managed rather than re-solved. And not without reason, they are often assumed to be intractable. Coping means avoidance of the activities that cause flare-ups and focusing on other concerns. This article will examine whether something more is possible and, specifically, whether the description and exploration of these moral issues can take us further than resigned acceptance or evasion through denial.

Competing Claims and Contrasting Perspectives

The context for that description and exploration is a maze of competing obligations and contrasting viewpoints. The legitimate claims of vulner-able patients, demanding caregivers, harried colleagues, and neglected friends or family are often entangled in a daunting variety of perspectives about how the moral choices between acknowledged duties are to be analyzed. Should the concern be with character or conduct, with rules or responsibilities, with individual needs or uniform treatment, with maximum benefit or minimal coercion?

Relative priorities among claims and the relative value of different perspectives are significantly dependent upon the particulars of the situ-ation. Significantly, but not entirely. Both the nature of nutrition support and the structure regulating its provision are important constraints on a

George F. Luthringer, "The Ethics of Ordinary Time," *Nutrition in Clinical Practice* 6, no. 3 (June 1991): 99–105.
Copyright 1991, the American Society for Parenteral and Enteral Nutrition. Reprinted by permission.
George F. Luthringer, an Episcopalian priest, served as chaplain and clinical team member
at a large medical center in Cincinnati, Ohio.

framework for moral decisions. Hence, both must be considered when examining the fundamental questions of relationship and orientation.

Questions of Relationship: Patient, Client, Team, and Self

The ongoing provision of good medical care often requires individuals and teams to negotiate and nurture a complex network of relationships. Nowhere is that more crucial to success than in nutrition support. Rarely the primary caregivers and always focused on the commonplace issue of feeding, competent teams recognize that positive responses to their assessments and prompt compliance with their recommendations depend largely on personal courtesy, persuasive communication, and demonstrated competence.

The subject of those assessments and the intended beneficiary of those recommendations is a patient, in most cases a very ill patient. By professional training, personal commitment, and social mandate, that patient's well-being is the sole concern of treatment personnel.

The reality is often somewhat different. The matrix of institutional responsibilities, professional bonds, and personal friendships within which all health care is delivered neither emerges nor disappears with any particular patient. Whatever the frictions and frustrations, competent treatment depends on functional relationships. Except in rare circumstances, to insist that nothing matters beyond the well-being of your patients is to burn down the house to stay warm.

In other words, precisely because they must be the primary concern of any responsible caregiver, patients cannot be the sole concern. Institutional interests, professional prerogatives, and personal sensitivities legitimately demand attention, not simply out of pragmatic necessity but because they present competing moral claims.

Even so, moral behavior cannot be reduced to "go along, get along." No caregiver can meet the common standards of professional responsibility—or maintain a sense of personal integrity—without openly confronting the self-centered and self-serving inclinations of colleagues when they threaten patient harm.

Neither can a caregiver ensure dedicated treatment by overriding, or dismissing as unimportant, the interests and needs of the others involved. Self-righteously waging war on the behalf of patients is self-defeating, because the patients themselves will be the first casualties. At best, that sort of moralistic posture will gain grudgingly offered benefits for current patients at great expense to the patients yet to come.

The tension created by legitimizing concerns other than patient well-being is the moral context for most patient care, certainly for consultant teams. Conflicting obligations "come with the territory." The important question is how they are managed.

Management requires guidelines that identify personal and institutional duties, suggesting how they are to be balanced. What, in fact, does one owe one's employer, one's colleagues, or one's self under these circumstances, and how are the inevitable conflicts to find a moral resolution? The answers, it turns out, depend significantly on the approach.

Questions of Orientation: Character, Commitment, Discretion, and Rights

To specify appropriate attitudes and behavior is the business of ethics or, to be more precise, normative ethics, what Socrates labeled "how we ought to live." This specification of relevant "oughts" and "shoulds" rests on important distinctions between competing ethical perspectives.

Those alternative viewpoints reflect important differences over the place of character, commitment, discretion, and rights in making moral choices. Is the focus to be exclusively on professional conduct, or is the primary concern to be with the personal character of that professional? Are guidelines to be grounded in general principles and consist mostly of rules, or should they be rooted in relationships and largely specify commitments?

Further, is the goal an objectively fair system in which all can expect the same treatment or an individually responsive structure within which discretion is allowed and encouraged? Finally, does one give primacy to achieving medical benefit or to respecting each patient's right to live as he or she wishes, to be the author of his or her own fate? Each of these issues must be explored. The answers that prove acceptable will shape the specifics of ethical response.

An Ethic of Doing Versus an Ethic of Being

In its western origins and for much of western history, the primary concern of ethics was with achieving virtue, with developing the traits of character that could be expected to produce moral acts. Only during the past 300 years has the focus shifted to principles and rules that could serve as guides to moral behavior. Now, for the most part, the assumption is that it is what we do, not who we are, that is of primary importance.

Rules are often no better as guarantors of moral decisions than is virtuous character. As surely as good motivations can produce grossly immoral behavior, rules can be coldly manipulated by those with disreputable intent. The nature of medical care makes rules particularly inadequate as moral standards, even though they are absolutely necessary.

The reason is that rules, like laws, serve best at regulating relationships between strangers or adversaries. Inevitably, many caregivers are indeed strangers, so patients need rules for protection. Yet no patient, in this time of enormous vulnerability, wants to be cared for by people who not only are strangers but who also accept no obligations beyond those of strangers—and who therefore must be feared as potential adversaries. The character of the caregiver alone ensures that the stranger will not act like one.

An Ethic of Justice Versus an Ethic of Care

Among the benefits of the feminist challenge to our cultural biases has been the stimulus to reexamine the basic assumptions and approach of traditional ethics. Fostered by Carol Gilligan's work in the late 1970's, an expanding critique of the accepted structure for moral decision-making developed in the eighties.[1] The existing system for analyzing moral problems was attacked as reflective of male interests in the public arena and inappropriate or inadequate for the characteristic concerns of women.

Many women, and some men, make their moral assessments by focusing on the responsibilities they take to be implied in their relationships. Most men, and a significant number of women, deal with moral issues by defining their rights under the established rules. Put another way, the central moral value of men is likely to be justice, and that of women, caring.

That this difference may reflect long-standing, culturally imposed roles, particularly for women, does not diminish its importance. Whatever the gender associations, it suggests that principles and abstract reasoning, by themselves, cannot provide satisfactory solutions to a large number of moral problems. Quite apart from considerations of character, these principles and their application are insufficient to the moral complexity of human life.

Nowhere is that more obvious than in treating those who are ill or injured. It is not by accident that we call this patient care. The essence of a moral response to the sick is caring—sensitive, personal attention to both the physical and emotional needs of specific patients. Justice may be necessary to ensure access, and even sufficient, in most cases, for substantial physical improvement. But justice, abstract and impersonal, doesn't heal. Caring alone can do that.

Equity Versus Equality

It is a basic principle of ethics that our actions must be impartial. One person is not to be treated differently from another unless there is a relevant difference between them, and the interests of all people affected by our actions are to be considered important. In general, people subscribe to that principle, but they are torn between its threat and its promise. They know about the pervasiveness of discrimination and the privileges given to those with influence, so they demand objectivity from their institutions. All must be prepared to justify distinctions made between one person and another in their treatment.

Yet there is outrage when the treatment is impersonal and vehement protest when uniform application of a rule makes things personally difficult. What is wanted, quite naturally, is both the assurance of fairness and the dignity of individual consideration. Each feels deprived when others receive special treatment, and all feel abused when they do not. None is of one mind.

The importance of that fact to caregivers lies in the uncertainty it creates with regard to discretion. To treat everyone identically brings charges of insensitivity, and to treat each person differently raises questions about favoritism. There is no escape from criticism.

There is a choice, however—a choice about whether or not to risk discretion and take responsibility for the inevitable inequality it entails. This is, in reality, a choice about whether to respond to patients' hopes or to their fears. The demand for all to be treated identically is a plea not to be discounted in relation to others. It is not a claim that equivalent medical conditions imply equal human need. Equality represents the minimum acceptable standard of fairness; equity is what we want—fairness in relation to our circumstances.

Medical Paternalism Versus Patient Self-Determination

Over the last 30-some years, there has been a well-publicized and often contentious revolution in progress about the appropriate relationship between caregivers and patients. In the language of ethicists, the struggle has been between the traditional beneficence model of health care, with its focus on appropriate medical care, and a contemporary model emphasizing autonomy, centered on patient values and goals. More simply, the fight has been over who makes the final decision about treatment.

By now, health care professionals who believe those decisions ought to remain their prerogative find themselves in a position comparable to that of smokers still convinced that restrictions of that behavior are unwarranted. They obey the new rules but feel depressed and resentful. For unreconstructed caregivers, the legal obligation to obtain informed consent is at best a nuisance and at worst a significant barrier to optimal care.

They have a point. Like democracy, patient autonomy looks good only when compared with the alternatives. It is time consuming to enable, cumbersome in practice, and vulnerable to irrationality. Worst of all, its beneficiaries are often uninterested in accepting its burdens. They do not want frightening details or confusing options, and they certainly do not want a doctor who may, in the end, seem all too fallible or uncertain.

A retreat to paternalism, though, threatens patient dignity as well as patient rights. No one must be forced to take charge when the need is to trust his or her caregivers. No one must be faced with the truth when he or she cannot bear to hear it. Yet it is never right to deny choice to those who wish to fashion their futures, and it is always right to preserve and enhance the capacity of a patient to choose.

The desire for control is a demand for respect. The patient, after all, must live with the consequences of treatment decisions; his or her values and life are at stake. The technical victories that bring such great satisfaction to health care professionals may be devastating to the persons for whom, in name, they were won.

By itself, however, patient sovereignty is not a reasonable answer to the problem of professional domination. The ideal answer is what the President's Commission has called shared decision-making, a process characterized by respect for the knowledge and skills of the caregivers as well as for the dignity and desires of the patient.[2] Within that context of mutual respect, the theoretical best for the body can become the actual best for the person.

A Provisional Stance

Given the competing claims and contrasting perspectives described thus far, what can be said, even provisionally, about a framework for examination of the typical moral dilemmas within nutrition support? With regard to relationships—concern for patient welfare is always paramount but rarely exclusive, and it is not only necessary but appropriate to consider the legitimate interests of the institution, of primary caregivers, of colleagues, and of self in ethical decision-making. With regard to approach—caring, character, respect, and discretion are required if morality is to be more than the cold and uncertain justice of rules and regulations, no matter how fair.

Some additional convictions have been implied: responsible moral behavior inevitably entails risks to self-esteem and professional relationships; the subtle manipulation and quiet deception so common in health care degrade many of the patients they are meant to serve; loyalty cannot be singular when reality is plural; boundaries are both necessary and treacherous; and the peril of acknowledging a rightful place for self-interest must be countered by a demand for objective limits on self-service.

Common Quandaries

Recurring dilemmas call for guidance. The seven dilemmas examined here were identified during several months of my participation in nutrition support rounds and from conversations with the professionals on a nutrition support team as well as observation of their work. Thus they capture repeated themes and ongoing concerns originated from only one team and are not a definitive list of all possible issues. Even so, they are likely familiar to most practitioners.

Owning Responsibility

Things go wrong; mistakes are made. The carefully considered recommendations do not work; the change in solution brings an adverse reaction. An important message is forgotten; infection control is neglected. No matter how strict the discipline, how exacting the procedures, or how skilled the practitioners, human imperfection sometimes wins out. What to do?

Among the options: admission, evasion, denial, and even cover-up. The ethical choice is obvious, but making it is hard. Taking responsibility turns out to be much more difficult than advocating it—for good reason. The price may be a lot higher than temporary embarrassment. Verbal abuse, public humiliation, diminished respect, and residual distrust are all potential consequences, not to speak of negative performance evaluations or lost professional opportunities.

It is fair, then, to ask why it is right to own up, especially if your fingerprints may be smudged. The quick answer is utilitarian: the long-term benefits normally outweigh the short-term costs. What is lost for the moment is often secured for the future. Given reasonable competence and apparent diligence, nothing is so reassuring as the knowledge that a colleague will not duck when something goes wrong. The courage to stand accountable frees everyone to focus on the problem, not the blame. Afterwards, it is possible to go on without lingering suspicion and resentment. It is over; there are consequences, but not unfinished business.

There is another answer, of course, but this one is harder to sell. It is that taking responsibility is a requisite for self-respect, not just acceptance, and self-respect may be crucial. One's standing with others is fragile if it surpasses one's view of one's self, but that, too, is pragmatic. The deeper issue is about basic values, about the relative worth of status and integrity.

Limiting Options

Early in their clinical training, most professionals learn that offering their patients fewer choices minimizes undesirable answers and reduces the time for consent. Pressured by too many demands, they are readily convinced by their experiences that less is better. Picking a home care provider is easier when the list is short; concerns about body image do not intrude when the access device is specified; setting up a home schedule goes more quickly if it is prescribed rather than tailored to the lifestyle of the patient.

What is lost if personal convenience and professional judgment replace patient choice? The most persuasive answer is compliance. Patients often pay little attention to the directions of those who appear indifferent to their feelings and circumstances. Even when their lives are literally at risk, they will frequently do as they wish, not as they were told. Only the most hardened or "burned out" among caregivers is not distressed by those responses. The emotional highs come from successes not failures, from help welcomed not help rejected.

At their most vulnerable, people still demand respect, in one way or another. They will suffer in defiance rather than submit to indignity. That suffering is the moral issue. Efficiency in patient care is suspect when the price is patient pain, even if self-inflicted. Limiting options is a kind of coercion, a blow to the mind if not the body. Worse, in practice the omission of relevant choices is rarely a means to patient ends and is almost always a means to the professional's—a reason to pause if not to desist.

Justifying Lies

Lies, too, are coercive but are much more disreputable. Bragging about manipulation is allowed, at least in moderation. Boasting about lies is gauche. Yet, the temptation is real, and yielding to it is common—with the best of intentions. "You need to talk with your doctor" isn't always enough, nor is smiling, unresponsive silence punctuated by an occasional nod of acknowledgment.

The questions about prognosis and the explanations of risk are perhaps the worst, but being faced with obviously false impressions from others is a close second. "The doctor said you're going home on Friday?" you ask the beaming face, hoping for a clarification that will take you off the hook. "Well, maybe," you respond cheerfully, knowing that it will be next week without the kind of miracle you have read about but never seen.

Sissela Bok suggests that there are two main reasons for lying to patients, neither of which is very convincing after scrutiny.[3] The first is that patients do not want bad news; the second is that the truth will harm them. Research supports neither. More likely, the health care professionals touting those justifications find it very hard to deal with the emotions surrounding bad news and project those difficulties onto their patients.

The "work of worrying," as Alexander Capron once noted in some comments about informed consent, is important to patients.[4] It is a time for reflection and decisions concerning the life that is and the death that is to come. For caregivers, in reaction to their own anxieties, to withhold the truth or offer pleasing falsehoods is usually to frustrate that work, diminishing the humanity of their patients. Yes, the truth can be frightening or distressing to patients; sometimes it overwhelms them for a while. The caregivers' task is to see them through it, not help them avoid it, and so to face it themselves as well.

Challenging Colleagues

Sharing bad news with patients is daunting; questioning the decisions of colleagues is hazardous. Curiously, a kind of ambivalence surrounds it. On the one hand, it is the primary check in a system with uncertain balances. If others involved in the care of a patient do not press their concerns about treatment issues, who will? At the same time, questioners who persist in the face of unsatisfactory answers are viewed as mutinous crew or traitorous colleagues. Even this mildest form of whistle blowing is appreciated more by the spectators than the participants.

In short, the system depends on people with strong egos or thick skins. To allow decisions to remain unchallenged when patient well-being seems threatened is to abandon a first-order moral responsibility. Many give in to their fear, but no one doubts what is right. Whatever the threat to professional relationships, to future effectiveness, or to anticipated advancement, one is not to keep silent.

At the same time, a smoldering wastebasket is not to be reported as a five-alarm fire. The ethical dilemma is about judgment, not just about fear. When is it one's duty to question authority and when is it one's duty to respect it? Both are important. To say, "It depends," is unhelpful. Of course it does: on the potential harm, on one's background and experience, on one's certainty about the facts, on one's possible bias, and on the likely consequences, among other things.

The central moral responsibility of professionals goes beyond the deliberate nurturing of a capacity for objective analysis. It includes the duty to develop the interpersonal skills required for that analysis to have influence. It is a moral failing as well as a relational deficiency to remain, over time, unable to make oneself heard when that is vital. If careless dressing changes do not stop after staff have been approached, they are not alone to blame. If the team does not really consider a claim that total parenteral nutrition is unnecessary, the outcome may reflect the style of the presentation and not its content. Successful interventions are rarely a matter of authority and intimidation, though the culture of medicine still values both. They are far more likely to depend on hard data, sound reasoning, personal courtesy, and unembarrassed persistence—equally possible for all to pursue.

Accepting Boundaries

Role relationships often complicate the honest questioning of decisions. Professional prerogatives within medicine are jealously guarded, and overlapping competencies foster boundary disputes. Even among professional colleagues, there are sometimes differences over whose assignment includes a particular task.

There is more to this than intergroup competition and inflated egos. For trained professionals, dignity is linked to independent practice and satisfaction is tied to expanding competence. Inherently, limits on discretion are insulting and limits on growth are frustrating. Both difficulties are magnified by the American belief that limits, in general, are not only unnecessary but harmful. Compliance is for wimps; testing and rebellion are the norm.

Not surprisingly, then, there is sometimes tension over who does nutritional assessments or specific elements of patient care. What attitude should one take if the concern is what is right? Tradition favors pride and assertiveness. Common sense prescribes a heavy dose of humility and generosity. It is hardly immoral for organizations or professional groups to battle over who ought to perform certain functions. In a democracy, there is no better way to resolve those disputes. Yet, to wage that war at the expense of one's patients is unconscionable.

The closer one is to the bedside, the less defensible a win-lose scenario. Morally, at least, competence is the issue and collaboration is the rule. The interest of the patient lies in having the job well done and in escaping the anxiety generated by warring caregivers. Mutual consideration and mutual restraint are virtues; stubborn demands for primacy and rigidity about roles are not. Boundaries are to be respected, not enshrined, and deference to skill is the final arbiter.

Apportioning Loyalty

The occasional struggle to define acceptable boundaries is a part of the larger and more pervasive issue of apportioning loyalty. How do professionals, when acting as consultants, distribute allegiance among the competing claimants? What commitments do they make to their patients; to their clients, the physicians responsible for those patients; to the other caregivers tending those patients; to colleagues in their primary disciplines; to other members of the consulting team; to the institution they serve; and to their own physical and emotional welfare or that of family and friends?

Admittedly, that recitation makes the problem sound worse than it is, but in the best of situations, strained relationships born of failed expectations can develop both rapidly and unexpectedly. Miscalculations and unintended slights can instantly erode vital support. Defending the behavior of a colleague to the nurse who felt abused may earn kudos within the team but a new coldness from the staff. Residents who have spent time with the team may then expect favored treatment when it should not be given.

The primacy of patient well-being conditions all other allegiances, although not identically. Ethics suggests that priorities be derived from the intimacy of the relationship and the nature of the bond. Acceptance of the consultant role is a commitment to deliver the expected services to one's client as well as to the patient. Only when loyalty to those caregivers threatens patient welfare can that commitment be subordinated.

Membership on the team implies commitment to both its purpose and its personnel. Only patient welfare and consultant obligations take precedence. Loyalties to one's employer or to one's professional group cannot be put before these commitments to patient, client, and team, unless there is violation of the law or a major threat from unethical behavior. Floor staff and ancillary service personnel are due respect as associates in providing patient care but have no claim to more than that.

The place of self, family, and friends apart from work is a function of the boundary established or negotiated between one's public and private lives. The reasonable expectation of health care professionals is that a full-time commitment to patients goes beyond 40 hours and entails some unanticipated sacrifices of personal plans. That leaves the line between moral obligation and institutional exploitation for individual definition, but wherever it is drawn, that line must recognize the just moral claims of partners and children on the time, energy, and attention necessary to sustain and nurture those relationships. For the most part, that is not possible unless time, energy, and attention are also allotted to oneself.

Serving Self-Interests

Concern with one's self and with one's private life is awkward for Americans, even though many seem preoccupied with their lifestyles. There is a seldom articulated understanding that an appropriate balance between personal and professional commitments is not only difficult to define in the abstract but troublesome to achieve in practice. After all, caregiving can be an addiction as much as a vocation—gratitude, admiration, and the "rush" derived from rescuing are in short supply elsewhere. It can nurture nobility or provide effective cover for less lofty pursuits.

No one is sure what can be claimed for oneself. Ethical justification of self-interested behavior is in short supply from mainstream philosophy and religion, at least apart from the few who assert that it is either our only moral duty or our sole psychological possibility. It is viewed as admirable to be ambitious but slightly disreputable to act that way. Achievements generate both praise and resentment. People are keenly aware that advancement and status are often won at the expense of others and that taking care of oneself can shift all too easily from discipline to principal occupation.

The moral goal is self-respect, the via media between self-effacement and self-promotion, between abandoning one's own interests and ignoring the interests of others. To see every patient every day may well be to do nothing else: to write no papers, to undertake no projects, to build no relationships. No ethical claim or moral commitment requires such a sacrifice. What both do require, in the aggregate, is that one's own interests do not take priority over obligations to others, and that in times of urgent need the others come first.

The Struggle for Integrity—Practical Wisdom and Muddling Through

What emerges from the attempt to define ethical responses to these recurring dilemmas in nutrition support is a humbling awareness of the obstacles to integrity. Under the best of circumstances, the effort required is considerable; in this setting, it is greater. Competence by itself can ensure neither effectiveness nor self-respect, and it is backed up by neither line authority nor role security—like all consultants, the team serves largely at the pleasure of its clients. Hence, both personal and professional integrity are crucial to the influence of the team.

Easy to say, but hard to live. No one can always be right by the rules, but by itself, following the rules makes no one right—sometimes a bit safer, but surely not right. None of us can meet all the demands on our time and energy, but meeting every demand signals fear not integrity. In the end, there are times we must choose between safety and commitment or between fear and self-respect. Further, surrounding those tests of character are tests of judgment. Conflicting duties are the rule, not the exception.

The will to be responsible and the courage to act decline with uncertainty. Yet, the balancing of moral imperatives is an art not a science. The materials used in that balancing are situational assessments and provisional decisions, rooted in experience as much as in logic and sustained by the acceptance of frailty and fallibility. In a different context, Harry Moody has described it as "muddling through"—words of praise, not criticism.[5]

No one would suggest that the moral problems in patient care should be exempt from disciplined reflection, but the messy reality of the complex ethical issues facing caregivers demands more than intellectual analysis. As Edmund Pellegrino and David Thomasma have written, "Medicine is itself ultimately an exercise of practical wisdom—a right way of acting in difficult and uncertain circumstances for a specific end, that is, the good of the particular person who is ill."[6]

The good is particular, like the integrity required to achieve it, not so much the result of principles learned as character forged. The good is particular, rooted in caring about patients who are known, not in abstract justice for strangers. The good is particular, characterized by a discriminating equity rather than a defensive uniformity. The good is particular, an enhancement of dignity, not the repair of a body.

For the caregiver as well as for the patient, the good is particular. It is created each day. There is always another chance. In an imperfect world of imperfect souls, one should not ask for more.

Notes

1. C. Gilligan, 1982, *In A Different Voice* (Cambridge, MA: Harvard University Press).
2. President's Commission for the Study of Ethical Problems in Medicine and Biomedical and Behavioral Research, 1982, *Making Health Care Decisions* (Washington, DC: Government Printing Office).
3. S. Bok, 1978, *Lying* (New York: Random House).
4. A. Capron, 1986, Keynote Address: Access To Health Care—Rationing Resources (Denver, CO: Center for Applied Biomedical Ethics).
5. H. Moody, 1986, "Fiduciary Paternalism—Autonomy in Long Term Care." Conference on Ethical Issues in Health Care for the Elderly (Memphis: University of Tennessee).
6. E. D. Pellegrino and D. C. Thomasma, 1988, *For the Patient's Good* (New York: Oxford).

CASE A

BENIGN MISCONSENT

"A consent must be voluntary, competent, and informed except in an emergency situation." This contention of Kurt Darr in his *Ethics in Health Services Management* is given particular elaboration: "To have an informed consent full disclosure of the nature of the condition for which treatment is proposed, all of the significant facts about the condition itself, and an explanation of the likely consequences and difficulties that can result from treatment and non-treatment must be explained by the physician to the patient." Darr's articulation fairly represents the macroethics approach to the informed consent issue. How does it play out in the micro dimension of healthcare?

The manager of a busy short-stay unit in a large medical center where, on average, 35 patients a day undergo some surgical procedure, often encounters situations that do not fulfill the above criteria. The following case describes a specific instance of this common microethics matter.

Mrs. Jones, a 39-year-old white female is admitted for surgery. Her medical history states that she has had intermittent bleeding of long duration and that it has increased over the past two weeks. Mrs. Jones is scheduled for a total abdominal hysterectomy, bilateral salpingo-oophorectomy. Ann Brown, R.N., a staff nurse, takes the consent form to Mrs. Jones to have her sign prior to going to the operating room. Ann asks Mrs. Jones if Dr. Smith has explained the procedure and requests that she read the consent before signing. Mrs. Jones says that her doctor has been treating her for a long time and knows what is best so she does not have to bother reading "all that technical stuff." Ann insists that

Mrs. Jones read the form before signing. When Mrs. Jones comes to the clause about sterility resulting from the procedure, she asks Ann what that means. Ann tells the patient she will have the physician come to talk to her to answer any questions she has before she signs the consent form. When Dr. Smith answers Ann's page, he tells her that he is scrubbed in the operating room and that Mrs. Jones knows all about the surgery, so just have her sign. He tells Ann that Mrs. Jones is his patient and probably doesn't remember half of what he told her. Ann then goes to the unit manager and asks what she should do. Ann says that she feels that Mrs. Jones does not really understand all of the implications involved in this type of surgery.

What should the unit manager do? It's a hectic day. She knows and trusts Dr. Smith. Patients routinely sign that consent form without discussion. And Ann has a history of sometimes being a little overeager. To quiet Ann, the unit manager goes down the hall to talk with Mrs. Jones. She realizes that the patient does, indeed, lack sufficient information to give informed consent. But an important budget meeting begins in five minutes. Dr. Smith is waiting in OR. What to do?

The unit manager quickly ponders the issue: What is the real problem? What are the true facts of the situation? What actions could she take? Who will the decision affect? Will important values be damaged? Mrs. Jones is scheduled to have a surgical procedure that will have numerous consequences for her future health. She does not seem to understand what these effects will be. Mrs. Jones came to the hospital to have surgery; this *implies* consent. No family member is with Mrs. Jones (her husband is out of town on a business trip and will not return until later in the afternoon). Dr. Smith says that he has explained the surgery to the patient. Hospital policy states that the physician is required to obtain consent. Customarily, however, most physicians write an order to obtain consent and the RN obtains the signature and signs as witness. Two registered nurses have concluded that Mrs. Jones does not have all the facts and is not familiar with all of her options. Mrs. Jones needs medical treatment. Hospital policy regarding obtaining consent is not being followed. Legally the medical center could be at risk if it were claimed that Mrs. Jones was not aware of the consequences of surgery. The patient's rights and autonomy are at stake. Staff's professional judgment is being questioned by the physician. The physician is being challenged regarding the relationship between physician and patient. Is the patient's family aware of the significant outcome of the operation? What is the ethical thing to do?

A significant number of people are involved in this situation: Mrs. Jones and her family, Dr. Smith, the medical center, and two registered nurses. The outcome will have some repercussions for all of these people. Personal, professional, and institutional values are involved here. For the patient and her family, the competence of the physician and the nurses, honesty, fairness, responsiveness, and her very dignity are involved. For the physician and nurses, efficiency, professionalism, loyalty, consistency, and legality need to be considered. The medical center has a responsibility to the community to provide healthcare that is in the best interest of all of its patients. Responsiveness to ethical issues that affect clients and staff is an important value of this institution. What to do?

The unit manager has some options. She could let Mrs. Jones sign the consent. She could insist that Dr. Smith come to Mrs. Jones' room and talk with the patient. She could explain the outcome of surgery to the patient herself. She could inform her supervisor of the problem and let him handle it. She could refuse to obtain the consent. She could report Dr. Smith to the hospital administrator. She could present the problem to the operating room/recovery room committee meeting for a clarification on the procedure to obtain consents.

The real problem may not be too complex. A patient is about to have a surgical procedure and apparently does not have enough information on which to base her decision. The facts of the dilemma as described are easily identified. Actions that can be taken by the manager can be narrowed down to yes, let Mrs. Jones sign, or no, do not let her sign until she receives more information. Subtle organizational constraints are influencing the options: responsibility for consent is clearly defined by hospital policy; but past experience has demonstrated that you do not have outright conflict with the physician staff without incurring consequences. The manager's action could have a negative impact on all of the actors involved if not handled properly. If Mrs. Jones does not sign the consent, surgery will be delayed or postponed, putting her health at risk. Dr. Smith will likely be angry and may well take some action that will be negative for the unit manager. The nurses, the manager, and others may have their professional values challenged. What to do?

The unit manager decides to telephone Dr. Smith to talk about the matter, thinking that a word from her might influence the doctor's understanding of the importance of the situation and help to resolve it. The phone call does seem to have positive results. Dr. Smith agrees to come to the short-stay unit and talk to Mrs. Jones. When he arrives, both he and the manager go to the patient's room. The doctor talks to the patient for about ten minutes and explains in detail what the surgery involves. He has Mrs. Jones sign the consent, and the unit manager witnesses it. Mrs. Jones goes into surgery seemingly knowing what to expect.

The unit manager later shares this experience with the staff to reinforce their understanding of informed consent and their responsibility in the process.

Questions for Discussion

1. Did the unit manager act ethically? How so?
2. What consequences of her action are possible or likely?
3. What was all the hand-wringing about in the first place? In the hubbub of everyday healthcare, with all of the paperwork involved, shouldn't well enough have been left alone? After all, isn't a cursory signing of consent forms the norm anyway?
4. On the other hand, wasn't the unit manager's response obvious? But suppose Dr. Smith was ornery; suppose the OR was already backed up? Suppose Dr. Smith refused to come out and again ordered her to get the consent?
5. How would you distinguish the macro issue of informed consent from the micro issue of actually obtaining it?
6. Evaluate the unit manager's follow-up action with staff.
7. The unit manager attempted to reflect on her own ethical responsibility and behavior instead of focusing on Dr. Smith's behavior. Is the dynamic of reflecting on one's own behavior different from that of reflecting on the behavior of someone else? Is it easier or more difficult?

Annotated Bibliography

Bok, S. *Lying*. New York: Vintage, 1979. A sensational and popular reflection on the "seemingly trivial" reality of microethics in general, including a chapter on healthcare in particular.

Cooper, T. *The Responsible Administrator*. Port Washington, NY: Kennikat, 1982. Written for the field of public administration, providing good insight for health administrators on the nature of responsibility in the micro dimension of the field.

Crawford, K. "How Ethical Dilemmas Are Resolved." *Journal of Long Term Care Administration* 22, no. 3 (Fall 1994): 25–29. Although focused on experience with ethics committees, nonetheless provides perspective on the issue of education for healthcare ethics.

Guy, M. *Ethical Decision Making in Everyday Work Situations*. New York: Quorum Books, 1990. An effort to probe the daily routine of managers.

Lipsky, M. *Street-Level Bureaucracy*. New York: Russell Sage, 1980. A probe of public service professionals in general that gets right at the nature of the micro dimension.

Thompson, D. "The Possibility of Administrative Ethics." *Public Administration Review* 45, no. 4 (November/December 1985): 555–61. A Princeton professor who offers insight to the nature of administrative ethics in any public service profession.

Worthley, J. "Ethics and Public Administration." *Public Personnel Management Journal* 15, no. 1 (spring 1981): 41–47. A framework for exploring the micro dimension of public service ethics.

ASPECTS OF MICROETHICS IN HEALTHCARE: DOGMA, DEVELOPMENT, AND DILEMMA

JUST WHAT *is* ethics in the micro dimension of healthcare? And, another thing, how does one *do* ethics there? To put it more properly, what is the nature of healthcare ethics and what constitutes ethical behavior in the micro dimension of our profession?

What Is Ethics in Healthcare?

In courses and workshops I usually ask participants to respond to these questions with the first three words that occur to them. The most often proffered response is "the right thing." "Ethics is about right and wrong," they explain, "and ethical behavior means doing the right and avoiding the wrong." "Integrity" is another big one on the response list. "Ethics is about integrity," they argue, and putting ethics into practice is a matter of being a person of integrity. The third most presented response is "values." Ethics is about values, and being ethical means upholding the basic values of healthcare.

A bit facetiously I then throw back questions like: How do we know what the "right" thing is? Just what *is* integrity anyway? And what, specifically, are these values you're talking about? I then routinely ask if I did the ethical thing at the beginning of the session when I delayed starting by seven minutes. The program was advertised to begin at 9 a.m., and most of the registrants were in their seats at that time. Realizing that six registrants were missing, that the meeting room was not easy to find, that no one at the university ever starts on time anyway, and that traffic jams probably were clogging nearby roadways, I waited until 9:07 a.m., at which time the last participant arrived breathless from rushing. Was it ethical of me to do that—to delay for the sake of a few and break the implicit contract of a 9 a.m. start that most of the participants had honored? Of more reflective urgency, is there any ethical significance to this meager matter in the first place? Moreover, as the last late participant enters the room, I usually glare at the latecomer, making it embarrassingly obvious that he or she is quite late indeed. Is that ethical? Does it have any ethical dimension?

At this point most of the participants laugh, thinking these questions absurd. So, annoyingly no doubt, I keep at it: "Is it okay, then, for me to begin and end our sessions whenever I please?" and "Wouldn't the ethical thing, the *right* thing, have been for me to start promptly at 9 a.m., no matter that some paid participants were stuck in traffic?" Whereupon most participants have to be wondering what in the world this all has to do with healthcare ethics!

So I tell them about my 3 p.m. doctor's appointment last week: about how I arrived on time, having rushed from an important business meeting, and was kept waiting until 3:25 p.m. before I was called into the examination room. I tell them about how irritated I was sitting there, about how my blood pressure shot up in a setting that is supposed to foster my health, about how I told the doctor—but only *after* he had treated me—how unethical I thought it all was, and about how baffled he was at my outrage. In view of this, I ask the students (rather loudly), "How *dare I then* make you all wait a full seven minutes and presume to teach ethics? What about the value of fairness to you who were here on time? What about efficient use of the program time for which you have paid top dollar? Am I a person of integrity when I agree to a 9 a.m. starting time, then proceed to break that agreement?"

One might imagine the heads now shaking in confusion and consternation as I suggest that healthcare ethics may be more complex, subtle, and multidimensional than we think at first blush; that it may involve seemingly silly and small matters; that it may be more about *ourselves* and our own behavior than about the ethics of others; and that a more sophisticated understanding of the nature of healthcare ethics is an essential first step in the quest to "do" ethics in our profession.

What, then, *is* the nature of ethics in healthcare? Is it about doing the right thing even in trivial situations? Is it about figuring out, with integrity, what the right thing is? Is it about dealing with conflicting "right" things? The answers, I suggest, are yes, yes, and yes. In my experience there are three major elements of healthcare ethics and—as argued in the previous chapter—two basic dimensions, macro and micro.

Healthcare ethics is, indeed, about right and wrong and doing the right thing, but this is only one ethics aspect of our healthcare reality. I call it **dogma**. One reality of healthcare is that some situations in professional life are clearly matters of right and wrong, and ethical behavior in such cases is simply a matter of doing the right thing. In these situations, ethical distress can arise when it is difficult to do that perceived right thing. This dogmatic aspect, however, constitutes only a part of the real-life experience of healthcare professionals; in fact it makes up a relatively small part of the daily routine of healthcare delivery.

In the macro dimension acceptance of a kickback for awarding a hospital contract is *dogmatically* wrong, and it is not difficult to figure out that it is unethical: section III, sub-paragraph C of the *Code of Ethics* of the American College of Healthcare Executives, for example, specifies this dogma (see Appendix A). In the micro dimension, stealing a bottle of pain relievers from the pharmacy is dogmatically wrong, and it is not difficult to figure it out: the Ten Commandments, for example, helps. Certainly, if the announcement or invitation to the seminar mentioned above had stressed that we start at 9 a.m. no matter what, then we might well argue that the right and ethical thing to do is dogma: start at 9 a.m. But how often do these dogma situations occur in your healthcare reality? For me, I must say rarely. Would that they occurred more frequently, because that would make ethics so much easier to figure out.

There is a second ethics aspect to the modern healthcare reality, an element that reflects a process more than fixed tenets like dogmatic ethics. We can call it the **development** element. Such situations arise in our healthcare reality when we sense that there is a right thing to do but have not yet been able to determine precisely what that right thing is. Ethical uncertainty results. In the macro dimension we have examples like the Karen Ann Quinlan case, in which high technology complicated our moral reasoning. It seemed there was a right thing to do but it took some time to develop the answer. Was it all right or not to pull the plug on this person? The doctors said no, the family said yes, but both with difficulty. So the case went to a judge who deliberated at length, and gradually the community came to a consensus on what is right. The consensus *developed*.

In the micro dimension gifts from suppliers have long caused some uneasiness among healthcare providers. We get to know some vendors well and even become friendly with them. We get invited to play golf with them; then they give us the cashmere sweater, then the case of champagne. Is it all right to accept? Is it the right thing to do? Is it ethical? Is it even relevant ethically? Healthcare professionals have felt confused by these situations believing, on the one hand, that there is something wrong here and, on the other hand, sensing a friendly harmlessness in it. So reflection on this matter has deepened over time and, as we know, many healthcare organizations and professions have now developed dogma that declares it to be unethical to accept a gift with a value of over X dollars. Under X dollars it's okay and ethical! In many healthcare organizations this sort of consensus is still in *development* and professional ethics committees continue to spend time dealing with it.

In the seminar case discussed earlier, the institution where I held the session may have developed over time, or may still be in the process of *developing* (albeit unofficially) the consensus expectation that all courses there begin the first session seven to eight minutes late. If that is the case, perhaps the dogma mandating an on-time start is not the right thing to do after all; in fact, we might argue that through an informal ethics development process a new dogma had been emerging, namely, "Thou shalt start late on the first session or be deemed unethical."

There is a third ethics aspect to modern healthcare reality. It involves those situations when one right thing—such as seeing my patient at the appointed time—competes with another right thing—such as responding to the needs of the previous patient by giving her the extra time she needs. These are situations for which there is no predetermined dogma, and for which no "right thing to do" can be developed. These are venues of enduring conflict characterized by the "damned if I do, damned if I don't" context. Their frame of reference involves what Donaldson and Dunfee call "bounded moral rationality."[1] If I respond to the current patient's need, the next patient is harmed by waiting; if I adhere to the set appointment and respond to the next patient, the current patient is harmed. What should I do? If I start on time at 9 a.m., the registrants caught in traffic are harmed; if I wait seven minutes the sitting patients are harmed. What should I do? We call this **dilemma** ethics, the third "big D" of healthcare ethics reality. In my experience it constitutes the largest reality of the daily routine of healthcare. We confront it constantly. In the micro dimension do I bend the rules all the time, just some of the time, or never? Do I clinically deal with all patients efficiently and fairly, or do I listen and talk, responding humanely, thus attending to fewer patients within the limited 24-hour day? Do I do something about the behavior of my colleague toward patients, or do I mind my own business and keep my mouth shut? Do I give some slack on lunch time to one subordinate whose work ethic I admire, or do I, in my union environment, treat all subordinates by the rules? And, by the way, in all of these kinds of situations, what is the *ethical* thing to do?

In the dramatic macro dimension, what is the ethical thing to do when my boss tells me, just prior to our Joint Commission inspection, to doctor-up some files we have been maintaining incompletely. It seems dishonest, but if we fail accreditation the hundreds of patients we serve may be harmed. And if I resist my superior's request my career could be harmed. So much of the accreditation requirements seem like "Mickey Mouse" things anyway. But my authority figure—the person with power over me—is asking me to do something deceitful. I'm damned if I don't and damned if I do. What is the ethical thing to do?

In the seemingly humdrum micro dimension, what is the ethical thing to do when a call comes in from an influential doctor while I am on another line with a patient? Should I put the patient on hold with a trite "could you hold a second," or should I put the doctor on hold until I finish my call with the patient? Is it honest to say "hold a second" knowing that the call will take at least many seconds, if not minutes? Is it fair to make the patient wait when she was there first on the phone? Is it a managerially competent act to put the doctor on hold? The doctor's call could be very important! Even if it is not, the doctor has influence over our operation—and my job! What is the ethical thing to do? What does such a "phone dance" have to do with ethics in the first place?

The matrix shown in Figure 2.1 depicts these three aspects of healthcare ethics.

From the aspect of *dogma*, ethics is about **doing** the right thing. This aspect sees reality as black and white, and ethics can be objective. We stress rules and principles and promulgate codes. We teach values and emphasize courage or moral fortitude. In the macro dimension dogmatic ethics is about the big concepts and their dictates for clearly significant situations. In the micro dimension it is about seemingly trivial things and more subtle situations. From the *development* aspect ethics is about **designing** the right approach for realities in which no rule yet exists but for which there can and should be a rule. Things are gray from this aspect, and ethics can be objectified. We stress cases and send them for judgment to a court or an analyst. We teach case studies and emphasize interactive deliberation by the best and the brightest lawyers, ethicists, and medical

Figure 2.1 Aspects of Healthcare Ethics

	Macro	Micro
Dogma		
Development		
Dilemma		

luminaries. In the macro dimension it is about dramatic reactions to stirring situations. In the micro dimension it is about seemingly simpler and less serious situations. From the *dilemma* aspect ethics is about **discerning** the responsible response to realities in which there is not one right answer but many in conflict. Things are opaque in this aspect and ethics is more subjective. We stress reflection and create options. We teach consciousness-raising analysis and emphasize the role and responsibility of *every* individual professional. An ethical dilemma in the macro dimension lies in clear and disturbing quandaries. In the micro dimension, the ethical dilemma lurks in choices initially less noticed and disturbing.

For me it is helpful to form analogies of these aspects of ethics in healthcare. Some years ago I regularly drove from Long Island to Rensselaerville, New York to give ethics workshops. Sometimes the weather was bright and clear, and getting to the site safely and punctually was simply a matter of departing on time, following the signs, obeying the speed limits, and paying attention. If I got lost or crashed it would be because I had failed to do what I knew I should be doing. If I arrived late, it was because I had left later than I knew I should. On those days, that drive was like dealing with the dogma aspect of healthcare ethics.

But I remember the first few times I made that drive to Rensselaerville. It was night time and, not being familiar with the route, I had to slow down, stop, read the map, and ask for directions. I remember trying some different routes to see which way was faster, safer, and easier, and asking people who had done the drive which route they had found best. After awhile I figured out the best way to get there and the amount of time I needed. Up until then the drive had been like dealing with the development aspect of healthcare ethics.

The operative reality, however, is that Long Island is close to New York City. Traffic is usually unpredictable and often congested. Getting over the bridges from Long Island can be slow. Rensselaerville is in the mountains; the roads there are narrow and winding. In the spring—when these workshops were scheduled—fog and mist are common. Moreover, having a hectic schedule, I was often delayed in getting on the road. More often than not, I was trying to arrive at my destination safely and on time in a situation of slow traffic and low visibility. I knew where I wanted to go, and I thought I knew the most effective way to get there, but on many of those spring days the drive was like dealing with the dilemma aspect of healthcare ethics. Should I slow down and be safe or do what it takes to get there on time? It was not so simple, it was not so clear; it certainly was not as easy as driving on those bright days with "dogma-right" conditions.

Literature abounds with help for the macro dimension. From the dogma aspect we have codes of ethics and works exemplified by Griffith's engaging book[2] and Gatewood and Carroll's useful article.[3] The development aspect offers a wealth of superb deliberations, such as Veatch's case studies[4] and Arras and Steinbock's issues.[5] And dilemmas have brought us the illuminating likes of Harron, Burnside, and Beauchamp.[6] For the micro dimension, however, we are not so enriched. Some professional codes of ethics are helpful at the dogma level in spelling out rules, and works like Glaser's[7] attend in part to the development aspect; but the micro issues of the dilemma aspect are all but ignored, and that's where this present book enters the picture.

The Reality Prism

Another way to conceptualize the aspects of ethics in healthcare is through what I call the PCV reality prism. Healthcare ambulances have PCV valves for their engines; healthcare ethics need PCV prisms for their deliberations. If we do not use PCV valves our ambulances will break down; if we don't use PCV prisms—or good facsimiles—our ethics will also tend to break down. Prisms are like eyeglasses: whether we are nearsighted or farsighted, without glasses we cannot see clearly. Our surroundings are blurred and distorted. But with glasses—a prism— we can see clearly. So, too, I am convinced, it is important that we professionals have and use "prisms" for a clear view of ethical reality. As William Kahn puts it in his agenda-setting analysis of business ethics research, a prism can "clear a person's vision, enlightening what is clouded."[8]

The ethical dimension of healthcare consists of three salient realities that need to be seen clearly, I would argue, if we are to be ethically mature. One is the actual influence, or **power (P)** , that healthcare professionals have in their work position. It is the basis of the ethical question, for as soon as my presence in a healthcare position affects other people, then the ethical dimension begins. Is that effect good or bad? The first step toward ethical maturity, therefore, lies in seeing clearly the influence or power that I in fact wield, and the effect it has on patients, subordinates, peers, my family, and others. The next chapter focuses the prism on that reality of power.

Second is the reality of expectations or **values (V)**. As a healthcare professional I am expected to use the power I wield in a way that maintains and supports the fundamental values of the healthcare enterprise. These expectations or values are the guides to the ethical use of power. Unless I see and understand them clearly, I am apt to get lost on the road of power. As Terry Cooper maintains: "Doing ethics involves thinking

Figure 2.2 The PCV Reality Prism

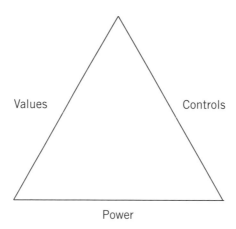

more systematically about the values that are imbedded in the choices we otherwise would make on practical or political grounds alone."[9] Chapter 4 thus focuses the prism on this reality.

Third, it is a fact that all sorts of mechanisms of **control (C)** permeate the environment of healthcare—mechanisms designed to direct the power of healthcare professionals along the road of expectations and values. What are these controls, how do they affect the everyday reality of the healthcare professional, and how do I deal with them? Clarity in this regard is equally important for ethical maturity, so chapter 5 focuses the prism here.

These three key realities of the ethical dimension of healthcare are depicted in Figure 2.2, the PCV Reality Prism. Notice that while there are three sides, it is one prism. Clarity is not achieved if one side of the prism is faulty. Notice also that the three sides interact with each other. The values side is directed at molding the power, which in turn is directed at realizing the values; the controls side is directed at limiting the power side by reflecting the values side. And so forth. The science of physical optics is actually helpful in understanding the nature of healthcare ethics reality.

How Does One "Do" Ethics?

In view of these aspects and realities of healthcare ethics how can one "do" ethics in healthcare? Historically, three approaches have dominated the quest. The classical or **philosophical** approach turns to the great tradition of thinkers and seeks to apply the principles derived from them to the ethical dimension. Most of our literature in healthcare ethics draws from this approach and employs concepts such as Kant's deontological "moral imperative," and Bentham and Mills' utilitarian theories. Guidelines such as "always be honest" and "do the greatest good with the least harm" emerge. Similarly, ethicists like Glaser[10] and Pellegrino and Thomasma[11] draw from theological as well as philosophical traditions to stress the beneficence imperative, "love thy neighbor." A practical manifestation of this approach is the recent presence on some hospital staffs of philosophy/theology experts. This approach has proved to be marvelous in clarifying principles for behavior, but limited in addressing the conflict that so often arises in practicing those principles.

A second approach turns to juridical systems for guidance in doing ethics.[12] In contending through courts, struggling to develop codes and statutes, and relying on specific rules and procedures, this **legal** approach has directly addressed the conflict problem. A practical manifestation of this approach is the delegation of most ethical questions to the counsel's office in many healthcare organizations. But, as Foster and others have argued, this approach can be debilitating: "The law in fact fosters a particular way of looking at and responding to situations that is essentially amoral in nature; in other words, there is created a general inability to judge right versus wrong. Indeed, all things are viewed as either legal or illegal."[13]

A third approach has been what I call **organizational.** Attention to theories of organization culture developed by researchers like Weick[14] and Pettigrew[15] has convinced many that principles of ethics can be better applied in realities of conflict by developing organization cultures that facilitate ethically mature behavior. Victor and Cullen, for example, focus on work climates[16]; Nash suggests that the use of mechanisms such as mission statements and procedural processes has made a difference in the ethical behavior of some major corporations.[17] Development of ethics committees and the presence of in-house ethics consultants in so many healthcare organizations is a clear manifestation of this organizational approach in healthcare. But ethics committees have proved to be subject to significant pitfalls and limitations.[18]

A more recently evident approach—the approach emphasized in this book—is what I call **phenomenological.** It is suggested by thinkers such as O'Neill, who finds that "while the work of professional philosophers and social scientists will doubtless provide the ultimate formulation of organizational and managerial ethics, the reflections of practicing managers can and should be an invaluable source of insight and realism;"[19] Leys when he argues: "The administrator, charged with discretionary responsibilities, has to make an indefinite standard of action precise and explicit;"[20] and Marilyn Ray in her emphasis on moral interaction:

"The method is an experiential one, a phenomenologic ethical inquiry."[21] Such a phenomenological approach stresses the actual experience of the healthcare professionals who deal daily with an ethical dimension on the front lines. It values the hard-earned insights of this experience and sees heightened consciousness of actual experience as the key to improving ethical maturity. It thus elicits recognition of the reality of power and the centrality of conflicting principles, values, and expectations. It highlights the importance of reflection and the professional necessity of reflective skill. Efforts in business, health management, and public administration master's programs to develop ethics courses rich in reflection demonstrate this approach. But these efforts have proved to be difficult and slow in developing.

Conceptually, different approaches to acting ethically can be portrayed with the matrix shown in Figure 2.3. We can all "do" ethics—most of us probably do—in box 1. With this approach we do our job the best we can in the daily hubbub of healthcare where there is never enough time, staff, or resources to do things the way we might prefer. We rely on *external* forces—whatever they may be—to put us back on the ethical track if we stray. We are thus ethically *passive*, but we respond when someone else calls the question, whether peer, prosecutor, or priest.

Some of us—I believe many of us—are in box 2 in our approach to ethics. We do not rely on external forces to keep us ethical. We rely on ourselves because, after all, we were brought up right. We are people of integrity and, therefore, we innately behave ethically. In our approach we need not reflect on ethics (Lord knows we don't have time!), and we certainly don't need some guru to tell us how to be ethical. We rely on the *internal* moral fiber that our moms and dads and others gave us. It is like being on automatic pilot. We know when things are right and when things are wrong. Our approach to ethics is deeply internal and instinctive or *passive*.

But most of us who subscribe to philosophical, legal, or organizational approaches to ethics are in box 3. In doing ethics we are *active*—we **seek** answers. But we look *externally*. We look to philosophers, to judges,

Figure 2.3 Approaches to Ethics

	External	Internal
Passive	1	2
Active	3	4

to ethics committees to tell us the ethical thing to do. And when they tell us, we do it. But we don't just wait for something to happen; we actively seek their enlightenment.

One can easily get "boxed in" to any of these approaches. Or we can attempt to do ethics, at least some of the time, in box 4. In this box we actively seek ways of dealing with the ethical dimension of our professional work, but *we* ultimately take the responsibility. We ultimately look to ourselves, engaging our minds, our imaginations, and our souls. We may get help externally—from our community, our guru, our rabbi, our lawyer, or our ethics committee—but we process their input *internally* to determine our behavior. We are educated people. We are professionals. We toil on the front line every day. We have the benefit of all those external advisors as well as of our intellectual skills and personal moral sense. We are the experienced professionals: drawing on our training, our experience, and our resources, we are supposed to know what best to do.

Notice the existential phenomena associated with each approach. In box 1, I can be confident and relaxed because, if I get it wrong, someone will correct me. Life is good. In box 2, I can be even more confident and relaxed because of my internal ethics thermostat given me by parents, God, and mentors. As a person of the utmost integrity I will always get it right. Professional life is a sense of good feeling. What, me worry? If I am in box 3 life is not so easy, but I find "relief from the grief" in the help of others. I get inspired by my good guy whomever he or she may be. After all, ethics is basically a matter of inspiration, isn't it?

No, it is not. Which is why more and more of us are finding our way, reluctantly or otherwise, into box 4. This box 4 approach to ethics is not easy. It takes work; life here is no cakewalk. In fact, rather than being a matter of inspiration, ethics here, as Dan Maguire brilliantly insists,[22] is a matter of perspiration! In focusing on doing ethics in box 4, this book, then, is dedicated to the task of getting us all to perspire more in our professional positions.

Summary

We ask, then, what ethics is and how one "does" it in healthcare. As you may have gathered by now, I contend that ethics is largely, although by no means exclusively, a micro phenomenon in the daily ordinary routine of healthcare professionals; and that performing ethically—"doing it"— requires active reflection and skillful analysis by each of us in the field. Ethics is largely—although, again I stress, not exclusively—about the seemingly trivial, about, as Sissela Bok superbly puts it, what may seem "harmless" to the professional but is quite significant to the client;[23]

about what Laura Nash views as "common, everyday problems that put [our] basic values on the line often without [our] noticing."[24]

Ethics in healthcare is largely about what Willa Bruce calls "third level questions."[25] The past century, she argues, has focused on the grand issues:

> The first level questions have been properly assigned to the political philosophers. The second level questions are under scrutiny and debate. Now is the time to examine what we might call the third level questions that face us as we stand at the threshold of the future. . . . Third-level questions are the deeper questions at the heart of administrative action. . . . Ethicists have become skilled at objectifying moral and philosophical arguments, but third-level questions personalize them. Instead of discussing a corporate body called "the Organization" or "the Government" or "Mankind," third-level scholars will wonder about "the person." They will ask what effect a decision has on the individual—on the least one, rather than upon the collectivity. They will ask us to search our hearts rather than our minds.

While I would amend her point to say "search our hearts *and* our minds," she offers a useful insight.

Consequently, I believe that ethics in healthcare needs to be much more concerned with *consciousness* than with *conscience*. And "doing ethics" has much more to do with raising my consciousness than with developing my conscience. The more conscious I am of what I am doing, of the values at stake, of the options I have, and of the dignity of every patient, subordinate, peer, and superior, the more likely I am to be ethically mature. And the less conscious I am, the less likely it is that I will behave with ethical maturity.

Ethics in healthcare is much more about integration than about integrity—it means systematically integrating principles with practice, intention with behavior, perception with action. It is, as Michael Harmon argues, about paradoxically integrating individual moral agency with communitarian answerability.[26] Indeed, it integrates the routine with the extraordinary, the micro with the macro. For if we are not ethically mature and skilled with the "little" things, how can we presume to be so with the big things? The proverbial "slippery slope of sin" is real.

Finally, to do ethics well we healthcare professionals need to be ethically "fit." We need to train, to work out, to lift the weights of conflict and run the track of reflection and analysis. The hope is that this book provides a good, rigorous, and sweaty workout.

Notes

1. T. Donaldson and T. W. Dunfee, 1994, "Toward a Unified Conception of Business Ethics." *Academy of Management Review* 19, no. 2 (April): 252–84.

2. J. R. Griffith, 1993, *The Moral Challenges of Health Care Ethics* (Chicago: Health Administration Press).

3. R. D. Gatewood and A. B. Carroll, 1991, "Assessment of Ethical Performance of Organization Members: A Conceptual Framework." *Academy of Management Review* 16, no. 4 (October): 667–90.

4. R. M. Veatch, 1979, *Case Studies in Medical Ethics* (Cambridge, MA: Harvard University Press).

5. J. D. Arras and B. Steinbock, 1995, *Ethical Issues in Modern Medicine* (Mountain View, CA: Mayfield).

6. F. Harron, J. Burnside, and T. Beauchamp, 1983, *Health and Human Values* (New Haven, CT: Yale University Press).

7. J. W. Glaser, 1994, *Three Realms of Ethics* (Kansas City, MO: Sheed and Ward).

8. W. A. Kahn, 1990, "Toward an Agenda for Business Ethics Research." *Academy of Management Review* 15, no. 2 (April): 316.

9. T. L. Cooper, 1990, *The Responsible Administrator*, 3rd ed. (San Francisco: Jossey-Bass), p. 6.

10. J. W. Glaser, *Three Realms of Ethics*.

11. E. Pellegrino and D. Thomasma, 1988, *For the Patient's Good: The Restoration of Beneficence in Health Care* (New York: Oxford University Press).

12. See, for example, J. A. Rohr, 1978, *Ethics for Bureaucrats* (New York: Marcel Dekker).

13. G. D. Foster, 1981, "Law, Morality and the Public Servant." *Public Administration Review* 41, no. 1 (January/February 1981): 29–34.

14. K. Weick, 1977, "Enactment Processes in Organizations," in B. Staw and M. Salancik (eds.), *New Directions in Organization Behavior* (Chicago: St. Clair).

15. A. Pettigrew, 1979, "On Studying Organizational Cultures." *Administrative Sciences Quarterly* 24, no. 4 (December).

16. B. Victor and J. Cullen, 1988, "The Organizational Bases of Ethical Work Climates." *Administrative Science Quarterly* 33, no. 1 (March): 101–25. This brilliant piece is reprinted in chapter 6.

17. L. L. Nash, 1990, *Good Intentions Aside* (Boston: Harvard Business School).

18. See, for example, B. Lo, 1987, "Behind Closed Doors: Promises and Pitfalls of Ethics Committees." *The New England Journal of Medicine* 317, no. 1 (2 July): 46–49.

19. M. O'Neill, 1992, "Ethical Dimensions of Nonprofit Administration." *Nonprofit Management and Leadership* 3, no. 2 (Winter): 202.

20. W. Leys, 1943, "Ethics and Administrative Discretion." *Public Administration Review* 3, no. 1 (Winter): 13. Reprinted in its entirety in ch. 3.

21. M. A. Ray, 1994, "Communal Moral Experience as the Starting Point for Research in Health Care Ethics." *Nursing Outlook* 42, no. 3 (May/June): 108.

22. D. C. Maguire, 1979, *The Moral Choice* (Minneapolis, MN: Winston).

23. S. Bok, 1979, *Lying* (New York: Vintage), p. 63.

24. L. L. Nash, 1990, *Good Intentions Aside* (Boston: Harvard Business School Press), p. 248.

25. W. Brace, 1995, "Ideals and Conventions: Ethics for Public Administrators." *Public Administration Review* 55, no. 1 (January/February): 115.

26. M. M. Harmon, 1995, *Responsibility As Paradox* (Newbury Park, CA: Sage).

READING

Although it was written nearly two decades ago, Daniel Callahan's perspective on and analysis of the nature of healthcare ethics remains among the best articulations of the state of the art. The vision is implicitly and rigorously macro—as indicated by his emphasis on policymaking—and that focus is still contemporary. Within that perspective, however, his analysis is illuminating, and his insights are directly applicable to our exploration of the micro dimension of healthcare ethics.

Early on, for example, he argues that ethical analysis can bring guidance to otherwise inchoate practice and behavior. While he is speaking of the macro ethical reality of healthcare, his emphasis on clarity is equally relevant to the micro reality. His contention that "ethical analysis almost always entails a tension between moral ideals" speaks to the concept of ethics as dogma versus ethics as dilemma. Chapter 4 of this book further probes this point. Callahan's discussion of the interaction of law and regulation with ethics anticipates our discussion of controls in chapter 5. His thinking on the locus of decision making—on whose judgment should prevail in ethically challenging situations—will be taken up again in chapter 5. Finally, his phenomenological argument that good ethical analysis begins with detailed understanding of the actual experience of healthcare professionals is fully embraced throughout this book.

CONTEMPORARY BIOMEDICAL ETHICS

Daniel Callahan

The resurgence of biomedical ethics has been a striking phenomenon of the past decade. Although ethics has, of course, always had a role in the practice of medicine, only in recent years has it become a subject of intense interest and controversy. Moreover, this interest has affected a variety of other fields as well, in particular, philosophy, religion, the social sciences, and law. The superficial reasons for the fresh interest are obvious and need not be elaborated on. Seen narrowly, they include a variety of difficult moral dilemmas facing medical practitioners, patients, and the health-care delivery system. Seen broadly, they encompass questions about the nature of health and illness, the goals of medicine, and procedures for decision making. These concerns have generated a large body of literature, a variety of organizations, new legislative and regulatory mechanisms, and considerable comment in the media.

My thesis is that after at least a decade of intense and fruitful activity, biomedical ethics must now move into a new phase, one that will force a rethinking of its role, its methodology, and its relation to other disciplines and institutions. It must do this not only for its own sake as a field still in the process of development, still groping for greater coherence and disciplinary integrity, but also to be of genuine service to medicine at its core, and not just when occasional moral puzzles arise or consciences are troubled. My working assumption is that only rarely can ethical analysis and prescription lead the way in social and cultural change. On the contrary, they ordinarily represent an attempt to organize inchoate and disparate practices and jerry-built and ad hoc principles (what are usually called mores) into a coherent and structured moral system. That system can then be used to provide clearer guidance to practice and behavior. This is not to say that ethics cannot or should not have a radical or reforming role; it can oppose current practices, point out a subversion of important principles, and espouse higher ideals. But that is a relatively rare situation. Its more normal role is to try to interpret and structure the flux of behavior, experience, and intuition, and from there to develop general moral visions and goals together with specific principles and rules to exemplify them.

Two conditions seem necessary for ethics to play that part effectively: in the first place, it must correctly grasp and understand the realities of

Daniel Callahan, "Contemporary Biomedical Ethics," *The New England Journal of Medicine* 302, no. 22 (29 May 1980): 1228–33. Reprinted by permission of *The New England Journal of Medicine*. Copyright 1980, Massachusetts Medical Society. Daniel Callahan is president of the Hastings Center.

culture and society; secondly, the principles and perspectives that it brings to bear must be effective in both their organizational and perceptive power. At a minimum, ethics ought to be of assistance in clarifying accepted general principles and particular moral rules. At the maximum, it ought to take the lead in proposing revised values, in helping to reform or extend the implications of existing rules, and in providing some means for resolving moral disputes. Ethical analysis almost always entails a tension between moral ideals—what we ought to do on the basis of moral values only—and the realities of personal, social, and political life that confound and complicate the pursuit of those ideals.

Let me try, first, to analyze our present situation. Why has there been a fresh interest in biomedical ethics? It is by no means a development that sprung full bloom from the heads of imperialistic or meddlesome moral philosophers or theologians, or from a guilt-ridden, anxious medical profession. I believe that it represents a confluence of forces, both internal and external to medicine. A variety of external causes are apparent: the rise in public concern about the behavior of all professionals, including physicians and biomedical researchers; intensified media attention, particularly when the media are drawn to situations of conflict and controversy; the sheer size and scope of a health-care system, heavily supported by public funds, that inevitably draws the attention of the public, courts, and legislatures; the general uneasiness and ambivalence about technology that has been a mark of the past two decades; discontent with a perceived lack of humaneness and quality in medical care; and the steady pressures on the health-care delivery system to deal with the whole range of human problems, many of which traditionally would not have been regarded as medical at all.

The internal reasons seem no less evident: a number of medical and technologic breakthroughs have created new moral dilemmas. There are problems in the care of the newborn and of the dying, in the use of psychotropic and other drugs to influence and change mood and behavior, in the development of an expanded scope of genetic knowledge and applied clinical applications, and in greater dilemmas of equity and distribution in the health-care delivery system. Had there been no external pressures at all, it is still likely that the internal pressures resulting from rapid technologic developments would themselves have created sufficient impetus for a renewed interest in biomedical ethics. Rapid technologic change forces a confrontation with received values and moral principles. The moral vision that gave coherence and guidance in the past under one set of social conditions appears threatened by new and disruptive conditions and what could be newer and more disruptive than immediately induced changes in mankind's ancient struggle with illness and death?

It is hardly surprising, then, that the literature of contemporary bioethics centers around moral dilemmas generated by emergent technologies. At the same time, it is important not to lose sight of the larger external cultural context, which has intensified, influenced, and broadcasted the impact of the internal pressures.

When questions of ethics are widely and heatedly discussed, it is a good rule of thumb to assume that some larger cultural process is taking place, of which a concern with morality is only one symptom. After a long period of very rapid advance marked by the development of antibiotics and the control of infectious disease, medicine has now settled down to a somewhat different pattern, marked by slower therapeutic progress, higher budgets, a more complex delivery system, and a closer interaction of medicine with other parts of the society. The moral problems of contemporary biomedicine have stimulated questioning of the fundamental goals of medicine, and they are also a reflection of that questioning. Although it might casually be assumed that, for moral purposes, the traditional goals of medical care can remain unquestioned, that would be a naive assumption. Moral problems eventually force a confrontation with goals. How can one talk seriously about the moral responsibility of the physician without eventually asking what the physician is supposed to provide? How can one discuss an equitable distribution of health-care resources without also struggling with the question of what resources ought to be delivered, to whom, and under what circumstances? How can one examine the rights of patients without, in the very process, asking what patients want or ought to want? How can one cope with finding the right balance between investing money in basic research and investing money in the delivery of health care without asking what, in both the short and long run, medicine ought to seek in the name of human welfare?

The inevitability of such questions helps to explain why the emergence of a fresh interest in biomedical ethics has been met by some resistance. To be sure, physicians and medical researchers have on many occasions been resentful of the new laws and regulations to which they have been subjected. They have correctly perceived that the public's discussion of ethics has been one important cause of that development. And they have not always been pleased to find lawyers and those called "ethicists" wandering about, often causing trouble, in territory that they once considered their private preserve. A tradition of empiricism and positivism in medicine, which has held "soft" disciplines in some disdain, has only heightened suspicion about the value of ethical discourse. Matters are not helped by constant confusing of ethics with moralizing, indoctrination, whistle-blowing, or mere taste. Nonetheless, despite all these reasons for skepticism, I suggest that the primary reason for resistance is simply that, if ethics is taken seriously at all, it must force an examination of fundamental goals and assumptions. That is never a very pleasant enterprise, whether the impetus comes from ethics, the law, or any other source. It is difficult enough to practice any complex discipline, even when agreement exists on its goals and purposes; there will still be some moral problems. But when moral problems are combined with uncertainty concerning professional purposes, the stage is set for considerable anxiety, suspicion, and resistance.

Yet uncertainty within medicine is not the only reason for interest in bioethics. The fact that academic philosophers have flocked to the subject says something also about contemporary philosophy. For some decades, especially during the 40's and 50's, philosophy was a narrow, dry, and technical field. Only recently has it come out of its deep slumber, as questions have been raised about the purposes of philosophy (internally and externally there as well). In that context, the problems of biomedicine have provided both interesting and difficult material to test the proposition that moral philosophy could, despite its sophisticated detractors, have something pertinent to say about human life. In that sense, not only is medicine itself being tested by ethics, but ethics itself is being tested by medicine.

How has biomedical ethics progressed and responded during the past decade? At the risk of considerable oversimplification, one can cite four broad currents, each jousting with the others for dominance. One current can conveniently be associated with the name of Joseph Fletcher, whose book *Morals and Medicine*[1] and other writings espouse a radical "situation ethics" and a rejection of fixed moral rules and principles. In deciding whether a defective neonate should be allowed to die, for example, we should be bound by no hard-and-fast moral rules; context and consequences alone should be decisive. Professor Fletcher's works have found a warm reception among many physicians, for whom the specificity and idiosyncrasy of individual clinical cases seem a dominant feature. By virtue of his rejection of what he calls "absolutes," he has been a congenial thinker for those who would emphasize the importance of moral flexibility and the dominance of context over abstract ideas. A second current is well reflected in the works of Paul Ramsey, beginning with *The Patient as Person.*[2] In contrast to Fletcher, Professor Ramsey has emphasized the importance of firm moral rules, has rejected the notion of a situation ethics, and has steadfastly urged adherence to traditional medical and religious moral principles. If Professor Fletcher's tendency has been to say "yes" to recent biomedical advances and the permissive liberal culture of which they are a part, Professor Ramsey's tendency has been to say "no" and to oppose to that culture principles that require drawing sharp lines.

Professors Fletcher and Ramsey were trained as theologians. A third current has been signaled by the entrance of a group of younger moral philosophers into medical ethics. Mostly trained in the dominant analytical school, they have tended to reject what seems to them the gross imprecision and crude utilitarianism of Joseph Fletcher and the rigid theological moralism of Paul Ramsey. As a consequence, they have been much more inclined to clarify and analyze problems and concepts than to propose moral solutions (which neither Fletcher nor Ramsey have ever hesitated to do). At the same time, their work has reflected in the language of secular philosophy the struggle between the strongly utilitarian biases of Fletcher and the equally strong principle-focused (often called deontological) proclivities of Ramsey. All, however, display in their writings the characteristics noted above concerning the role of ethics: they attempt to interpret present realities and to propose a scheme of moral order for those realities.

A fourth current is represented in the works of those who have tried to find both a different language with which to talk about ethics and a different way of framing issues. This tendency can be seen in an emphasis on virtue, as in the case of Alastair MacIntyre; covenant, as in the case of William F. May; or fidelity, as in the case of James M. Gustafson. All share some degree of resistance to what has been called "dilemma ethics," that is, a reduction of the moral life to problems of resolving particular moral dilemmas.

If one can discern various schools and currents in ethics, all drawing on old and deep streams in Western philosophical and religious thought, one can also discern some general developments that have had a profound effect on recent biomedical ethics. Perhaps the most important is the increasingly strong interaction between ethics, law, and regulation. One of the most important trends of the past decade has been the rapidity with which ethical debate has been taken to court, has been the subject of legislation, and has stimulated regulatory activity. One need only mention the Karen Ann Quinlan case, the Saikewicz case, human-subject regulation, the regulation of recombinant-DNA research, and so on, to signal that development. It has had two important consequences: an excessive emphasis on the language of individual rights, and a blurring of the distinction between law and morality.

More than one social commentator has noted the excessive tendency in recent American society to use and overuse the language of "rights." It is not difficult to understand why that should be the case. On the one hand, it is a language very congenial to courts and to the political process;

it is the kind of language that, if successfully carried through, can ensure concrete victories and immediate change in the social and political arena. On the other hand, it is a congenial language because it focuses for the most part on individuals, rather than on society as a whole or on the welfare of an entire community. Thus, it is a language that plays directly into the hands of American individualism and also reflects the absence of any strong communal language with equally effective social force. Terms such as "the public interest" or the "common good" do not seem to have a political bite equal to that of claims to individual entitlements. As much as many in the field of ethics and other disciplines can well deplore an obsessive focus on individual rights at the expense of other moral values, its favored status in the political arena has brought questions of rights to the fore. If the most prominent example is the debate on abortion between the "pro-life," and the "pro-choice" forces—the right to life of fetuses over the right of women to their own moral choices—analogies abound in most other moral debates.

A second consequence of the increasing interaction between ethics, law, and regulation is a blurring of the appropriate role and boundaries of each of them. The simple fact is that court decisions, legislation, and governmental regulations make a decisive difference in our country in the ways in which people actually behave and, beyond that, in their perceptions of both the positive ideals and the negative constraints of morality. Perhaps one of the most harmful fruits of a permissive society dominated by the language of individual rights is that it is very hard for a large number of people in our society to make any sharp distinction between the different demands of law and morality. In principle, it is easy enough to distinguish between what the law may or should allow or prohibit for the sake of public order and what the requirements of personal morality may or should allow. But as the debate over abortion, regulation of psychotropic drugs, or care of the dying patient indicates, the language of principled personal or social morality is one that leaves many uneasy. It is far easier simply to talk about the right of individuals to make their own decisions or about the establishment of public procedures to adjudicate among contending values and interests than it is to talk about what individuals ought to do when they make personal moral choices. The latter is, helter-skelter, left to the realm of taste, caste, and subjectivity.

Nonetheless, it should be evident that both personal and social values are constantly being shaped. A common allegation against formal ethical analysis is that little if any progress is ever made in the field; nothing gets decided and disputes are endless. But that allegation makes sense only if one expects a clean-cut, decisive resolution of ethical conflicts here and now, with one side accepting the arguments of another side or one view becoming so rationally persuasive that all instantly adopt it. That happens infrequently. Nevertheless, if the past decade has made anything clear, it is that a number of ethical disputes have been resolved, although in ways that can best be seen only retrospectively. One can think of any number of arguments over the past decade that resulted, finally, in at least a rough and broad consensus—for example, the debates over whether it is appropriate for the government to regulate research on human subjects, over the appropriateness of a brain-death criterion for the pronouncement of human death, and over whether physicians should always strive to keep every patient alive regardless of the patient's condition. All those debates have subsided, and the only arguments remaining turn on comparatively minor squabbles concerning what the resolution of the debate actually means. (What, for instance, does "informed consent" really mean?) Even the earlier fight about "socialized medicine" (a term little heard these days) has changed considerably. Practically all those who argue over the issue of national health insurance and government-funded medical aid for the poor and others acknowledge the need for a better distribution of health-care resources. Most people are prepared to agree that there are profound inequities in the health-care delivery system. The debates now concentrate on the best means of achieving a better distribution of care and services, whether through a market mechanism, through direct government control of the health-care system, or through some combination of the two. Only that very hardy perennial, abortion, seems resistant to a general moral consensus. But even in that case, one should recall that the abortion-reform movement only began in the 1950's, that the 1973 *Roe vs. Wade* decision made a real difference in the availability of legal and safe abortions, and that the practice of abortion is now common throughout the country. In short, life does not stand still in ethics any more than anywhere else. The experience of the past decade should indicate that the question is not whether ethical conflicts get resolved or ethical questions answered, but how well they get resolved and how good the consensual answers are.

A distinction is in order at this point. Many broad ethical agreements can and have been reached recently in the absence of any agreement on the theoretical principles and foundations at stake. A theological rationale for ceasing to treat a dying patient can be very different from a secular, humanitarian rationale; yet the theologian and the secular humanitarian may achieve complete accord on appropriate standards of action concerning the dying patient. What I want now to contend is that the next round of ethical problems may be far more resistant to practical consensus than those that captured attention during the past decade.

They will be resistant precisely because they will much more directly force a grappling with theoretical issues of morality and medicine, and they will, more than ever, reveal the shortcomings of the language of "rights," of individualism, and of merely procedural solutions to problems of deep principle. Let me try to sustain that thesis by focusing on a central problem of contemporary medical ethics, the doctor-patient relation, and also focus on just that moral principle concerning the relation that seems the most obvious and easily defended.

In a recent article,[3] Dr. Carleton B. Chapman was critical of the traditional code of medical ethics of the American Medical Association and also of the new code presently [*sic*] being debated. Along with other critics, he notes that "nowhere does one derive a sense of primary and dominant concern for the patient." He urges that "the profession should put its unwritten patient-centered ethic into written form and officially affirm the profession's commitment to it. . . . Once the professional relation between physician and patient is established, the physician must put the patient's interests, welfare and rights above all other considerations." As important as his recommendation is, it is simply not clear that it can do full justice to the emerging ethical situation.

At the least, the principle of a patient-centered ethic will have to be placed in the context of a number of other contemporary moral principles and social realities. The main problem that I would raise is whether it is desirable to elevate any single moral principle to a position of overriding importance. If one can assume that Dr. Chapman is correct in asserting that a patient-centered ethic has always been implicit (and I think he is), it does not necessarily follow that it should always take precedence over other moral principles or considerations. Instead, it should be asked whether the very idea of a single-value morality can be adequate to a fully balanced professional ethic. Some examples may help to make my point clear. In the law, the most important moral principle has traditionally been the interests of the client; in journalism, the right of the public to information; and in medicine, the welfare of the patient. But in each case, it has become obvious that other values are now becoming more important—values that, although they do not by any means lead to rejection of the importance of those principles, force them to be set alongside others that are perhaps no less important. It is increasingly recognized in journalism, for instance, that the right of citizens to privacy, to confidentiality, and to their personal reputation can be as important as any right of the public to information. An earlier journalistic ethic held that a reporter could use any means available, at whatever cost to other moral principles, to get a good story. And why not, if the only moral principle of consequence was the right of the public to information? In the case of the law, it is increasingly recognized that, however important the interests of the client, there can also be other interests—justice, fairness, and the protection of the system of law. No longer can the idea of the "adversary system" or of the "lawyer-client privilege" mechanically be invoked as a reason for violating other, more general moral rules.

In medicine, it is clear that many physicians must now serve legitimate interests and values in addition to those of individual patient welfare. Those in the field of public health are charged with the welfare of whole groups of individuals, as are those who serve in administrative roles. Even the physician in private practice must consider on occasion the welfare of a family and not necessarily only that of a single patient in that family. Difficult decisions of allocations of resources must sometimes be made. Which patients, and under what circumstances, should be served when not all can be served equally well? There are, in fact, many imaginable circumstances in which a physician's duty to the public, to a family, or to a valuable policy could take precedence over obligations to an individual patient.

None of this is to deny the value of a patient-centered ethic. But can it always be the inevitably superior value? I doubt it, at least in some circumstances. The more complex issue is that ways will have to be found to balance that ethic off against the legitimate interests of the public, to adjudicate conflicts of other moral principles with those of patient welfare, and to define just what, in the end, is in the interest of the welfare of individual patients. In the face of scarcity and the necessity for allocation decisions, it would no doubt be noxious to make individual physicians bear the full weight of making such decisions, and thus force them to choose between and among patients. Nonetheless, it is evident that for judicial and financial reasons, the trend is in the direction of limitations on what physicians may do in the name of individual patient welfare, e.g., unlimited diagnostic tests at the expense of third-party payers.

It should remain the deepest desire of the physician, even in that context, to serve individual patient welfare. But the external structure of medical practice under the present health-care delivery system will inevitably force limits on what physicians may do for patients and restrict the choices that they can make. It will not do to say that the interests of individual patient welfare are to be dominant unless clearly superseded by other moral considerations. That would tell us little of real moral value. Eventually, only a deeper analysis of the relation between the good of individuals and the good of communities will be helpful; this analysis will only be obfuscating if it sees communal welfare as nothing more than the aggregate welfare of individuals (a weakness of the concept of the "public interest").

Paradoxically, in the face of bureaucratic and economic pressures it may never have been more important than it is now to stress the necessity of a patient-centered ethic; it is perhaps as important to stress other values that physicians ought to serve as well—social, family, and communal values. That sets the stage, unfortunately, for far more difficult ethical choices and dilemmas for the physician than were required earlier, and analogous demands are creating the same situation for lawyers and journalists.

At just that point, some fundamental assumptions about the nature of medical ethics must be reexamined. The mark of an older medical ethics was a strong focus on the moral dilemmas of the individual practitioner. That was a pattern very much in keeping with the dominance of professionals, with the individualistic ethos of our culture, and with the perceived need, in a pluralistic society, to allow individuals to make choices in consonance with their own consciences and professional judgments. It presumed as its model that of one physician treating one patient, the necessity for some qualified or expert individual to make a final choice, and the general belief that there could be no fixed answers to specific moral dilemmas. The most important recent change has been to call that model into question. As the Karen Ann Quinlan case made perfectly clear, individualistic solutions can simply be impossible when there are sharp contradictions in the values of individuals. No one suggested that either the physicians or the parent in her case were acting in anything less than a virtuous manner. The parents had one set of reasonable values—their claimed right to make the decision—and the physicians had another set of reasonable values—their claimed right to make the decision. The matter had eventually to be taken to court; there was no way that problem could logically be solved in the context of an ethic centered on the individual consciences or qualifications of the various actors.

Although pluralism needs to be respected in this country, a great number of biomedical advances have indicated that some general solutions and binding group norms need to be worked out that are of more than a consensual or procedural kind. Not all issues can be left in the hands of individuals. Important developments in recent biomedicine have been expensive high technology, a massive system of third-party payments, and rapidly increasing economic pressure on medicine. Together, they have made evident mainly by omission, that ethics has had much more to say at the level of individual decision making than at the level of policymaking. Those in ethics have had little to contribute to the general discussion of the allocation of resources, the development of a just health care delivery system, or the adjudication of the rights and claims of different competing groups. Moreover, having attempted to deal with them myself, I can say that those problems seem to me infinitely more complex than those that many of us in the field of biomedical ethics cut our teeth on. By contrast, an issue such as the definition of death is relatively simple and discrete. The just allocation of health resources is far more complex—calling into question a wide range of group values and interests, and of conceptions of the nature of American society, and a far greater array of experts from different fields. There is not one problem to be solved, but perhaps a dozen, and the difficulty of solving all of them simultaneously—which seems to be the ridiculous requirement—strains all the capacities of those in ethics and in every other field as well. Yet those are and will be the important moral problems of the future. To be sure, there will still be difficult individual life-and-death decisions and hard individual choices for physicians and other health-care workers, for patients, and for families. But on a national scale those decisions are going to be overshadowed by large structural moral and political decisions. It is these decisions that will eventually shape the individual decisions.

Looking back over the recent history of biomedical ethics, I think it is fair to say that biomedical ethics has elevated and improved the general discussion of morals and medicine. It has brought greater clarity, some degree of resolution in many areas, perhaps some minor degree of improvement in medical care, and a generally increased sensitivity to the moral dilemmas of medical decision making. On the other hand, so rapid have been the changes within the past decade in the delivery of health care that the ethical deliberations have barely been able to keep pace. The increasing necessity to make social and policy decisions for large groups, indeed, for the whole population in some cases, raises fresh and extraordinarily difficult moral problems. It will force biomedical ethics to move into the mainstream of political and social theory, beyond the model of the individual decision maker, and into the thicket of important vested and legitimate private and group interests. The language of "rights" is not likely to be up to that task, unless there is a better language for the rights of an entire group, nor is a focus on the intricacy of individual decision making likely to be of much help.

At this point, I can only offer some items that need to be put more squarely on the future agenda of biomedical ethics. The most important is the necessity for a closer working relation between those in ethics and those in medicine. At least part of that agenda is in the process of development. Those in ethics have learned, mainly by hard experience, that they will make little sense to practicing physicians if they are not fully aware of the experience and details of clinical practice. It is simply not enough for those in ethics to roll up to the bedside the ghost of Immanuel Kant, John Stuart Mill, or G. E. Moore and provide instant moral diagnoses. It is hardly better to do the same with the writings of John Rawls. If the ultimate strength of ethics lies in its capacity to develop coherent modes of ethical analysis and comprehensive moral systems, it needs at the moment far greater skill in penetrating the often confused dynamic of the clinical setting. Only after a detailed analysis of the actual experience of the clinician (or a patient trying to work out a moral choice) can it be in any position either to invoke traditional theories or develop new ones.

If that is true of clinical medicine, it is even more true of health-care policy. One can at least talk with an individual physician or patient; experience can be evoked, and some understanding reached. That is not so with large-scale policy issues. Matters of policy are rarely decided by individuals. Policies are shaped by a variety of actors and are implemented by still others. Only in rare cases can any individual be said to have the crucial decision-making power. The unfortunate temptation in that situation for those in ethics is to retreat to a global analysis, one heavy on general principles, high theory, and ideal solutions. If the tendency of the policy maker is to be too sensitive to constraints, too willing to compromise, and too easily intimidated by special-interest groups, the opposite seems the case with many in ethics: constraints are ignored, compromise eschewed, and interest groups bypassed. Contemporary biomedical ethics is learning only very slowly the way to do ethical analysis and to foster moral values within a political system marked by limits, which means that most ethical and moral solutions will be second-best solutions. The idea of an "applied ethics" is growing, and that idea must encompass not only the individual decision maker but the policy-making process as well.

If those in ethics must learn to work more closely with those in medicine, they must also learn to do so with those in the law and the social sciences. The relation between ethics, law, and regulation cries out for more careful analysis. If it is true, as I have suggested, that many in our society now hopelessly confuse the different demands of law and morality, then it is imperative that the differences between them once again be sorted out. If personal morality comes down to nothing more than the exercise of free choice, with no principles available for moral judgment of the quality of those choices, then law will inevitably be used to fill the resulting moral vacuum. If individual standards and self-restraint cannot be counted on, then regulation will be used to ensure an acceptable standard of public behavior. As much as we might appreciate the value of individual autonomy, it is not likely that we will allow someone else's exercise of autonomy to endanger or diminish our lives.

The troubled relation between the law and ethics is matched by that between ethics and the social sciences. The latter are now commonly looked to for the data and information necessary to formulate policy. The techniques of linear programming and of cost-benefit, risk-benefit, and systems analysis have become the common tools of the medical-policy analyst. Although it is well recognized that those tools are laden with value judgments, anything but neutral in their premises and uses, little attention has been paid to the moral problems inherent in their use. Since policy formulation and implementation require an enormous amassing of data, nothing seems more necessary for the future than greater clarity about the ethical issues at stake. Short of pointing out the problems, those in ethics have had little to say of a positive, helpful nature, and those in the social sciences, willing enough to concede the moral problems in a general way, continue to practice as usual. And why not? They have been offered no alternatives.

I have suggested only an agendum here. As in the other issues touched on, progress can be expected—that is, something will happen that will represent a change. The challenge now is to make certain that the change is indeed progress and that the solutions are worthy ones.

References

1. Fletcher JF. Morals and medicine: the moral problems of the patient's right to know the truth, contraception, artificial insemination, sterilization, euthanasia. Boston: Beacon Press, 1954.
2. Ramsey P. The patient as person: explorations in medical ethics. New Haven: Yale University Press, 1970.
3. Chapman CB. On the definition and teaching of the medical ethic. N Engl J Med. 1979; 301: 630–4.

CASE B

TO ADMIT OR NOT TO ADMIT

The following report presents and analyzes a situation involving nursing home admissions. At the macro level public policy has determined that biased, preferential admissions procedures and behavior are forbidden. It is dogma that all applicants for admission to nursing homes are to be treated equally and fairly. The micro level presents some difficulties in dealing with the dogma. Specifically, this case examines the dilemma confronted when a nursing home is screening patients for an admission.

The executive vice president of the adjoining hospital is urging the administrative director of the nursing home to give priority admission to a private-paying patient despite an official open admissions policy. The policy in place states: *It is the policy of the Bonhomme Nursing Home Co., Inc. to admit and treat all patients without regard to race, creed, color, national origin, sex, handicap or source of payment.* Nevertheless, it has been common practice of the nursing home—and of other nursing facilities in the area—to seek private-paying, non-Medicare/Medicaid patients because of the financial benefits that ensue. These patients are routinely given priority over government-supported patients who may have been on the waiting list for months.

Scenario

Mrs. Midas, a native-born prominent citizen of the community, is currently a patient at Community Memorial Hospital. Mrs. Midas is 86 years old and has been diagnosed with arteriosclerotic heart disease and chronic pulmonary disease. Prior to her hospitalization, Mrs. Midas lived independently in her own home, receiving services from the Visiting Nurse Association. Mrs. Midas has been hospitalized several times during the past year. In consultation with the hospital discharge planner, the nursing home administrator is informed that Mrs. Midas' son and daughter are interested in pursuing nursing home placement, but only at the Bonhomme Nursing Home. The patient and family have signed a consent form giving the hospital permission to send out referrals to area skilled nursing facilities. The family states that the patient has considerable assets and would be a private-paying resident. The family is aware that although they have a preference for the Bonhomme Nursing Home, it is the hospital policy (and for Medicare patients, a regulation) to refer the patient to all area skilled nursing facilities to increase their chances of getting placed. However, since Mrs. Midas is a private-paying patient, the family and patient can refuse bed offers that are made from facilities they are not interested in, unlike Medicare or Medicaid patients who cannot refuse a bed offer without losing their Medicare/Medicaid benefits.

The preadmissions committee composed of the nursing home administrator, the social worker, and the director of nursing, review Mrs. Midas' application and medical record, and add her to the waiting list. Chronologically there are approximately 60 people ahead of her on the waiting list. The committee is informed by the administrator that the executive vice president of the hospital has instructed him to give priority for the next available bed to Mrs. Midas.

Dilemma

Should the nursing home administrator follow the directive of the executive vice president despite the official policy and the length of the waiting list? Or should he adhere to the procedure of working down the list and screening patients until a "suitable" patient is found? What is the ethical thing to do?

Familial and Patient Factors

The private-pay patient's family is eager to get her placed and settled in a facility. Upon interviewing the patient, the social worker discovers that—contrary to what the family is saying—Mrs. Midas has ambivalent feelings regarding nursing home placement. Although she is agreeable to placement, there appears to be little patient understanding and preparation on the part of the family. The patient has many valid personal questions and fears that have not been addressed, and is concerned about her assets, the breaking up of her home, and loss of her independence.

The family apparently is no longer able to provide the necessary care for Mrs. Midas at home and is experiencing feelings of guilt. The family expresses several concerns: not knowing how to properly care for the patient, having no time for a life of their own, and having no time for their families.

In screening the Medicare/Medicaid candidates involved in this situation, the patients and families seem sincere and genuine. Although these patients express many of the same fears regarding nursing home placement, many have no homes or no families to assist them. Some of these patients are confused and experience short-term memory problems. Some recognize family members but are easily disoriented to time and place, most likely due to their long hospital stays. Several of these patients would be candidates for programs at a skilled nursing facility as opposed to lying in a hospital bed hoping for placement and becoming more debilitated.

Medical Factors

All of the patients screened and interviewed require skilled nursing care and thus cannot be discharged to a lower level of care. Also, none of the patients has any known history of psychological problems, nor are any of them receiving special medication or using special equipment. However, the preadmissions committee finds that one of the Medicaid patients screened exhibits a great deal of motivation and would likely benefit most from nursing home placement.

Organizational, Fiscal, and Political Factors

Some salient organizational dynamics are at work in this situation. Although the hospital and nursing home are separate entities, they are governed by the same board of directors and the executive vice president oversees the operation of both facilities. Under this setup, the administrator of the nursing home is responsible to the executive vice president. Within the past three years, the hospital has experienced severe financial setbacks and it remains in the throes of a scandal involving embezzlement. The hospital has hired a consulting firm to oversee its operations for the next three years. The new hospital executive vice president was hired through this firm. Understandably, in view of the financial situation, administrators are anxious to increase revenues. Admitting a higher-paying private patient over a Medicare/Medicaid one makes financial sense.

In terms of loyalty to the organization, the nursing home administrator is no fool. He knows what is at stake; he knows about being a team player; he knows about his own job security and future in the organization. And he knows the stated policy and regulatory expectations.

Further complicating the present situation is the insertion of outside political influence. The community's mayor has written a letter to the executive vice president asking that Mrs. Midas be given priority.

Reflective Ramblings

In reflecting on the situation the nursing home administrator writes the following in his journal:

> Honesty is a multifaceted value affecting many people in this particular dilemma. There is honesty to myself, honesty to the organization, and honesty to the patients. In this situation honesty to myself and to the patients, as opposed to the organization, could result in serious reprimands from above. Being honest to myself and to the patients would mean proceeding with the regular admissions process as opposed to giving priority to a private-paying patient. But I would run the risk of reprimand or even the loss of my job. If I were to act in a dishonest manner, my actions would be looked upon as favorable within the work arena. What should I do? I lean toward accepting the private paying patient because 95 percent of our current resident population is Medicare/Medicaid and only 5 percent are private-pay. At other facilities, the ratio is reversed. My loyalty to the organization stems from a sense of duty and service. Given the financial situation and my experience here, I appreciate the needs of the institution. At this time it is essential that the organization be efficient in all its operations. We can no longer afford to operate in an inefficient manner. It could result in the closing of one or both of the facilities, loss of jobs, displaced patients/residents, and the loss of two valuable services to the community. These losses could not be sustained by the community and would be economically detrimental to the area. Given this situation, an ethically efficient approach for me as the administrator would be to give priority to the private-pay patient thereby maintaining the hospital and nursing home optimum funding with little or no known negative impacts to any of the patients. Any ethical implications that may occur would be minimal compared to the ethical implications that could result from inefficiency—like loss of jobs, for instance, and/or the closing of the facilities.
>
> At this point in time the hospital and nursing home administrators need to be concerned about the finances; therefore, it is timely that we seek out private-paying patients not for profit, but simply for survival. This could change in time when the facilities become more financially stable. Therefore, in the light of these hard economic times, private-paying patients should be given priority. It is ethically acceptable to act in this manner, but only if we are open and willing to change should the financial situation change.

Questions for Discussion

1. Do you agree with the administrator's decision and reasoning? If not, what do you suggest, and what is your reasoning?

2. Is the thinking manifested in this case simply justification for dishonesty, unfairness, and self-service?
3. When organizational survival is in conflict with the values of honesty and fairness, what is the ethical thing to do?
4. What appears to be the administrator's approach to doing ethics? What approach would you recommend?
5. What does this case suggest about the intersection of macro policy ethics issues with micro administrative ethics issues?
6. The nursing home administrator could have directed his ethical deliberation at the responsibility of the executive vice president instead of at his own ethical responsibility in the situation. What differences, if any, are there between analyzing the former and probing the latter?

Annotated Bibliography

Aroskar, M. "Anatomy of an Ethical Dilemma: The Theory, the Practice." *American Journal of Nursing* 42 (April 1980): 658–59. A good, brief, and rare look at a micro-level dilemma in healthcare.

Arras, J., and B. Steinbock. *Ethical Issues in Modern Medicine*, 4th ed. Mountain View, CA: Mayfield, 1995. An excellent macro view of ethical realities in healthcare.

Foster, G. "Law, Morality and the Public Servant." *Public Administration Review* 41, no. 1 (January/February 1981): 29–34. Offers an insightful critique of ethics as dogma alone.

Gatewood, R., and A. Carroll. "Assessment of Ethical Performance of Organization Members: A Conceptual Framework." *Academy of Management Review* 16, no. 4 (October 1991): 667–90. Presents a tool for evaluating ethical behavior in terms of right-wrong dogma.

Glaser, J. *Three Realms of Ethics*. Kansas City, MO: Sheed and Ward, 1994. Part one a sensational approach to dilemma reality; most of the cases macro level, however.

Griffith, J. *The Moral Challenges of Health Care Management*. Chicago: Health Administration Press, 1993. In probing the professional and organizational dimensions of healthcare ethics, an important companion to our book focused on the individual healthcare professional.

Harrington, S. "What Corporate America Is Teaching About Ethics," *The Executive* (February 1991): 21–30. Offers a framework for conceptualizing managerial ethics from the perspective that good ethics is simply good business.

Harron, F., J. Burnside, and T. Beauchamp. *Health and Human Values*. New Haven, CT: Yale University Press, 1983. Among the best at articulating the values horizon of dilemma ethics and offering approaches to moral reasoning; focuses, too, however, on the macro dimension.

Kuhn, W. "Toward an Agenda for Business Ethics Research." *Academy of Management Review* 15, no. 2 (April 1990): 311–28. A very helpful overview of the study of managerial ethics.

Nash, L. *Good Intentions Aside*. Boston: Harvard Business School Press, 1990. A practical and insightful analysis of the ethical dimension. Although focused on organizational ethics, much is relevant to our interest in individual ethics.

Purtillo, R., and C. Cassels. *Ethical Dimensions in the Health Care Professions*. Philadelphia: Saunders, 1981. Although dated, an excellent and rare effort at probing some micro dimension issues for healthcare professionals.

Ray, M. "Communal Moral Experience as the Starting Point for Research in Health Care Ethics," *Nursing Outlook* 42, no. 3 (May/June 1994): 104–109. Presents an overview of current approaches—largely macro and dogmatic—to nursing ethics study.

Willbern, Y. "Types and Levels of Public Morality." *Public Administration Review* 44, no. 2 (March/April 1984): 102–108. An interesting perspective on categories of ethical reality in public service.

POWER AND THE HEALTHCARE PROFESSIONAL: THE BAD THINGS THAT WE GOOD PEOPLE DO

WHAT IS professional power? Do we, as individual healthcare professionals, have any? How powerful is each of us? And what does that have to do with ethics? This chapter reflects on these questions in a quest to raise our consciousness of the power reality in the daily routine of the practice of healthcare.

When these questions are raised, I find that professionals typically deny that they wield power: "The administration has power, the boss has power, the medical director has power. But not me. I wish I did." Dennis Thompson claims that a professional "ethic of neutrality" causes professionals to underestimate the power they actually exercise.[1] A bit more cynically, Michael Lipsky maintains that denying power is a common way to limit responsibility: "[Professionals] seek to deny that they have influence, are free to make decisions, or offer service alternatives. Strict adherence to rules and refusals to make exceptions when exceptions might be made provide . . . defenses against the possibility that they might be able to act more as clients would wish."[2] A fifteenth-century monk, Thomas à Kempis, offers a more philosophical explanation: "We blame little things on others and pass over great things in ourselves; we are quick enough in perceiving and weighing what we suffer from others, but we mind not what others suffer from us."[3] In any case, we do seem to place restraints on awareness of the power we wield as professionals, and that may be the major obstacle to raising our ethical maturity. So let's focus the PCV reality prism, introduced in the last chapter, on the subject of this chapter: power.

What Is Professional Power?

First, when we say "professional power" what are we talking about? Simply put, it is the ability to influence or affect the life of another person by virtue of the professional position we hold. It is not about affecting people by virtue of who we are personally, how big we are, how loud our voice, or how charismatic our personality—although these kinds of things can be involved. Power primarily concerns the *influence* stemming from the professional position we hold. It is the ability to have an *impact* on the state of being of a person—physically, mentally, emotionally, psychologically, spiritually—in the context of the professional role. In professional literature it is often referred to as "discretion." It is about *dependence*; as Kabanoff astutely articulates it: "A has power over B to the extent that B depends on A to supply B with outcomes or resources that B values and for which B has no alternative source of supply."[4] In Ed Pellegrino's view, it reflects *inequality*, and he suggests that the power imbalance between patient and physician must become the root of a new medical ethic.[5] In Karen Lebacqz's brilliant illumination, it bespeaks *vulnerability* and unnatural intimacy: "The intimacy that arises between professional and client is not the natural intimacy of sharing living space and common necessities through time, but an *imposed* intimacy. It is an intimacy given with some reluctance to secure some end."[6] It involves, in Linda Trevino's words, *behavior* "affecting the lives and well-being of others."[7]

But what has this power thing to do with ethics? In a word, **everything**. John Rohr argues that such power is "at the heart" of the ethical issue and "should form the basis of our approach to ethics."[8] I agree. Michael O'Neill notes that "Confucianism reminds us that any time power enters a human relationship, ethics must follow."[9] I agree. And Lou Gawthrop eloquently maintains that Athens left to the future of civilization "a code that fixed ethical responsibility squarely on the shoulders of anyone who presumed to affect the lives of others."[10] I agree wholeheartedly! The professional power that we wield is the foundation of the ethical dimension of healthcare. Indeed, this book could aptly be subtitled, "A Reflection for the Powerful."

Yet, remarkably, the reality of professional power has been probed very little in the ethics literature or in professional studies. As Davis correctly describes the situation: "Writers . . . characteristically recognize the role of discretion and explore all around the perimeter of it but seldom try to penetrate it."[11] And, as Mark Lilla rightly observes, "the task for which students are now unprepared is the responsible use of the discretion with which they find themselves."[12] This situation is alarming if one agrees, as I do, with Rohr and others that it is always dangerous when the powerful are unaware of their own power.

So, let us reflect. *Why* are healthcare professionals powerful? Why is it allowed? The short answer is so that we can get the job done, so that we can heal people and care for people and comfort people. Power is there for all good reasons, and power is essential if healthcare is to be delivered. The problem is not that power is bad, but that the good reasons for having it can nonetheless produce bad results. Therefore, any useful reflection on power is not about the bad things that bad people do, but rather about the bad things that we good people, we healthcare professionals, can easily end up doing.

There are two key reasons, I think, that help explain how and why we can end up doing some bad things. One is a natural result of being powerful: it is not, as Lord Acton presumed, that power corrupts; rather it is, as Will and Ariel Durant observed, that "power *dements* . . . lowering the guard of foresight and raising the haste of action."[13] A second reason is suggested in the movie, *Edward Scissorhands*. Edward is created with hands and fingers made of the finest and sharpest cutlery. Endowed with these special hands he is able to do some wonderful things. He cuts and trims lawns and shrubs and makes them magnificent. He grooms animals and styles peoples' hair in beautiful ways. He is very powerful. Then he falls in love, and with his special hands he reaches out to caress his love and, instead, his fingers cut her face and she bleeds. His wonderful power is, like ours, also dangerous; and if we, like Edward, are under-aware of our power, we, too, can unwittingly harm the very people we love and seek to serve.

What makes a healthcare professional powerful? What is our equivalent of the cutlery hands of Edward Scissorhands? From where does the power of a healthcare professional come? What is the source? It is the professional position in general, certainly, but Raven and Kruglanski[14] offer more specific insight to facilitate our understanding. They identify six "power bases" related to professional positions. One is *coercive* power. The power of coercion stems from fear of what we can do to people from our position. We can hurt particular patients with the needle if we don't like them. We can make them wait. We can reprimand our clients and staff. We can assign a C grade instead of a B. This power basis tends to make clients and subordinates treat us with deference and comply with what we do and want. They allow us to get away with a lot, to be powerful over them, out of fear for what we can do to them.

A second basis they identify is our *connective* power. They need us to refer them to the hospital they want; they need us for a reference to get the job they want; they need us in order to get access to what they need or want. They put up with us, allow us power over them, comply with our whims in order to gain favor with us or to avoid disfavor, because they need a particular connection and we are their option.

A third power source is our expertise, or perhaps more accurately, our *presumed* expertise, skill, or knowledge. Because they believe we possess expertise that they need, they listen to us, they defer to us, they do what we say, they put up with us. Bernard Barber thus argues that professional knowledge is not just professional but is "powerful knowledge."[15] I doubt that students would read a boring 400-page book I recommend simply because I ask. But if they believe they had better read it to pass the final exam, or to obtain the skill they need for a new job, then they are likely to put up with a boring assignment. If they believe I can perform a surgical procedure to relieve their pain, patients are likely to defer to me and to put up with a lot from me—even when I demean them by being half an hour late for our appointment. If I lacked the surgical skill they need, they would probably leave at the appointed time; but, needing my skill, they will probably wait and quietly endure my insulting tardiness or over-scheduling.

Another power source Raven and Kruglanski suggest is *information*. Because I have needed or desired information, or access to it, clients are likely to be nice to me even when I'm a jerk. Because I know how to get their Medicare processed, patients defer to me. Because I know which hospital has the best xyz unit, the patient listens to me, even when I babble.

A fifth power basis the authors identify is *rewards*. If patients or subordinates defer to me and comply with what I say, they believe that they will be rewarded. As the doctor I will take good care of them and maybe give them preference. As the healthcare professor I will give them the benefit of the doubt and assign an A. So they allow me power over them.

Finally, there is power stemming from *legitimacy* or authority. Simply by virtue of being a doctor, nurse, or technician licensed by the state, or an administrator designated by the hospital, or a professor tenured by the university, I am deferred to. I am in a position of authority both legitimate and institutional, so people allow me power over them.

These are some explanations of the phenomenon of professional power. In identifying them we can reflect further on the results of this—what power has to do with ethics.

Three Levels of Power

Conceptualizing three levels of power can help clarify the nature of the power we wield. Figure 3.1 depicts the nature of these power levels. The first level is macro—the power of the organization or the profession of which we are a part. It is well known and thoroughly studied: the power of "the bureaucracy," the power of "the medical profession," the power of "the system." From the nineteenth-century writings of Max Weber, who warned that "the power position of a developed bureaucracy is always overtowering,"[16] to the more recent analysis of James Burnham that the managerial profession rules modern life,[17] the phenomenon of **macro power** has been well understood and appreciated. What has not been so well recognized is that organizations and professions are in reality conceptual figments of the imagination—they don't *really* live and breath. Macro power is, therefore, not something that is ethically practical, although it certainly is something about which it's fun to ethically theorize. What is real and meaningful, what does live and breath, are the individual people who together comprise what we call organizations and professions. It is in fact the power that they wield—**micro power**— that produces, in concert, macro power. And micro power is ethically practical; it is something we can deal with.

Micro power, that second level of power to consider, has not, as already suggested, been very well probed. In noting this Brass and Burkhardt, in their pioneering research, observe that "the macro-micro split is exemplified in the distinction between potential power and power use."[18] An example of this distinction could be the hospital ethics committee, a macro entity with renowned potential power; however, as Lo cryptically but correctly implies in his otherwise macro-level study of ethics committees, it is the *micro power* of each committee member that is meaningful in terms of impact: "If committee chairpeople are forceful

Figure 3.1 Levels of Power

Type	Characteristics
Macro power	Organizational
	Impersonal
Micro power	Individual
	Official
	Direct
	Specific
Subtle micro power	Individual
	Indirect
	Unofficial
	Generic

leaders who control discussions, they may unintentionally discourage frank debate and disagreement."[19]

This second conceptual level of power is about the specific and direct, visible and official actions that we all take in our professional positions. It is more about the *effect* we have than about affect. For example, as individual doctors we have the power to prescribe drug A or drug B, or to prescribe nothing at all; and we can discuss possible side-effects or forget to. As nurses we have the power to insert the IV needle—in the left arm or the right one—in a hurry or carefully. As technicians we have the power to run the magnetic resonance apparatus, to do it abruptly or with explanatory conversation. As administrators we have the power to establish scheduling procedures that maximize patient waiting time or that attempt to be patient friendly. And as healthcare professors we can assign five books or one to the class of busy working professionals, and we have the power to give an A grade or a C, or to give an incomplete and invite the student to redo the course project. As supervisors we all have the power to hire William or Willa, to assign task x to Mary and the easier task y to Mike, to grant Harry's vacation request but delay Hillary's.

These are all examples of fairly visible routine and direct powers that healthcare professionals wield. They illustrate power that goes officially with the job. They are job-specific and comprise what I refer to conceptually as this second level of power. All of us can raise our level of power consciousness simply by personally listing those kinds of powers that we use every day. The list can be soberingly long and terribly important if Davis is right when he asserts that the exercise of these powers "may mean either beneficence or tyranny, either justice or injustice, either reasonableness or arbitrariness."[20]

With that list we can then reflect on the impact that the use of each of these powers has on the patient, the peer, the subordinate, and so forth. For example, unadvised of possible side effects of the drug I prescribed, my patient might well experience physical pain and emotional anxiety—because of what I did and did not do. My IV patient might wince at the pain prick I produce in hurriedly inserting the IV, or might not even notice the insertion when I do it carefully and skillfully despite the hectic day. My MRI patient can be petrified or calm depending partially on how I administer the MRI. Mrs. Smith can wait 45 minutes to see the doctor and miss her hair styling appointment because of the scheduling I administer. My assistant can learn and develop professionally because I assign new tasks—or can get stale because I give him only repetitive things to do. And my student, to whom I give a C+ instead of a B-, is out $1000 tuition which would have been reimbursed by her employer had I assigned a B grade.

As we reflect on these sorts of things, our power consciousness can become higher and we can be more clear in asking questions about our professionalism, our responsibility, our options, our microethics. It can at first be a bit disconcerting when we realize the extent of the impact and influence we have over real people, and the routine, subconscious way in which we might tend to wield that power.

This then gets us into a third level of power. Let's call it **subtle micro power**. Unlike the second level, it tends to be indirect and unofficial, generic instead of specific. It is more about the *affect* we engender while the second level is more about our effect on our surroundings. It stems from such ordinary and seemingly inconsequential functions as advising, questioning, reporting, complaining, informing, applauding, rebuking, cautioning, and retarding—behaviors that healthcare professionals are in a position to do or not to do many times every day. Ironically, it is suggested by the great legal scholar, Kenneth Culp Davis. Power, he argues, "is not limited to substantive choices but extends to procedures, methods, forms, timing, degrees of emphasis, and many other subsidiary factors."[21]

For example, in treating a patient a doctor can *advise* the person on the pros and cons of various medications, diets, and exercise regimens; can partially advise on them; or can choose not to advise but to simply prescribe. Visible, direct micro power is wielded in treating the patient and prescribing measures. The subtle micro power lies in *how* the doctor chooses to use that visible micro power, in what she or he does in the process of administering clinical care. In assisting the doctor, while using her or his official micro power, a nurse can directly *question* the doctor's approach to a patient, can question nonverbally with a puzzled glance, can choose not to question at all, can bring it up privately or in the presence of others, can do so insistently or softly. An administrator can *report* suspicion of on-the-job alcohol consumption by a provider, can wait a week for another occurrence, or can decide not to report it. I can *applaud* my busy healthcare student for a superb class report or I can just return it with an "A" and no comment; and I can applaud her publicly in class, privately after class, with great enthusiasm, or with matter-of-fact understatement. A senior physician can *inform* a junior colleague on strategies for getting tenure at the medical college, and not so inform another colleague.

All healthcare professionals are commonly in positions to *initiate* action or not to; to *caution* a peer, patient, or subordinate strongly, gently, or not at all; to register a *complaint*—on tardiness, for example— to do so aggressively or meekly, or not at all; and, of course, to act now or *delay*, to see the friendly patient first and the obnoxious patient after; to put talkative Tom on hold and take another call; to process a claim today or tomorrow, to review the literature on that new procedure next week, next month, or never. This power to delay can sometimes get very subtle indeed. In an insightful cover story some years ago, entitled "When Doctors Play God," *Newsweek* magazine slipped in—in the midst of an otherwise macro power analysis—a micro power example of delay: nurses, the article suggested, routinely walk instead of run when a terminally ill and suffering patient takes a serious turn for the worse.[22]

What is the impact of carrying out such routine and frequent role activities, of exercising this subtle micro power? What, indeed, *is* the big deal? Compared with the consequences of pulling the plug or not, of deciding who will get to use the dialysis equipment next, of telling the patient of a terminal illness or not, are not the consequences of these more routine activities dwarfed? And don't they have much less significant ethical implications if, indeed, any at all?

I submit not. Although the consequences can certainly be much less direct, apparent, and engaging, they surely can be critical for an individual patient, colleague, or subordinate. Consider the patient who, unrebuked by his doctor for smoking, contracts lung cancer; or the same patient who, rebuked but not advised of means, quits and becomes unbearably edgy and abusive to his family and develops an ulcer. Consider the colleague who, unreported by me for drinking on the job, performs an improper procedure that results in infection, a lengthier hospital stay, and higher bills; or the same colleague, reported for drinking on the job, who quits the staff of my inner-city hospital increasing the shortage of doctors there. Consider the subordinate who, uninformed by the supervisor about the personnel department's informal procedures, misses the chance for a promotion while another, informally informed by the boss, gets the higher-paying job. And consider the impact on all of us when the efficiency-minded practice administrator schedules us so that we sit an hour or so in the waiting room: our blood pressure goes up, we become irritable, we miss our business meeting, and we receive a speeding ticket while rushing to get back to work. Ridiculous? Perhaps, but our life and its effect on the "affect" of other people is altered by the way a healthcare professional has used or failed to use his or her seemingly inconsequential micro power over us. Are ethical implications not present in such scenarios? Is the question of ethical responsibility relevant here? The American Heart Association has offered a response: "Ethical practice in the profession may well stem more from sensitive awareness of one's self and how one is actually impacting on persons and situations than from any specific knowledge."[23]

Two significant aspects of these kinds of micro situations seem germane to ethical discourse. One is the thousands of them that appear on the job. Exercising power of this sort comes with the career of healthcare professional, and not exercising such routine power can clearly have untoward consequences—just as exercising it can. Because the exercise of power in this dimension is so common, apparently ordinary, and expected, an understandable and natural tendency may be not to recognize it as power at all, or to dismiss any suggestion of its ethical implications as picayune or unrealistic given the hectic conditions of healthcare delivery. Yet precisely because it is so routine and extensive, this third level—subtle micro power—may encompass the largest area of professional power and, therefore, the power reality most in need of reflection and consciousness-raising. Because it can be so subtle, however, it can also be the most difficult of the levels to broach.

Willbern is helpful in this regard. Especially in service professions like healthcare, he argues, "attitudes and the tone and flavor of official behavior are morally significant."[24] For example, one official behavior of a nurse is the insertion of an injection needle. This typifies the visible and direct micro power of nurses, and they clearly have an ethical obligation to be clinically skilled in such a procedure. But what about a nurse's attitude, tone, and flavor in the official act of needle insertion? Does it make any difference? Does it have any ethical significance? One of my first lessons in reflecting on these questions was given, unwittingly, many years ago in a Navy hospital in Japan. As a patient there, I distinctly remember two nurses who served on my ward. One—I think we called her Hardhearted Hilda or something like that—would administer injections with such clinical skill that we hardly knew we were being punctured. She never missed the vein and the job was done in seconds. But she barely said anything except "give me your arm," never looked us in the eye, and maintained a facial expression resembling that of Zeus. The other nurse, Lt.(jg) Mellow Mary, was not nearly as clinically expert as Hilda at needle injections. She got the job done but we would usually notice a little tingle in the arm, and once or twice she missed the vein and had to repeat the procedure. But, in the process of injecting us, Mary would look us in the eye, chat with us about how we were doing, and so forth. She surely took more time to make the rounds than did Hilda. She was probably less efficient; but the difference in impact on us patients was enormous. We even talked to each other about how much better we felt when Lt. Mary was there. With Lt. Hilda we felt intimidated, vulnerable, even denigrated. She might as well been injecting oranges or grapefruits instead of human beings, let alone naval officers. With Mary, on the other hand, despite the higher level of imprecision and physical pain, we somehow felt good, we felt dignified, we felt better. The difference in "effect" impact of clinical and official micro power between these two nurses was distinct if only marginal; the difference in "affect" impact of unofficial, subtle micro power was enormous, at least to us who were the subjects (in Hilda's case the objects) of that micro power.

Is there an ethical dimension to this little anecdote? Was Hilda more ethical because she trained harder, was thus more clinically skilled, and caused less physical pain? Was she more ethical because in being so efficient she was able to serve more patients and, incidentally, reduce hospital costs? And was Mary, in contrast, less ethically mature? Or was Hilda ethically responsible for our feeling demeaned and was she ethically less mature than Mary who, despite our vulnerable condition, made us feel valued and important as people? We did no studies at the time, but is it possible—as it did seem to us—that because Mary made us feel better we actually got better sooner, thereby reducing hospital costs? In that way was Mary actually more efficient than Hilda and therefore more ethically mature in the productivity sense too? To us patients, there was no doubt: Mary was a professional nurse, Hilda was a machine. The nursing super-visor may well have favored Hilda. As for Hilda—who was, by the way, an extremely good person trying to do her job professionally in very stressful circumstances—I doubt that she was aware at all of the nonclinical impact she had on us. So whose ethical analysis do you embrace? Sissela Bok argues strongly, and I agree with her, that the one whom power directly affects has the more accurate perspective on the situation.[25]

A similar dynamic occurs in my graduate healthcare ethics classroom when I exercise my micro power, as The Professor, in trying to do the job of teaching professional ethics. The purpose of my direct, official micro power in class is to lecture, to speak, to question, to respond toward fulfilling my ethical responsibility to teach, to help students—who are paying a tidy tuition—in the development of ethical skills. Toward that ethical end, patterns of my classroom behavior have evolved, mostly in the genre of subtle micro power. Have we all not experienced from our own healthcare professors, for example, some ethically interesting classroom dynamics of subtle micro power similar to the following?

When discussions get lively many hands go up to respond, to par-ticipate, to question; careful about the limited class time available, and knowing there is neither time nor teaching need to recognize all of the hands, we typically and rather arbitrarily recognize people who are likely not to talk too long, or we call on someone who has said nothing and whose hand is not raised. Is that ethical? How does the healthcare student *feel* when we thus continuously fail to give him or her a chance to speak? And then, when the person we recognize has finished speaking, we often give her or him a blank stare as we call on someone else. Is that ethical? And how do you feel when you are the recipient of that blank stare or snide professorial facial expression that nonverbally suggests that you said something stupid? How do you feel when the professor walks right up to you, stands in front of your desk and peers down at you as you struggle to remember a good answer? Is the professor just a jerk or a wielder of subtle micro power denigrating you in the name of helping you learn? The professor is, of course, using these and other techniques because, having acquired "wisdom" from years of professorial experience, he or she has figured out how to get graduate students to pay attention, to work harder, to develop better professional skills that—God Almighty well knows—we surely need more of out there in the field. Is it not, after all, the professor's sacred ethical responsibility to make sure that healthcare students get their money's worth and graduate with the professional skills presumed of the holder of a master's degree? Or is it? And if a little perspiration in the classroom motivates students, is not the professor's described use of subtle micro power not only effective teaching but highly ethical? Or is it?

Isn't this similar to a doctor's attempts to inoculate a screaming and squirming dog-bitten child so that the boy won't get rabies and die? Doesn't the doctor exercise his or her subtle "information" micro power by telling the boy "This won't hurt"? Lying to the child is the ethical thing to do, isn't it, because the doctor's official inoculating micro power is involved in the noble effort to save the child's life? Or is it?

Characteristic of these kinds of scenarios is a second significant element of the exercise of subtle micro power. It is what I call the "chain reaction" trait. Whereas actions at the macro level, such as turning off the respirator, have a direct result and a fairly clear cause-effect relationship, actions at the micro level do not. This is particularly true at the subtle micro level. Instead, the exercise or non-exercise of micro power often forms merely a part of a series of events, circumstances, or activities, and in such a way that the effect of the micro power exercise on the final result is unclear and often invisible. Indeed, the healthcare professional may never know what eventually will happen. The impact is indirect. Because of this it is much more difficult to recognize any ethical implication of the action or choice. More to the point, it is fairly easy to disclaim any responsibility, ethical or otherwise.

Consider the case of urging the patient to quit smoking mentioned earlier. Influenced by the provider's words, he does quit, does become edgy and abusive as a result, does get divorced a year later, and does develop a nervous disorder. Did the healthcare professional's use of micro power—the reprimand—cause a chain reaction that led to those later events? Did it make a difference? Should the professional have exercised other micropowers—such as advising of alternatives, monitoring progress, applauding efforts? Does this clinician share any responsibility for those later events? It may not be altogether clear.

And remember the case of Hardhearted Hilda. One of our fellow patients on the ward was a marginal basket case owing to his battle experience. He was down on himself. Hilda did all the right clinical things for him and his physical wounds healed. But in dealing with him so efficiently, in treating him like the proverbial grapefruit, she seemed to reinforce his self-perception as a failure. Many weeks after discharge from the hospital he killed himself. Did Hilda, by the chain-reaction effect, share any ethical responsibility for his action? I'm sure she never knew what happened to him, and would have been devastated if she had known. She was devoted to making him well. But, as a professional healthcare person wielding considerable micropower, subtle as well as visible, did she bear some ethical responsibility for the chain of events? Or is this very question absurd?

And what about the case of me, the Pompous Professor who, in the name of helping a student become a better professional, glares down at the student as he or she struggles to remember an answer to my question. The student has worked hard at the clinic all day. This is a respected professional trying to become even more skilled through graduate healthcare education. And I put this person down, albeit subtly. Thus disturbed, he or she returns home after class and takes the frustration I have contributed to out on a young daughter with an ornery disposition. Do I have any ethical responsibility for the harm done my student's child? The student will probably come to class more prepared next time, so there was indeed a method to my madness. But was my teaching behavior ethical given the outcome for the daughter? Or is this suggestion of chain-reaction responsibility absurd? The answer may not be altogether clear.

What about the boy the doctor was trying to save, in part by deceitfully telling him that the painful rabies needle would not hurt? The boy lived. Ninety-nine more times he heard healthcare professionals tell him unwitting lies like "this won't hurt." Now he has grown into an adult. He lies to his clients. He lies to his spouse. He lies to his friends. Is it preposterous to ask if the doctor who once saved him from rabies holds some ethical responsibility for the pattern of deceit this person developed? Is it preposterous to suggest that when the imposing figure of a doctor lies to me as a means of achieving an end, he teaches me how and why to lie, albeit subtly and indirectly? Is it ridiculous to suggest that a professional might be professional enough to achieve short-term ethical responsibility without contributing to long-term ethical harm? How can one fruitfully reflect on these kinds of questions?

Dramatic illustrations can help. A classic illustration is Stanley Milgram's famous experiments with electric shock. An American whose relatives were all but wiped out in the Holocaust, Milgram dedicated his life to figuring out how such a thing could happen. Among his efforts were experiments involving "teachers" and "learners."[26] Under the pretense of trying to advance the noble science of education "teachers"—initially college students but later people from every background and situation—were asked to read a list of word associations to a "learner" and then to quiz the learner on the list. The teacher was told that the experiment was trying to determine if "stimulus-response" techniques, in particular the effect of punishment on learning, work for education.

The experience scenario plays out consistently as follows. On arriving at the experiment site, the subject is met by the experimenter and a pleasant confederate who is actually an actor. The above-described bogus purpose of the experiment is explained, and the subject is given a small "wage" for participating. After a rigged drawing the "lucky" subject wins the role of teacher and the experimenter's confederate becomes the learner. The learner is strapped into a chair—giving the appearance that he can now not get away—and electrodes are attached to his arms. When asked if the electric shocks will harm the learner, the experimenter responds: "While the shocks may be painful, they will cause no permanent tissue damage." The teacher is instructed to read the learner a list of word pairs, to then test him on the list, and to administer punishment—an electric shock whenever an incorrect answer is given.

The teacher is given a sample shock of 45 volts—which is the only *real* shock ever given—and the discomfort is severe enough to cause the teacher facial contortions. The teacher is told to increase the intensity of the shock one level on the shock generator for each error. The generator has 30 switches escalating from a low of 15 volts to a high of 450 volts. The experiment starts routinely, but by the fifth switch the confederate begins to grunt in "pain." At the tenth level, 150 volts—more than three times the sample with which the teacher has personal experience—the learner cries out, "Let me out of here! I don't want to do this anymore!" The teacher usually gets increasingly agitated, turning to the experimenter and asking what to do. "You must continue" is the response. By 270 volts the learner is letting out agonized screams. At 300 volts he stops answering the questions and the teacher is told to consider no answer as an incorrect answer. From 330 volts on there is no response or scream. Because they are separated by a large screen preventing them from seeing each other, the teacher does not know whether the learner is conscious or even alive.

Representative of Milgram's observations during the experiments is the following: "I observed a mature and initially poised businessman enter the laboratory smiling and confident. Within 20 minutes he was reduced to . . . a point of nervous collapse. At one point he pushed his fist into his forehead and muttered 'Oh God, let's stop it.' And yet he continued to respond to every word of the experimenter, and obeyed to the end."[27]

What does this have to do with our reflection on the micro power of healthcare professionals? As described, aren't the experiments *emotionally* shocking? Isn't it amazing that anyone normal actually continued to participate once they heard the grunts and screams? On the contrary, the shocking and dramatic aspect of these experiments—and their relevance to our micropower reflection—is that the vast majority of people not only continued administering the shocks but continued to the full 450 volts. And these were not people from the local penitentiary or insane asylum. They were people like us, drawn over the years of the experiments, from every social, economic, religious, and ethnic group possible. They did protest, sweat, complain, and exhibit considerable disturbance during the exercise, but they nonetheless administered the full level of shock, even when the "learner" screamed and stopped responding, even though they themselves had personal experience of the pain of the electric shock, and even though they were, in fact, free to stop at any time.

How could they do it? Or, more precisely—and this is the real relevance of our reflection—how could *we* do it? Although I, like the reader, cannot imagine myself ever participating in such horror, the experiments suggest in the strongest terms that I am fooling myself and am resisting an avenue to raising my awareness of the power I wield. For when I get to the point of being able to acknowledge that I am probably one of those "teachers," that I probably have a strong proclivity to use my micro power unwittingly in shocking ways, then I can seriously begin to reflect on how and why, and to develop skills and methods toward minimizing that proclivity.

When interviewed afterward and asked how and why they did what they did, the "teachers" all—just like Hilda and that pompous professor— offered very good reasons: "I had a job to do." "It was approved by the university." "You [the experimenter] are a PhD, an expert in this stuff, and you told me to shock the guy." "It's good for society; it will help us educate better." These are good people doing bad things for good reasons. How often do I "zap" my patients, students, and subordinates for good reasons? How many volts is making a student feel stupid equivalent to— 30 volts or 300 volts? How many volts is the deceitful "this won't hurt" expression equivalent to? I know that when the doctor makes me wait 30 minutes after my scheduled appointment, the wait is equivalent to at least 225 volts of pain to me!

Four aspects of the Milgram experiments are particularly disturbing and, consequently, fruitful for reflection. One is the fact that the shockers had a major benefit that we usually do not have, and *still* they administered the shocks: they knew they were causing pain because they could hear it. When I inflict my denigrating facial expressions or my burdensome reading assignments on students, I seldom hear the pain. They usually don't scream and rarely do they dare to complain. When Hardhearted Hilda demeaned those naval officers, not one moaned about it. This suggests to me a somewhat scary situation: if the "teachers" administered shocks *despite* hearing the pain, how much more likely are we unwittingly to zap our clients when we don't have the benefit of hearing or seeing the result of our subtle behavior?

Second is the structural aspect of the experiments. Like us in our professional work, the shockers were recruited and paid to do a job. They were trained in how to do it, and they were supervised by an expert in authority. The goals behind the structure were as lofty as ours in healthcare, namely, to help humankind be better. And the setting of the experiments was very clinical, just like our settings tend to be. Noting these structural realities Sabini and Silver, in their incisive analysis of Milgram's work, give us cause to pause and reflect: "Ordinarily, assuming the benevolence of the organizations of which we are a part, we do not trouble ourselves with questions of moral responsibility for the *routine* doing of our job."[28]

Third is the phenomenon of self-perception that emerges with the experiment participants and with us, the experiment observers. This phenomenon is the ease and clarity with which we view the power behavior of others, yet the difficulty we have in seeing the same power behavior in ourselves. Throughout his experiments Milgram interviewed cross-sections of people for whom he described the experiments. Inevitably, everyone claimed they would stop administering the shocks at some point. Milgram, then, assuming that most people would be reluctant to admit that they would administer the full level of shocks, asked samples to predict how far other people would go. The average prediction was that one person in a thousand would continue to the end. But, in fact, the vast majority of actual participants administered the full 450 volts. Moreover, when participants later realized what they had done, it so contradicted their self-image that Milgram had to provide extensive post-experiment counseling for these very upset "teachers." Similarly, without exception, when observers view cinematic re-creations of Milgram's experiments, they are horrified at the behavior they see and deny that they themselves could ever so behave. But the experiments are conclusive in suggesting that the behavior we are seeing is our very own behavior.

Fourth, the phenomenon of non-use of micro power is remarkable. The glaring issue in the experiments is the extensive use of direct, official micro power to shock with increasing intensity some innocent people called "learners." But is it not equally disturbing, and amazing, to realize that hardly any of the "teachers" used their extensive subtle micro power in the process? They all had the subtle power to determine the length of time to hold the shocking lever down; deciding on "just an instant" would have minimized the pain for the learners. Yet most of the teachers, unwittingly, held the lever down much longer, thus extending the pain. They all also had the subtle power to question, to ask the learners if they were all right. In the experiments hardly any teachers used this micro power. And all of them had the subtle power to request the experimenter to check on the well-being of the learner under shock. Amazingly, few requested this. They all had the power to inform the learner, through voice inflection, of the correct answer. None did. So, just as the Milgram experiments suggest the tendency to use micro power in ways that cause pain or negative effects, so too do the experiments suggest a strong tendency to underuse subtle micro power in ways that ease pain and lessen negative effects.

How often, for example, has the doctor's office *informed* you that the doctor is a half-hour behind schedule or *questioned* you on whether you would prefer to reschedule instead of waiting? How often has that healthcare professor smiled while glaring at you or questioned you about the reasonableness of the course workload? Hardhearted Hilda, of course, is a *par excellence* exemplar of the non-use of subtle micro power.

A second helpful dramatization for reflecting on micro power is Ken Kesey's *One Flew Over the Cuckoo's Nest*, brought to video with Jack Nicholson's and Louise Fletcher's Academy Award–winning performances. It is a wonderful book and a sensational movie for reflection because of its stark portrayal, both humorous and tragically real, of the power of the healthcare professional. It offers a rich opportunity to see ourselves in the likes of Dr. Spivey, the hospital administrator; Nurse Ratched, the ward manager; and Randall McMurphy, the de facto ward "therapist."

We see the stark differentiation between the uniform-clad professionals controlling a clinically antiseptic environment, and the vulnerable, pajama clad, controlled patients. We see the role of fear in conditioning the behavior of well-meaning professionals. We see the focus on safety, order, and control—so understandable in difficult healthcare settings—to the detriment of human dignity. We see the personable Dr. Spivey interviewing patients while he reads their charts for the first time. He does not extend them the courtesy, let alone the dignity, of having prepared for the interview. He obviously is not familiar with their records. In the movie we watch an apparently compulsive, controlling, and mean-spirited Nurse Ratched as she exercises subtle micro power with wonderfully realized stares, voice tones, and body language. We see her expression as she "zaps" patients through actions like taking their cigarettes "for their own good." We even witness clinically administered shock therapy while the skilled technicians lie with assurances that "this won't hurt you." We see McMurphy in subtle ways give dignity to the otherwise denigrated patients. And we see the results of McMurphy's reckless use of his micro power in contrast to Ratched's rigid use of hers.

The book and the movie actually are seldom useful for ethical reflection because Kesey keeps us on the outside looking in. From that vantage we clearly see Nurse Ratched's misuse of micro power. We hate her—and even cheer when McMurphy tries to strangle her. From the outside we are watching a bad healthcare professional doing bad things, and we quickly condemn her. The book and the movie become fuel for ethical reflection when, but only when, we step inside and see ourselves in Nurse Ratched, when we consider her a good healthcare professional who has become, unwittingly, a doer of bad things.

To make this step, it can be helpful to reflect hypothetically on the "ethical goodness" of Nurse Ratched: Mildred Ratched had experienced mental illness in her family. When she completed nursing school she wanted to dedicate herself to the care of the mentally ill just as all of us have dedicated ourselves to healthcare. She thus chose a specialty and took a job in a field that few healthcare professionals will take up—to work where the patients are crazy. Her strong dedication led her to a place of great need but where few of us would choose to go. Then, like we have, she entered a facility with structures, an organizational culture, with rules and procedures that had evolved over time. During her first year Mildred was much like McMurphy. And, like us, she tried to change some things. More than once she was put in her place by supervisors, sometimes formally but usually in subtle, informal ways. Like us, she cared about each patient and reached out to some of them. After 18 months at the facility she exhibited symptoms of stress and was advised by her doctor to ease up. Peers had already told her she was getting too involved with the patients. Life on the ward is just too difficult, they cautioned her, to treat each patient too individually. But her dedication continued. During her second year one patient suddenly became violent and beat her up. She continued to ease the rules, though not as much, to accommodate individual patient needs. At the beginning of her third year another patient she was helping tried to rape her. After that she came to understand more pragmatically the fragility of life on the ward.

She became more cautious, more attentive to the rules and procedures. Shortly after, two of her favored patients were severely beaten by three newly arrived deranged patients.

In short, Nurse Ratched became experienced with the daily routine of healthcare in the mental health setting. Her peers socialized her; her experience seasoned her. Gradually, this dedicated healthcare professional grew into a veteran who knew clearly the primacy of safety for patients, visitors, and staff; who knew personally and daily the fear of the ward environment; who realized the wisdom of rules and procedures; who had figured out her own physical, emotional, mental, and psychological limits on the job. The Nurse Ratched we read of in the book and see in action in the movie is this experienced Mildred who still cares deeply for her patients ("I'm not going to let anyone hurt you," she says with conviction) but who carries out this concern in a context of experience and organizational culture, and *without skilled ethical reflection*. She has not developed an awareness of her micro power so she is without a clue about what we see so clearly in her behavior. Maybe just like all of us before we pay attention to ethical reflection.

Implications

In this chapter we have attempted to focus the reality prism on the phenomenon of power in the healthcare professional, particularly the reality of subtle micro power. This effort suggests that ethics in healthcare does not so much concern the bad things that bad people do as it does the bad things that we good people do for seemingly good reasons. Bill Kuhn's extensive research of business ethics comes to a like conclusion. Professionals are not vicious people given to astigmatism, he finds. Rather, myopia sets in unannounced: "They are so busy processing the day's volume of demands that it is hard for them to step back from it."[29] Nurse Hilda could, undoubtedly, relate to that, as could the rabies doctor, the scheduling administrator, Nurse Ratched and, of course, that pompous professor. Laura Nash's studies concur: "Good managers can be fooled by their own good intentions."[30] Michael Lipsky offers a more practical explanation. Professionals, he finds, "develop conceptions of their jobs, and of clients, that reduce the strain between capabilities and goals, thereby making their jobs psychologically easier to manage."[31]

That line between capabilities and goals can be a very fine line indeed. Without a well-focused prism a good professional can easily cross the line from micro power that dignifies and nurtures to that which denigrates and consumes—the line that is key to distinguishing ethical from unethical behavior. Indeed, it is the fineness of that line and the difficulty of seeing it that leads Kuhn to define professional ethics as "a kind of corrective vision."[32] The importance of developing skills—in having a professional prism—for raising awareness of the professional power we wield cannot be overstressed. But, as Karen Lebacqz in concert with Pellegrino, puts it, traditional professional ethics is not adequate "because it does not take sufficiently into account . . . the implications of the power gap between professional and client."[33] Precisely. So we have to figure it out ourselves. This chapter tries to help with the reflection necessary to do that.

Notes

1. D. F. Thompson, 1985, "The Possibility of Administrative Ethics." *Public Administration Review* 45, no. 5 (September/October): 556.

2. M. Lipsky, 1980, *Street Level Bureaucracy* (New York: Russell Sage Foundation), p. 149.

3. Thomas à Kempis, 1920 edition, *The Imitation of Christ* (London: Collins).

4. B. Kabanoff, 1991, "Equity, Equality, Power and Conflict." *Academy of Management Review* 16, no. 2 (April): 422.

5. E. Pellegrino, 1979, *Humanism and the Physician* (Knoxville, TN: University of Tennessee Press), pp. 117–23.

6. K. Lebacqz, 1985, *Professional Ethics: Power and Paradox* (Nashville, TN: Abingdon Press), p. 111.

7. L. K.Trevino, 1986, "Ethical Decision Making in Organizations." *Academy of Management Review* 11, no. 3 (July): 601.

8. J. A. Rohr, 1978, *Ethics For Bureaucrats* (New York: Dekker), p. 50.

9. M. O'Neill, 1992, "Ethical Dimensions of Nonprofit Administration." *Nonprofit Management and Leadership* 3, no. 2 (winter): 208.

10. L. Gawthrop, 1982, "Where Does America's Day Begin?" *Public Administration Review* 42, no. 4 (July/August): 300.

11. K. C. Davis, 1971, *Discretionary Justice* (Urbana: University of Illinois Press), p. v.

12. M. Lilla, 1981, "Ethos, Ethics, and Public Service." *The Public Interest* 63, no. 1 (winter): 16.

13. W. Durant and A. Durant, quoted in C. M. Kelly, 1988, *The Destructive Achiever* (Reading, MA: Addison-Wesley), p. 3. Italics are added for emphasis.

14. B. H. Raven and W. Kruglanski, 1975, "Conflict and Power." In P. G. Swingle (ed.), *The Structure of Conflict* (New York: Academic Press), pp. 177–219.

15. B. Barber, 1980, "Regulation and the Professions." *The Hastings Center Report* 10, no. 1 (February): 34.

16. H. H. Gerth and C. Wright Mills (eds. and trans.), 1946, *From Max Weber: Essays in Sociology* (London: Oxford University Press), ch. 8.

17. J. Burnham, 1942, *The Managerial Revolution* (New York: Day).

18. D. J. Brass and M. E. Burkhardt, 1993, "Potential Power and Power Use: An Investigation of Structure and Behavior." *Academy of Management Journal* 36, no. 3 (June): 441.

19. B. Lo, 1987, "Promises and Pitfalls of Ethics Committees." *The New England Journal of Medicine* 317, no. 1 (2 July): 48.

20. K. C. Davis, 1969, *Discretionary Justice* (Urbana: University of Illinois Press), p. 3.

21. Ibid., p. 4.

22. M. Clark, 1981, "When Doctors Play God." *Newsweek* (31 August): 49.

23. American Heart Association, Committee on Ethics, 1980, "A Perspective on Teaching Medical Ethics," p. 6.

24. Y. Willbern, 1984, "Types and Levels of Public Morality," *Public Administration Review* 44, no. 2 (March/April): 105.

25. S. Bok, 1979, *Lying* (New York: Vintage), p. 21.

26. For details of the experiments see S. Milgram, 1963, "Behavioral Study of Obedience." *Journal of Abnormal and Social Psychology* 67 (3): 371–78; 1965, "Some Conditions of Obedience and Disobedience to Authority." *Human Relations* 18 (1): 57–76; and 1974, *Obedience to Authority* (New York: Harper and Row).

27. Ibid., 1963, 377.

28. J. Sabini and M. Silver, 1982, *Moralities of Everyday Life* (New York: Oxford), p. 63.

29. W. Kuhn, 1990, "Toward an Agenda for Business Ethics Research." *Academy of Management Review* 15, no. 2 (April): 317.

30. L. Nash, 1990, *Good Intentions Aside* (Boston: Harvard Business School Press), p. 244.

31. M. Lipsky, *Street Level Bureaucracy*, p. 141.

32. W. Kuhn, "Toward an Agenda . . . ," p. 317.

33. K. Lebacqz, *Professional Ethics . . .* , p. 135.

READING

Although it was published in a government journal half a century ago by an unlikely philosophy professor at a little known midwest college, the following article is among the few probing reflections on professional power (he uses the term "discretion") available to healthcare professionals today. Wayne Leys brings the rich tradition of philosophy to bear in probing professional ethics as "an exploration of insoluble problems." Although clearly concerned with the macro dimension—and focused on government organization—Leys' insights are helpful as well for understanding micro power in healthcare. Particularly salient is his challenge to the notion of ethics as a matter of "definiteness" or dogma. In making his point he distinguishes among technical discretion (i.e., power), such as that given medical experts like doctors and nurses; discretion involving vague criteria, such as the best use of our limited time for patients; and discretion involving rival criteria, such as caring for the patient *and* maximizing cost efficiency. In arguing against the prescriptive tendencies of philosophers, Leys sets a clarifying light on the reality of administrative power. He concludes with a cogent caveat germane to microethics reflection: in using our routine power in the work day, "uncongenial values" undoubtedly exist for each of us. As a consequence it may be significant to consider if there is something important we are not thinking about. This book is dedicated to helping us think about it.

The article is worth the concentration it requires, although you may want to read it selectively. Leys the philosopher does a remarkable job of making theoretical concepts practical and managerially relevant. While the discussion is included to expand our reflection on micro power, the author's analysis of values fittingly sets the stage for the next chapter as well. In absorbing this reading, be attentive in translating "government administrator" to "healthcare professional" and "legislature" to "board of trustees."

ETHICS AND ADMINISTRATIVE DISCRETION

Wayne A. R. Leys

Despite the growing importance of administrative discretion, it is a subject which is usually approached negatively, i.e., from the standpoint of the lawyer or judge who is interested in the *limits* of discretion. We have a large literature dealing with legislative restraint and judicial review. Much of this literature may be as necessary in the development of good administration as the negative criticism of rule-making and planning which greeted popular legislatures in the eighteenth century, when it was feared that those bodies would use their new powers tyrannically or foolishly. But we cannot expect administrators to act wisely if their only guides are statements of what they must *not* do. Those who are given discretionary powers must ask how the quality of discretion may be improved. Yet, as recently as 1939, Professor Leonard D. White, in his *Introduction to the Study of Public Administration*, remarked that the study of administrative discretion had never been undertaken from the administrative point of view.

As an addict of philosophy I cannot lay claim to the administrative point of view. Notwithstanding this handicap or advantage, I want to open the discussion. In view of the fact that ethics is the art (some say, science) of making wise choices, it would seem to be relevant to the problem of increasing the wisdom of administrative choices. Plato, Aristotle, Cicero, Bentham, and Kant, among others, tried to articulate moral principles for the guidance of legislators. Cardozo wrote an intelligible treatise on moral principles for judges who find that they have considerable discretion in certain cases. Why shouldn't ethics, the age-old quest for standards of conduct, help the administrator? The administrator is also looking for standards.

Some Unpromising Approaches

Executives in government probably feel that they could use some suggestions for the development of good standards and good judgment; but, influenced perhaps by none-too-enthusiastic memories of certain courses in college, they may doubt that ethics has any practical suggestions. If I take issue with this doubt, it is not that I regard everything that is called ethics as particularly relevant to the problems of administrative discretion.

Wayne A. R. Leys, "Ethics and Administrative Discretion," *Public Administration Review* 3, no. 1 (winter 1943): 10–23. Reprinted by permission of the American Society for Public Administration (ASPA), 1120 G Street NW, Washington, DC 20005. All rights reserved. The article is abridged. Wayne Leys was professo of philosophy at the Central YMCA College in Chicago.

I am not going to undertake a critical discussion of professional codes of ethics, such as the code adopted by the International City Managers' Association in 1924. Excellent as these precepts are for some purposes, they throw little light on the question of what to buy with the playground fund. There may be fifty ways of spending the money that are, all of them, compatible with the admonition to be diligent, above-board, free from avarice, and loyal to superiors. Professional codes of ethics do not contain the principles that we are looking for, because they prescribe standards for the administrator's *own* conduct. When we ask how his discretionary powers may be used wisely, we are asking about the standards which an administrator ought to prescribe for *other* people—citizens, departments, corporations, subordinates.

Another kind of ethics which is relatively unimportant for our problem is moralizing about the power of sin. Any observer of government must regret certain actions which have been, in his opinion, victories of selfishness and stupidity over the public interest. But where such conflicts are clearly recognized, the damage has already been done. We have been outvoted, or our own desires have prevailed over our conscience and we have had to act before we could resolve a mental conflict. Of course, we may ask what we ought to do next in such an imperfect situation; but that is quite a different topic from the contemplation of what might have been.

> If, of all sad words of tongue or pen
> The saddest are, "It might have been,"
> More sad are these we daily see:
> "It is, but hadn't ought to be."

The kind of ethical analysis which is profitable relates not to such closed questions but to the open questions, the as-yet-undecided questions of policy. I refer to the questions in which it is not yet clear what course of action will be both successful and in the public interest. The commissioners who are still puzzled as to what freight rates are fair, the directors who have not yet determined the standard by which milk shall be judged pure, the executives who have not yet decided which location for a public enterprise is in the public interest or what favors are legitimate public services: these men are confronted by the live kind of options which the great moral philosophers faced when they asked, *What* is good? It so happens that the philosophers spent part of their time discussing another question, viz., How great is the power of good will when we know what is good but are restrained by impulses and old habits? In answering this latter question the philosophers usually sermonized. Unfortunately the sermons are better known than the philosophers' analyses of the problem of setting up standards. The sort of ethics which may improve administrative decisions is concerned with the discovery of standards for right action rather than with the exhortation to do what has been already declared right.

Have the famous Occidental philosophers agreed upon anything concerning the standards for wise action? If I say, "Yes," it may seem that I am trying to speak for a roomful of prima donnas, for nearly every philosopher has started out by "refuting" his predecessors. The contentious aspect of the philosophical tradition is emphasized by the current academic custom in my field of carrying the student "through a hypercritical maze of ethical theories in order, finally, to convince him of the author's own particular theory as to the ultimate end of conduct" (I use the words of Professor Roland Warren). Philosophers are an argumentative lot, but their disputes often turn on "fine points." When we compare the philosophers with the lawyers, the merchants, the priests, and the politicians, we find the philosophers usually standing together. They are distinguished from other groups by the questions with which they are preoccupied and, especially, by the way in which they formulate the questions. If "the technique or treatment of a problem begins with its first expression as a question," as Suzanne Langer remarked in her *Philosophy in a New Key,* and if philosophers are unique in their phrasing of questions, they may occasionally have some very practical suggestions for solving problems that are faced by the nonphilosophical. Indeed, I believe that the history of philosophical ethics can be viewed as an exploration of insoluble problems, some of which, by rephrasing, have been transformed into answerable questions.

What have the philosophers to contribute toward the development of standards in those areas where the administrators are granted much latitude by the legislature? Their first (and perhaps their only) contribution is a criticism of the administrator's conception of his problem. In the section that follows I shall state and criticize the late Ernst Freund's view, which seems to be widely accepted among public administrators and legislators. According to Freund, the problem of the official endowed with discretionary powers is to increase the definiteness of legal standards. I shall try to show why the use of "definiteness" in formulating the task baffles those who ask how administrative sagacity may be increased. Then I shall restate the problem and indicate the sort of answers that may be expected with the help of the ethical disciplines.

Standards and Administrative Law

Political scientists and lawyers commonly treat administrative discretion as the consequence of indefinite terminology in legislation. The legislature is supposed to supply the public official with standards of conduct by which he can determine whether citizens are to be coerced, cajoled, or let alone. If the legislative standard is definite, the administrator has no discretionary power, but only the ministerial power of determining the facts in the case. If, on the other hand, the legislative standard is not precise, the administrator must use his own judgment in deciding exactly what rule the citizen is to obey, and, in some cases of violation, just what is to be done about the unruly person.

Professor Ernst Freund took this view of the situation and did much to popularize it in the United States:

> When we speak of administrative discretion we mean that a determination may be reached, in part at least, upon the basis of considerations not entirely susceptible of proof or disproof. A statute confers discretion when it refers an official for the use of his power to beliefs, expectations or tendencies instead of facts, or to such terms as "adequate," "advisable," "appropriate," "beneficial," "competent," "convenient," "detrimental," "expedient," "equitable," "fair," "fit," "necessary," "practicable," "proper," "reasonable," "reputable," "safe," "sufficient," "wholesome," or their opposites. These lack the degree of certainty belonging even to such difficult concepts as fraud or discrimination or monopoly. They involve matter of degree or an appeal to judgment. The discretion enlarges as the element of future probability preponderates over that of present conditions; it contracts where in certain types of cases quality tends to become standardized, as in matters of safety.[1]

Freund tried to distinguish gradations in the freedom of administrative discretion. Although he made the attempt several times, he was apparently never quite satisfied with his results. In his article on "The Use of Indefinite Terms in Statutes"[2] he describes three grades of indefiniteness:

> It is possible to distinguish roughly three grades of certainty in the language of statutes of general operation: precisely measured terms, abstractions of common certainty, and terms involving an appeal to judgment or a question of degree. The great majority of statutes operate with the middle grade of certainty.

He describes the middle grade as follows:

> Abstractions of common certainty may be furnished by words of popular usage, by technical terms, or by circumscribing definitions. No general rule can be laid down as to which of these serves statutory purposes best, although a good deal might be said about the illusory certainty of some technical terms, and of cumulations and qualifications sanctioned by traditional practice. Every common abstraction has its "marginal" ambiguity, which mere elaboration of definition cannot altogether remove.

A banking law which directs the banking commission to refuse a charter unless a new bank has a paid-in capital of at least $15,000 falls into the first grade of certainty or definiteness: the standard has precisely measured terms.

The second grade of legislative definiteness may be illustrated by a law which empowers the Bureau of Immigration to refuse admittance to a mentally defective person: "mentally defective person" is an abstraction of common certainty.

The third grade is exemplified in a statute which empowers a commission to compel an employer to take "appropriate" measures to keep his premises "reasonably safe and sanitary." The language calls for a judgment and raises a question of degree.

In his later and more systematic treatise Freund recognized an even greater freedom of choice that is conferred by statutes that are indefinite to the extent of not mentioning the conditions on which an official shall act. Thus, a permit may be required for a parade, but the police are not told on what basis they shall determine whether a permit shall be issued. Occasionally a statute will emphasize the discretion of the official by saying, "He shall have absolute . . . (or free) . . . discretion, and there shall be no appeal."

James Hart distinguishes four grades of administrative discretion. He uses the names (1) discretionary, (2) judgment passing, (3) fact-finding, and (4) ministerial. This is a somewhat different classification, but the extremes of complete freedom of choice and no freedom are similar to Freund's version.

Freund based his generalizations upon grants of regulatory power. Whether he would have adopted a different analysis if he had studied the discretion conferred upon officials of government corporations and service departments, I do not know. But it is clear that his emphasis in dealing with discretion is upon the indefiniteness of legislative standards. Where the legislature has been indefinite, the administrator must somehow become definite. It is impossible to prove just what the legislature meant. A question of public policy has not been completely decided by the legislators, and the enforcer of public policy must complete the decision. It follows that if we want wise public policies, we must have wisdom in the executive as well as among those who are called lawmakers.

These are the terms in which a student of administrative law phrases the need for ethical acumen and sound judgment. The administrator, charged with discretionary responsibilities, has to make an indefinite standard of action precise and explicit. How can he develop a definite standard?

Now let us evaluate Freund's analysis. It would be unbecoming of an amateur to question the accuracy of Freund's vast knowledge of administrative law, and my remarks should be construed as a conflict between the philosophical and the legal points of view rather than as an attempt on the part of a legal novice to find fault with a legal master. To one who is accustomed to philosophical modes of thought Freund's three or four grades of definiteness in legislative standards do not seem to have improved greatly the organization of his knowledge. In particular, I question his conception of the administrator's task as that of arriving at a definite standard. It may be recalled that Freund even suggested that the normal process would be for the legislature to enact the standards which the administrator should succeed in defining. Administrative discretion would thus be the means of eliminating the need for administrative discretion in the future.

To say that definiteness or susceptibility of proof is an inadequate criterion of a good standard may be to state a trifling proposition. Let me say it. Of course, I do not believe that Freund meant to imply that definiteness is a *sufficient* test of good administrative standards; but his failure to specify other tests gives an undue emphasis to "definiteness," as witness such a statement as the following:

> It appears from the foregoing that the normal function of an administrative order is to make a generic statutory prohibition or requirement definite.

The entire tradition of philosophical ethics is against acceptance of definiteness as an adequate criterion of good judgment. While Socrates and Kant and Bentham were constantly engaged in the work of definition, the popular standards to which they were opposed had only too much definiteness. And the philosophical standards which the philosopher rejects are usually definite. But he considers them to be definitely bad. The doctrinaire man is definite. The shrewd villain is definite in his standards. Something other than definiteness is lacking.

The crucial philosophical criticism of Freund's analysis is that it gives a misleading appearance of simplicity to the concept of definiteness. Philosophical controversies have long since sensitized students of philosophy to the indefiniteness of "definiteness." "Indefinite" may mean (1) "vague," "without limits," or it may mean (2) "ambiguous," "capable of referring to several set limits but not certainly specifying any one limit."

The indefiniteness of definiteness accounts for the difficulty of using Freund's classification of standards. It is doubtful whether any two observers could agree in assigning a hundred miscellaneous statutes to the three pigeon holes which he suggests. Where, for example would you place an old Wisconsin statute which required "joints, knuckles, and jacks of tumbling rods of all threshing machines to be *securely* boxed"? To judge the exercise of administrative discretion merely by the definiteness which the administrator gives to an indefinite statute is to oversimplify the discretionary problem. Is the administrator confronted with a really vague and unexplored subject? Or is he faced with a choice which the legislature has been unable or unwilling to make, a choice between two or more definite standards?

Legislative bodies are indefinite in their language for more than one reason. At times their failure to be specific or clear is an oversight. Again, it may be a recognition of their own lack of skill and experience. It may indicate the existence of a subject which can never be dealt with in general rules. Sometimes, the legislators do not feel that they can afford to spend the time required to hit the nail on the head. In all of these cases "indefiniteness" is probably vagueness.

On the other hand, the legislature may beat around the bush because it cannot muster a majority in favor of a clear-cut standard. The indecisiveness of the language then indicates the existence of several standards about which there is no vagueness at all. The statute is passed either in the hope that an administrative agency can settle a quarrel or from a desire to evade the issue. Pendleton Herring makes it clear that the vague language of statutory instructions for the Tariff Commission and the Federal Trade Commission did not imply a lack of definite standards which might have been applied in these fields.

> Congress has to an increasing extent escaped the onus of directly settling group conflicts by establishing under vague legislative mandates independent regulatory boards. . . . Upon the shoulders of the bureaucrat has been placed in large part the burden of reconciling group differences and making effective and workable the economic and social compromises arrived at through the legislative process.[3]

Where the legislature passes the buck in this way the problem is not a merely technical question of making vague standards definite. If the administrator becomes definite before something else happens, his rulings will be regarded as more unsatisfactory than if he, too, remains indecisive and ambiguous. "Moral gesture" legislation amounts to an instruction to do nothing specific, but most "pass-the-buck" legislation is an instruction to resolve the conflict between groups who want definite but rival standards to be legalized.

From the standpoint of administrators and administrative law there are many other observations to be made concerning discretionary powers and the improvement of their exercise. For our purposes, however, the significant points are: (1) the emphasis upon indefinite statutory language as the means of conferring discretion, and (2) the judgment of administrative success by the definiteness of standards supplied in such cases. A preliminary criticism of this diagnosis has called attention to two meanings of "indefiniteness": (1) "vague" and (2) "ambiguous." Particularly where discretionary powers are granted by ambiguity, it is doubtful whether "definiteness" is an adequate criterion of discretion.

Standards and the Philosophical View

The philosophical analysis of the problems of choice differs from Freund's. Its fundamental distinction is not between definite and indefinite standards. The philosopher is mainly concerned with the distinction between general (or abstract) standards, on the one hand, and specific standards, on the other hand. He wants to know whether you act on a general principle or only on an immediate, concrete rule. Some people suppose that "definite" is equivalent to "particular" whereas "indefinite" means the same as "general" or "abstract." This is not true. "You must not make that stairway too steep" is not general, though it is indefinite. "Educational facilities for the two races shall be equal" is definite, though it is quite general.

Dewey and Tufts stated the philosophical distinction in their *Ethics* as follows:

> Rules are practical; they are habitual ways of doing things. But principles are intellectual; they are the final methods used in judging suggested courses of action. . . . The intuitionist . . . is on the outlook for rules which will of themselves tell agents just what course of action to pursue; whereas the object of moral principles is to supply standpoints and methods which will enable the individual to make for himself an analysis of the elements of good and evil in the particular situation in which he finds himself.

Freund recognized this distinction, but he was interested in general principles that should serve as standards in the work of the legislator. He made little use of the distinction between general principle and detailed rule in his study of the standards which the legislature provides for the administrator.

Rules of action, which tell you just what acts to commit or avoid, are illustrated by the Biblical commands: "Neither shalt thou commit adultery," "Thou shalt make no covenant with the Jebusites," "These are the beasts which ye shall eat: the ox . . . etc." The more general type of moral principles can also be found in the Bible: "Whatsoever ye would that men should do unto you, do ye even also unto them." The Golden Rule does not tell anyone *what* he should do, but only supplies a test which presumably should be applied to all plans of action.

In philosophical ethics the discussion often begins with the statement of detailed rules of action, but rather quickly moves to the level of general principles. Thus, Book One of Plato's *Republic* opens with the statement of several specific rules, such as, "Return borrowed property"; then Plato turns to the more general principles of justice: "Do good to your friends and harm to your enemies," "Seek the happiness of the whole state," and "Let everyone do that for which he is best suited."

Of course, an ethics which supplies criteria of action rather than detailed rules of action runs the risk of mistaking a general criterion for a plan of action. The "visionary" moralist has decided that good will is the proper motive or that peace is the desirable result of conduct, and then he has forgotten that he still needs an institutional plan for carrying out his intention or achieving the result that he prizes.

The philosopher's interest in general principles does not imply a desire to live without detailed plans of action. Plato knew it was impossible to act-in-general. But general principles offer not only a bird's eye view of life but also the possibility of studying the wisdom of contemplated actions. Until deliberations reach the level of generality, alternative courses of action can be compared only in dogmatic fashion. Let A say, "Five dollars a day is a fair wage," while B contends that five dollars is not a fair wage. Unless A and B agree to appeal to general principles, all that they can do is to oppose the authority of one rule of action to the authority of another. Or, to put it another way, A can claim that his plan is endorsed by better men than the men who endorse B's plan. A may admit that he is the better man whose intuition gives authority to the five-dollar plan. Or more modestly, he may claim that his plan is approved by God, the prophet, the Pope, the philosopher-king, or mother. In this case, the rule of action is right because an expert says so. If the expert's qualifications are challenged, the debate must degenerate into name-calling or an appeal to force.

This is an explanation why many philosophers have refused to believe that any given act is either right or wrong in itself. If thought and talk about conduct are to be more than dogmatic assertions, a plan or rule of action cannot by itself be accepted as an ethical standard.

Criteria of Action as Standards

As soon as appeal is made to general principles to settle the wisdom of conduct, attention is directed to a statement that does not tell anyone what to do. The general principle merely states a criterion by which to test detailed rules of action.

Many criteria of conduct have been proposed in the course of the last three thousand years. Usually they specify either a motive or a result which an act must have in order to be acceptable. Some of the criteria have been institutional, e.g., the requirement of loyalty to state, family, church, or property, or the requirement that actions preserve and promote these institutions. Other criteria have not referred directly to institutions, and perhaps they are the best known ethical standards: the preservation of life, peace, my pleasure, security, health, abundance of food and possessions, aesthetic enjoyments, friendship, good will, harmony, equality, or freedom.

Many moral philosophers went no further than to articulate one of these criteria. If they were asked, "Why should I seek my own pleasure?" or "Why is equality worth striving for?" they could only answer, "I cannot doubt it, and, begging your pardon, you are a fool to ask such a question." One ethical criterion was their ultimate standard, and they usually claimed that they were satisfied on the point by an indubitable intuition.

Although the philosophers all hoped to find a single acid test of sound judgment, most of them recognized in one way or another that no one criterion of action is entirely adequate for testing the value of conduct. It is quite possible to evaluate any action with, say, the standard of equality; but action that stands the test of equality may be deficient from the standpoint of freedom or happiness or loyalty to the family. No doubt, every well-known ethical criterion, when taken as an absolute, can be used to justify bad conduct. Thus, "It is right to help a friend. Therefore, I did right in overlooking Smith's donation of government property to his friend." Or, "It is a man's duty to support his family. Therefore, Jones did right in defrauding Miller, for the proceeds were used to buy shoes for the baby." Or, "It is a good thing to protect health. Therefore, the commissioner should prohibit all fairs and conventions, for they increase the probabilities of an epidemic."

Such sophistry ignores the qualifications attaching to the principles to which appeal is made; each principle is treated as absolute. Reasonable men, on the contrary, find a conflict between criteria. They say, "Health is good, *other things being equal*," knowing full well that other things are frequently not equal.

Methods of Ranking Criteria

Moralists who recognize the conflict of values try to find some method for deciding which is the higher value. Much work remains to be done before these analytical methods will be readily applicable to the complicated problems of government.

At the present time I am inclined to classify ethical methods accordingly as they look away from the immediate choice situation or not. When the disciples of Socrates or Jesus find themselves torn between loyalty to country and love of peace or between regard for health and love of excitement, they are apt to look beyond their immediate circumstance. They ask what they would prefer in other situations, and thus seek by generalization to determine the permanent and universal *ranking* of values. In my language, they try to determine which criterion should always and everywhere be the ultimate test of action, and in which order other tests should be applied. Critical questions are propounded to direct the mind away from obsession with the practical alternatives as they appear in the immediate situation:

a. What is always and everywhere good?
b. What could we do without?
c. What would I want if I were in the other fellow's shoes?
d. What do I usually prefer?
e. What will seem insignificant in twelve-months or as soon as I am out of my present predicament?

Having assigned to values, ends, or criteria an order which seems permanent and universal, the moralist determines which of his immediate alternatives is consistent with this general value order. His motto is to put first things first, and not to treat ends as means. But this motto is meaningful only because he has previously engaged in an ethical generalization. He has looked away from his own conflict of the moment and decided what *in general* is most worthwhile.

The second method of comparing rival values may be called utilitarianism (although I include here not only Mill and Bentham, but also the pragmatists and part of Aristotle). The utilitarian does not attempt to assign permanent places in a general value series to health, life, country, home, etc. Rather he assumes that there is no point to saying once and for all that the enjoyment of food is more or less important than the enjoyment of friendship. He values both kinds of enjoyment and tries to secure both of them as far as possible in each choice situation. The question is, Which action will secure more of these goods and which will secure less in the present circumstance? He concentrates attention upon the immediate choice and its possible consequences. He asks such questions as these:

a. What are the pros and cons, the advantages and disadvantages, of the various alternative actions?
b. What are the pleasures and what are the pains consequent upon the alternatives, and how do they compare in number, duration, intensity and extent, certainty and propinquity?

c. Have I thought of all the consequences of the contemplated actions? Have I thought of everything that I value in this particular situation and its eventualities?

d. Which alternatives would I regard as extreme actions and which would seem to be the golden mean?

Having taken steps to apply all relevant tests to the contemplated choice, the utilitarian tries to pick the alternative that entails the most advantages and the fewest disadvantages. In my language, he prefers the conduct that satisfies the greatest number of criteria to the greatest degree. For this purpose he concentrates attention upon the immediate discretionary situation and its possible repercussions.

Utilitarianism is still a philosophical method of handling value-conflicts, although it fixes one's gaze upon the immediate situation rather than upon a universal hierarchy of values. It insists upon an analysis of the values involved in one's present decision, and applies a general value principle, i.e., that one should prefer the course of conduct which realizes the most values and the fewest disvalues.

Neither the Platonic type of ethics nor the utilitarian says that a particular act, such as raising the tariff, is always right or always wrong, The Platonist will say that some value like good will or harmony is more important than the personal profit of a few; then he will examine the immediate situation to discover whether raising the tariff is a rule of action by which personal profit would nullify good will or harmony. The utilitarian will ask *how much* benefit is conferred upon the protected industry, how much indirect benefit accrues to the nation, how much ill will is generated, how much loss is incurred by other industries, etc. Then he will adopt or reject the tariff rule according to its net benefit or detriment.

This brief restatement of ethics is incomplete, but it will bring to mind the differences between the philosophical approach and Freund's approach to the problem of standards.

Another Classification

The legal and the philosophical analyses of discretion may be juxtaposed by asking what kind of standards (from the standpoint of ethics) Freund was talking about. The "indefinite" legislative standards might be rules of action; again, they might be criteria for evaluating rules of action.

Obviously, the granting of discretionary power always involves some indefiniteness with respect to the rule of action. Even if the status and identity of the actor and the conditions under which he must act are completely specified, at least the description of what he is expected to do must be vague or ambiguous; otherwise, the administrator would have no choice to make. In order to arrive at a useful classification of discretionary powers, therefore, we must ask whether the criteria of action are indefinite; and, if indefinite, whether they are ambiguous or vague.

We shall distinguish three classes of discretionary powers: (1) technical discretion, which is freedom in prescribing the rule but not the criterion or end of action; (2) discretion in prescribing the rule of action and also in clarifying a *vague* criterion—this is the authorization of social planning; (3) discretion in prescribing the rule of action where the criterion of action is *ambiguous* because it is in dispute—this amounts to an instruction to the official to use his ingenuity in political mediation.

1. No discretion as to criterion.

This class of discretion is, in ordinary language, merely the choice of means to an end which is not in question. The legislature leaves it to the experts to hit upon the kind of action that will obtain a desired result. How the result is obtained is, within limits, a matter of indifference to the law-making body: it is the area of discretion for the administrator.

Typical of this grade of discretion are many of the delegations of power to regulate the processing and sale of food products. The criterion is not in dispute: it is the health of the consumer as far as science and the arts can achieve it without making costs prohibitive. Sometimes the regulating officials not only prescribe the rule of action but actually invent the rule, as in the famous case where scientists in the employ of the government worked out a new method of cleaning and canning blueberries.

Discretion is also limited to choosing the means of reaching a predetermined result in the regulation of insurance companies. The criterion or end is the solvency of the companies and the protection of the policyholders. Other examples are the rule-making powers of industrial and mining commissions with respect to safety, and the licensing powers in such trades as those of barbers, dentists, keepers of foster homes, and warehousemen. Technical discretion is likewise illustrated in the governmental services, e.g., the freedom with which military administrators act is limited by the avowed purpose of national security and victory in war. The protests over the Eisenhower-Darlan agreement are an interesting evidence of the technical character of military discretion.

In the history of ethics when the rule of action is all that is in question, we find that appeal is made to the judgment of an expert. The expert sets the standard. Moral philosophers have usually identified some expert-in-general, such as God, the priest, or the philosopher. In public administration it is interesting to note that the expert is an expert-in-particular. If the administrator is not himself a man of specialized training or experience, he will very likely hold hearings or take the recommendations of the appropriate specialists: bacteriologists, social workers, actuaries, the American Standards Association, or the American Bankers Association. Of course, experts don't always agree. Many arts are far from perfection. When the criterion is not in question, the chief difficulty in adopting a wise administrative standard is that of finding an occupational or scientific group which has attained at least semiprofessional status. Insofar as health, safety in employment, solvency, etc. are definite and agreed-upon criteria, there may be *relatively* little trouble about standards in the sense of rules of action. It is not always possible to give an absolutely precise interpretation to the legislative formula, such as eventuated in the first Illinois mining law which required "a sufficient supply" of pure air in mines and which was translated into the prescription that air currents moving at a stated velocity follow a specified route. But such indefinite language as "reasonable diligence" and "reputable practices" will be capable of satisfactory definition if there is an organized art or trade, and *if* the criterion of action is not controverted. As we shall see presently, it is in situations where the criterion is not agreed upon that expert opinion loses its effectiveness and acceptability in setting standards (rules of action).

2. Discretion regarding a vague criterion. Legislative power is delegated in a few fields where the legislature and the public find themselves unable to define either the rule or the criterion of action. These are the subjects on which most of those in the community do not know even the results which they desire. For a time, at least, the administrator may be free not only to choose the means but also the end of action. The legislative standard is indefinite in the sense of being vague.

The most common example of this type is in public education. The wayfaring man is able to tell, quite roughly of course, whether his child is sick or well, prosperous or poverty-stricken, safe or injured; but when is his child well educated? Although the pursuit and encouragement of school work has become almost a religion in this country, most of the friends of education have had only vague notions of what they desired. The first constitution of Massachusetts enjoined legislatures and magistrates to "cherish the interests of literature and the sciences and all seminaries of them." The Nebraska legislature enacted a bill in 1864 regulating the establishment of colleges and universities with an object "to promote the general educational interests and to qualify students to engage in the several pursuits and employments of society, and to discharge honorably and usefully the various duties of life." Other state school laws have been even vaguer as to the controlling purposes of the school system. If the criteria or objectives sound definite, the appearance of definiteness quickly disappears when we ask about the relative importance of literature and the sciences, or the relative merits of general and vocational education, or just what constitutes vocational success.

It is true that the Morrill Acts prescribed the curricula for the land grant colleges and that many state legislatures require or prohibit the teaching of certain subjects. Statutes declare the ages of compulsory school attendance and sometimes the minimum requirements for teacher certification. But it is doubtful whether the eighteen states that require the teaching of American history had a much clearer conception than the thirty states that do not require it of the precise and complete contribution of this study to the life of the child and the state. In any event, the teachers of history and their superintendents have had difficulty trying to decide what they should accomplish. The criterion being vague, the school boards, regents, and superintendents were often free to prescribe the governing objectives. This explains, in part, why educational literature is replete with discussions of the aims of education.

Of course, legislatures have occasionally set both a definite rule of action and a definite criterion in school legislation. Tennessee's legislature prohibited the teaching of evolution; nine states have laws directing instruction in the humane treatment of animals, and thirty-three states require the school officials to *supply* instruction concerning the effects of narcotics, stimulants, and alcohol. It should be observed that as the educational administrators define the aims of education they sometimes arouse a part of the community to the definition of opposite aims. But school administration is probably the best example of discretionary powers conferred by vagueness of the legislature as to criteria.

There are other administrators besides the school men who receive this type of discretionary power. Boards of censorship, heads of government enterprises like the TVA [Tennessee Valley Authority], city planning commissions, professional licensing authorities, and library boards may be mentioned in this connection. Where the legislative criterion is really vague, the official has the broadest kind of discretion, the discretion of an accredited social planner.

Faced with the necessity of choosing an objective, administrators may proceed in hit-or-miss fashion; they may seek the definition in ethical and political literature; or they may themselves use such methods of ethical generalization and specification as we described in an earlier section. Judging by the history of public education, I should say that the greatest danger faced by the official at this point is "professionalism" in the bad sense of the word. By that I mean a tendency to fall into the habit of judging proposals by their effect on departmental expansion and convenience, regardless of what is *said* to be the guiding principle. At least, the educational world is shaken periodically by charges that school officials, blinded by bureaucratic loyalties, fail to sense the emerging value possibilities of our civilization.

3. Discretion limited by rival criteria.   The third brand of discretion is the kind which Herring discusses in his book on *Public Administration and the Public Interest.* The legislature directs the administrator to regulate or license in the "public interest" or to see that someone serves the "public necessity and convenience." The language is indefinite, but it does not stand for a vague criterion of action. Rather, the public or the legislature is divided in favor of two or more sharply defined objectives.

Illustrations of discretion under these conditions engaged most of Herring's attention. The Tariff Commission received indefinite standards because the importers and consumers judged tariffs by different criteria than did the domestic manufacturers. The Federal Radio Commission was not told to require the use of the radio primarily for education nor was it told to encourage the use of radio primarily for amusement and advertising, for the simple reason that both purposes had strong support. The Bureau of Home Economics got into trouble over Circular 296 because the Department of Agriculture was conceived by some as promoting the farmer's prosperity and by others as promoting the health of the community.

More recently, the President and the State Department have come in for heavy criticism on account of the agreements which they negotiated under the Reciprocal Trade Agreement Act. The Supreme Court has declared that the President must be allowed a greater degree of discretion in international affairs than in domestic matters, and the Act in question explicitly conferred the power to reduce tariffs "wherever he finds existing import restrictions are unduly burdening or restricting American foreign trade." Yet it is safe to say that whatever the President might or might not have done under the Act, he would have been charged with an unwise exercise of discretion. If the cattle men and the distillers had been satisfied, we may be sure that at least the editors of the *New Republic* would have been dissatisfied. The trouble here is not a vague standard expressed in vague language, but many definite standards unable to come to anything but a vague agreement, which is hardly any agreement at all. . . .

The discretion of the administrator in the presence of two well-defined but hostile criteria is hardly more than authorization to do what he can to settle a conflict. The administrator guides or echoes or resists a political process in which there must eventually be some synthesis, victory, or compromise of divergent objectives. In so far as administration is subordinated to sheer political power there will be no opportunity for rational deliberation. Nevertheless, many of the policy decisions are determined at least partially by hearings and by public discussions. To that extent, the administrator can attempt to guide the deliberations of himself and interested parties in a rational manner. To that extent, he may be aided by the philosophers' methods of resolving the conflicts between antipathetic criteria. Because the administrator is meeting a problem of ends rather than a problem of means, the administrator who is merely a technical expert may be incompetent in this situation. Our analysis therefore supports the plea for general administration.

It is not always easy to identify the competing criteria. No group likes to admit that its criterion of right action is merely its own desire for pelf. I believe that Dexter Keezer was referring in part to this difficulty when he wrote:

> If the Administrator of the NRA could have appealed to a broad array of well-digested facts bearing upon the issues involved in the drafting of codes, this lack of balance between the powers of employers, wage-workers and consumers as pressure groups might not have been of major consequence.[4]

As I interpret the NRA [National Recovery Act] conflicts, it was not merely the absence of well-digested facts that made it difficult for the administrator to lift the issues above the arbitrament of unadorned pressures: it was also the absence of a clear and honest statement of the criteria represented by the competing pressure groups. The problem was to give every value a hearing which, at the same time, should be a grilling. But some people were busy disguising the values.

After the issues have been clarified so as to reveal the rival objectives, the administrator who is fortunate enough to preside over a semirational deliberation will probably employ one of the calculating or ranking methods by which philosophers have sought to resolve the conflicts between values. He will probably try to get the partisans to appreciate the criteria urged by their opponents. If he can get either side to say, "There is something we didn't think of," he will have gone far toward the avoidance of a foolish decision. A study of the amendments and repeals of rulings by our wartime agencies reveals a number of cases where the administrator and the interested parties had simply failed to appreciate the magnitude of the interests adversely affected by the original rulings. I am thinking not merely of economic interests that were ignored, but also, in cases where decisions were inspired by economic considerations, of adverse effects upon the recreational and educational side of community life.

An acquaintance with the ethics of Sidgwick, of Aristotle, of Hartmann, or of Dewey is no guarantee of wisdom in administrative decisions, but the leading principles and methods of these philosophers are articulations of the ways in which uncongenial values may be recognized and given a preference that will stand the criticism of experience. Ethics can at least give the administrator an enlarged vocabulary with which to discuss the subtle elements in a conflict of values.

The law sometimes specifies methods of comparing antagonistic values. This is the root meaning of "due process of law," although courts were for a time inclined to give "due process" a narrow construction which meant little more than testing action by its effect on property rights, regardless of other criteria. Occasionally the courts are quite voluble in specifying the "considerations" that are to be weighed in arriving at an administrative decision.... Although the criteria thus imposed upon the administrator are often vague, they are the most abstract type of legal principle and remind one of the terms in which philosophers talk about the problems of choice, i.e., they suggest a method for resolving the conflicts between rival criteria, which, in turn, are the basis for selecting detailed rules of action....

Conclusion

I have tried to bring the administrative and the philosophical points of view into a mutually beneficial juxtaposition. The task was difficult because of differences in occupational vocabularies. If I have taken liberties with both languages I hope that neither the philosophers nor the administrators will be outraged by my malapropisms, but will generously make efforts of their own to bridge the word chasm that separates the two fields. Philosophers can certainly profit from a knowledge of administrative problems, and I have been told that administrators need some philosophical insights.

The philosophical criticism of current administrative and legal views of discretion is that the administrator puts too much stress on achieving definiteness of standards. My own first reaction to the problem of discretionary powers is that Freund's classification according to definiteness should be supplanted or complicated by some other distinctions. I have suggested a three-fold classification which distinguishes:

1. Merely technical discretion, where the legislature has stated or assumed that the administrator knew the results which it desired;
2. Discretion in social planning, where the legislature doesn't know exactly what it ultimately will want in the way of results; and

3. Discretion in the work of reconciliation, where the legislature has, in effect, asked the administrator to break a political deadlock. . . .

Notes

1. *Administrative Powers Over Persons and Property* (University of Chicago Press, 1928). p. 71.

2. *Yale Law Journal* 30 (1921): 437–55.

3. P. Herring, *Public Administration and the Public Interest* (McGraw-Hill Book Company, 1936), p. 7.

4. Quoted by Herring, p. 245.

CASE C

TO PUSH OR NOT TO PUSH

At the macro level dogma is clear: professionals are to treat patients with dignity. But in the micro dimension how should a healthcare professional deal with a physician who is observed acting in a degrading manner with patients? What power does the healthcare professional have in such situations? Should one confront the doctor or not and, if so, how intensively and when? The following case, typical of Dr. Down's routine behavior, concerns such a situation.

After an interdisciplinary team meeting at a public psychiatric hospital, Sherry, a patient on the ward, asks to speak with the team claiming an emergency. She enters the conference room appearing much as she always does—neatly but a bit provocatively dressed. Although calm at first, as she continues to speak of her "incident" she becomes increasingly upset with halting speech and teary eyes. Sherry informs the staff that she has been assaulted by one of the lawn maintenance workers at the hospital. She tells a story that apparently differs slightly from a first report (to the nursing staff), although in only a few details. It is unclear whether her memory is inadequate for the retelling of a made-up story, or whether the story is true but her anxiety is contributing to her forgetfulness about some of the details.

The team leader, physician Donald Down, has a strong reaction to this woman. Not only does he not believe her; he proceeds to berate her in front of the team. Throughout the meeting the woman becomes increasingly upset. Dr. Kathy Kind, the clinical psychologist on the team, is outraged at the physician's behavior but is uncertain about what, ethically, to do.

Background

The physician and the psychologist worked together for two years on another ward where Kathy, not Donald, was the team leader. In that situation the physician was congenial and not verbally abusive toward patients. In the current position of greater authority, however, with another physician friend on the team and with additional responsibilities, pressures, and stress, his behavior is different. On this ward, there is little congeniality between Dr. Kind and Dr. Down, as the psychologist has occasionally disagreed with the physician's opinion on clinical matters. On the previous ward Down rarely attended the team meetings, thus avoiding potential conflict.

Although Dr. Down is not especially liked among his colleagues, the other physicians would likely react negatively to the psychologist if they perceived that she was not giving the physician full respect. Kathy fears being classified as a troublemaker, a label that might make future dealings with the physicians difficult.

Although Dr. Kind does not know for sure, it is possible that in his many years at the hospital Dr. Down has experienced similar accusations by patients himself, or has seen colleagues or other co-workers suffer the consequences on their reputations of an investigation. Similarly, perhaps he is currently in the midst of a false malpractice charge in his evening private practice.

In this particular instance, the physician has overtly broken no law or hospital procedure. He does, in fact, exercise his official micro power by following through with having the woman examined. An incident report is filed by the head nurse, and Dr. Down does write a note in the chart regarding the meeting.

One can hypothesize possible organizational factors that may have affected this physician's behavior. Perhaps feeling pressured and over-whelmed with work himself, he was concerned with wasting staff time on an investigation of what he guessed were false allegations. Another organizational factor was his standing in the hospital. He had been transferred to the community-oriented ward after several years on another ward where staff had tried to get rid of him. The unit chief there had frequently expressed her frustrations in dealing with this physician, but felt that there was little she could do about his behavior except to get him transferred. He apparently had some support in the upper echelons.

Still another organizational factor was the ambivalence of the other team members. Although they frequently complained about Dr. Down when not in his presence, they did not assert themselves at the team meetings. The one team member who had once confronted him found her dealings with him to be so exhausting and demoralizing that she dealt with the situation by requesting a transfer to another ward.

A fiscal factor may also have contributed to the physician's demeanor. Budgetary cutbacks had resulted in freezes on hiring in many departments, resulting in increased workloads. The clinical psychologist was also affected by this concerning her own job. Depending on how far she might push Dr. Down—if in fact he did have friends in high places accounting for the difficulty in getting rid of him over the years—he might have the connections to influence her tenure.

An important fiscal factor was the difficulty of attracting physicians to work at this hospital. In comparison to the going rate for physicians elsewhere, the salaries at this hospital were low. This made it difficult for the system to attract good doctors in the first place, and the fairly good ones who did come seldom stayed long. Thus, on an organizational level, and affected by fiscal realities, the organization perhaps would risk its accreditation and subsequent funding if it did not retain the minimum number of physicians required by state regulations. This was a constant worry in the facility. Furthermore, Donald Down did not have the language problem that affected many of the staff physicians and, to his credit, he was one of the few physicians at the facility who was fully board certified.

Principles number 3 and 6 of the "Ethical Principles of Psychologists" are germane. Principle number 3 regarding moral and legal standards stipulates that "as employees or employers, psychologists do not engage in or condone practices that are inhumane or that result in illegal or unjustifiable actions." It is unclear from this statement whether *not* acting is in effect condoning what the clinical psychologist considered to be an inhumane action in this situation. Principle number 6 pertaining to the welfare of the consumer states that "when there is a conflict of interest between a client and the psychologist's employing institution, psychologists clarify the nature and direction of their loyalties and responsibilities and keep all parties informed of their commitments." Moreover, the Preamble of the Code declares that psychologists should "make every effort to protect the welfare of those who seek their services" and that "psychologists respect the dignity and worth of the individual and strive for the preservation and protection of fundamental human rights." By not exercising some moral reproach, would Kathy Kind be condoning the physician's behavior and abandoning the patient to denigration? Would she be guilty by omission despite good intentions?

Controlling influences in Sherry's case include Dr. Kind's professional code, the law, hospital procedures, Kathy's boss, other clients, colleagues, fellow team members, and the physician. Dr. Down's idea of Dr. Kind doing her job competently and professionally might be that she keep quiet and defer to him. This expectation might conflict with other values and expectations of the rest of the parties involved. Whose judgment should prevail in this case? The psychologist's? The physician's? The team's? The unit chief's?

Options

Several workable options for dealing with the situation occur to the clinical psychologist:

1. Walk out of the meeting.
2. Do nothing.
3. Do nothing at the meeting but request a transfer from the ward.
4. Do nothing at the meeting but later report the physician or complain to higher authority.
5. Do nothing at the meeting but later offer support to the patient.
6. Do nothing at the meeting but later talk to a third party whom the physician respects and who may be able to influence him to treat patients with more dignity.
7. Do nothing at the meeting but later speak with the physician.
8. Do nothing at the meeting but later use behavior modification techniques to try to change the physician's behavior.
9. Intervene in the meeting with the patient by offering the patient support and focusing on procedures.
10. Intervene in the meeting with the physician by confronting him verbally or subtly as with a disapproving glance or by focusing on the facts and procedures to follow.
11. Suggest to the administration a workshop for physicians on relating to patients and/or on ethics and values.
12. Enlist team support to take a stand against the physician.

Dr. Kind realizes she has many micro powers—some official, some subtle.

Consequences of the Options

The clinical psychologist, Dr. Kind, later documents her analysis of these options for future reference as follows:

> Regarding the potential consequences of these various alternatives, doing nothing at all would be the most unacceptable to me. Doing nothing would preserve none of the values I consider important with the exception of respecting the authority of the physician. It would result in the negative consequence for me of feeling that I did not stand up for my values. The patient would likely perceive me as supporting the physician, and this would damage the positive

relationship we had been developing. Still another negative effect would be probable continuance of such behavior by the physician. And, as a professional, I would not be upholding the ethical principles of the field. The only possible positive consequence might be that Dr. Down would perceive my silence as support, which could then improve our relationship.

Doing nothing at the meeting and then later asking for a transfer is my second least-favorite alternative. Negative consequences would be continuing abusive behavior toward patients by the physician. This option would perhaps be in my best interest but not the patients'. In terms of my self-respect, I would feel that I abandoned the patients on the ward and that they would have one less buffer from the physician's behavior. A positive consequence for me would be the reduced stress that could in turn have a beneficial effect on my work. A slightly positive consequence for me would be in terms of self-respect in that I would feel I had taken a stand regarding my values, in particular that I did not approve of this behavior and would not work with someone who was so denigrating. However, although the physician and team members would know why I left, the physician in fact would probably be happy to have me off his back.

Another power which I hesitate to exercise is to take the patient out of the meeting. This step would have the most negative consequences for me since it would be overstepping my authority on the team and could jeopardize my job. It is questionable whether this would be the most professional way of handling this situation, although in the short run it would get the patient out of the situation. In the long run, it would just serve to increase the physician's rage, which would likely be taken out on the patient. Also likely is that working with him would be even more unpleasant and difficult. Advantages are that I would be upholding my values of loyalty to the patient, fairness, respect for her dignity, but at the probable cost of her continued mistreatment in the long run.

Walking out of the meeting myself is still another power I have. This option would show some assertiveness, and some loyalty to the patient. However, it would show only a neutral amount of loyalty to the patient and result in only a minimal amount of self-respect. Fairness and justice, however, would not be upheld by such a move. A positive consequence is that it would represent for me a way to stand up for my values, and would make a statement. A negative consequence that may indirectly affect the patient involved is that such action might increase the physician's anger, which could then be taken out against the patient. Another negative consequence would again be my feeling of abandoning the patient.

Another possible consequence of this alternative is the physician reporting my action to the unit chief. However, the repercussions of this would most likely be minimal, since the unit chief is an ally.

A more acceptable alternative for me would be to do nothing at the meeting, but to talk later to Dr. Down. Positive consequences would be maintenance of my self-respect since I would feel that I stood up for the patient's dignity. How to approach him, however, brings to mind a number of different options. I could try to approach him in as assertive a manner as I could. I could try to instill in him a curiosity regarding the patient's condition and try to convey the impact his interrogation had on the patient. I might say something like, "Dr. D., I realize that you don't believe Sherry in the least, and I think it may be interesting to try to figure out why she would lie, if that is the case; but I was also concerned that coming across so strongly to her was not getting anywhere in terms of finding the 'truth'." As I write this, I can feel Down's rage at his feeling of being criticized, and I can hear his backlash against me and a strong self-defense of his actions. He is not likely to be receptive to this sort of moral reproach, even if it is related in the gentlest possible manner. Based on my knowledge of his past reaction to confrontation, especially with women, he would likely become defensive—more angry, accusing, and insulting. Thus, although in the short run this approach may have positive consequences for me, in the long run the effects would be quite negative: the patient's rights would not have been protected, and the physician's behavior may actually become worse. The values of justice, fairness, and the patient's best interest therefore would likely not be upheld.

Four additional interventions that I thought of also involve doing nothing at the meeting, while still attempting to change the physician. One would involve recommending a workshop for physicians on relating to the patients. Disadvantages of this alternative are that it would not have a short-term effect on Sherry, and I could be seen as being on the doctor's side, thus affecting my rapport and relationship with this patient. An intervention that might have a possibility of success—in terms of the goal of having the physician begin to treat this patient and others with more respect—is to talk to a third party whom the doctor respects. The head nurse and the ward psychiatrist have the best relationships with Dr. Down out of all of the team members. Although they are often treated disrespectfully as well, he would handle criticism from them better than from the rest of the team members. Nonetheless, changes resulting from this approach are not all that likely, and if they do occur, they are likely to be short lived. Advantages of this approach are that it would result in less risk of increasing Dr. Down's anger than if I approached him.

Yet another intervention that would involve trying to influence this physician, but in a slightly more direct manner, would be to interact with him after the meeting. Instead of confronting him, I could instead try to "build him up" in the hope that the result would be his greater capacity to respect the patients. For example, I could praise him for something he did competently, empathize with his difficult workload, or offer to help him with team scheduling. A drawback to this approach is that if there is any change at all, it will be long term, and will not have an impact on the patient in this particular case. Furthermore, it would conflict somewhat with my value of honesty, since this approach would be discordant with my feelings regarding the doctor in addition to being a bit manipulative. Moreover, this approach showed only fair results in the past when employed by the head nurse. Advantages of using this approach are that it would uphold his authority and his dignity.

I do have the power to intervene during the meeting by offering support to the patient, by empathizing with how upset she seems, and by focusing on the need to obtain the facts of her report so that an investigation can be made. I can also offer to meet with her some time after the meeting if she wishes to talk about the incident. Positive consequences of this approach are that it would show concern for the patient's dignity by treating her with respect and responsiveness and would sustain my professional responsibility to protect the patient's rights.

A final option might be to do nothing at the meeting, but to complain about and/or report the physician later. The alternatives within this option involve a verbal or written complaint to either the unit chief or others in the administration, possibly even the medical director. I consider this option to be most likely to have an impact on this physician since I would expect him to respond to an authority with the power to dispense punishment (or negative reinforcement) for inappropriate behavior. Therefore, in the long run this approach could have a positive impact. Politically, within the chain of command, the person to bring this up to would be the unit chief. This would be the easiest for me to do since she is an ally. However, in the past, she has demonstrated little inclination to act. If nothing were done, a last resort could be to ask her what other steps may be useful and to tell her that I would be sending a memo to the medical director. Possible negative consequences of this approach would be development of a reputation as a "troublemaker" within the hospital, if indeed this physician has allies in the administration. Perhaps a safer alternative for myself, and possibly even more effective, would be to try to have a written complaint signed by the entire team. However, based on past experience with the same physician and team members on another ward, this is unlikely.

These alternatives could also be used in combination, such as making a complaint while also intervening to support the patient during the meeting. The advantage of such combined options is that it increases the likelihood of protecting more of the values at stake. The combined approaches that I would feel most comfortable with involve intervening at the meeting with support to the patient as well as talking to her again after the meeting. I would also try to talk to a third party. I would avoid speaking directly with Dr. Down due to the anticipated negative consequences. I would, however, show some subtle form of moral reproach during the meeting as well as at future meetings when patients are denigrated.

One of the most effective steps that I feel I can take in the long run is to report the incident, in writing, to the unit chief—and I can try to get the signatures of all of the team members as well. If nothing comes of this, I can then consult with my supervisor and the department director to determine who else in the chain of command would be appropriate to send a complaint to. Since they are more familiar with the hospital's political structure than I am, and since I have come to respect their opinions, I would defer my judgment to these individuals in this case.

Another approach that I can use to effect long-term change is to recommend seminars for the physicians on relating to patients; and I can use behavior modification techniques to try to make a small dent in Dr. Down's behavior. The advantage of this combination of approaches is that it will uphold my values to the greatest degree possible, given my goal of minimizing negative consequences.

Questions for Discussion

1. Does the clinical psychologist demonstrate ethical maturity or immaturity? How so?
2. Is "minimizing negative consequences" the mature way to deal with ethical dilemmas?
3. How powerful is a team member in such situations? What constitutes ethical responsibility in using or not using such power?
4. Distinguish official micro power from subtle micro power in this case. Which are being considered and which are being neglected by the clinical psychologist?
5. Were the clinical psychologist to analyze the ethical behavior of the physician team leader, would her analytical process be existentially different from the reflection on her own behavior?
6. Whose judgment of the responsible response to the situation should Dr. Kathy Kind follow?

Annotated Bibliography

Bok, S. *Secrets*. New York: Vintage, 1984. Wonderfully explains the role of information in a professional's maintenance of power over clients/patients.

Brass, D., and M. Burkhardt. "Potential Power and Power Use." *Academy of Management Journal* 36, no. 3 (summer 1993): 441–70. Discusses the micro/macro power distinction.

Caro, R. *The Power Broker*. New York: Vintage, 1975. A brilliant articulation and analysis—through examination of the career of Robert Moses—of the power possibilities of public service professionals.

Davis, K. C. *Distributive Justice*. Urbana: University of Illinois Press, 1969. Although written as a law school text, its opening chapter is conceptually among the most profound discourses on micro power.

Kabanoff, B. "Equity, Equality, Power and Conflict." *Academy of Management Review* 16, no. 2 (summer 1991): 420–32. Articulates useful insight on the nature of micro power.

Kelly, C. *The Destructive Achiever*. Reading, MA: Addison-Wesley, 1988. A wonderful analysis of different uses of power by managerial professionals.

Kelman, H., and V. Hamilton. *Crimes of Obedience*. New Haven, CT: Yale University Press, 1989. A sophisticated analysis of the power of authority and of ethical means for dealing with it.

Lebacqz, K. *Professional Ethics: Power and Paradox*. Nashville, TN: Abingdon, 1985. Written for ministerial professions, one of the most realistic and well-written insights available on the nature of micro power.

Lipsky, M. *Street Level Bureaucracy*. New York: Russell Sage, 1980. A brilliant, starkly realistic portrait of the micro power of the public service professional.

Lo, B. "Behind Closed Doors: Promises and Pitfalls of Ethics Committees." *The New England Journal of Medicine* 317, no. 1 (2 July 1987): 46–50. One of the few pieces that reflects on the role of the individual member of ethics committees in healthcare, that is, on the micro dimension.

Rohr, J. *Ethics for Bureaucrats*. New York: Dekker, 1978. Provides, in chapter 2, an enlightened commentary on the generic micro powers of public service professionals.

Sabini, J., and M. Silver. *Moralities for Everyday Life*. New York: Oxford, 1982. By far the best probe of the subtlety of micro power in print.

Warren, K. *Administrative Law*. St. Paul, MN: West Publishing, 1982. In chapter 3, a sound insight to the nature of administrative power.

MANAGING VALUES: FROM CONFLICT TO RECONCILIATION

I F ONE thing has characterized the study and analysis of professional ethics in general, and healthcare ethics in particular, it is a focus on values. Indeed, a review of the literature, graduate curricula, codes of ethics, and training materials suggests that the most prominent feature of the ethical dimension of healthcare *is* values. Take a look at your own professional or organizational code of ethics. While some contain lists of things to avoid and possible conflicts of interest, *all* are filled with statements of values: honesty, integrity, fairness, dignity, and competence are the pervasive words, and healthcare ethics is clearly identified with these concepts. Let us focus the reality prism on values and try to see what's there.

Expectations and Expecters

Would that healthcare ethics were simply a matter of upholding the values so eloquently expressed in our codes—ethical life would be so much easier. Unfortunately, when we focus on the reality of values, we find several salient challenges that complicate the situation. One is that there are many sources of values aside from just our peers, organizations, or professional associations, and they tend to express their values not in nice words written on sacred scrolls but in hard core demands. There are our clients, our subordinates, and our bosses, there are judges and lawyers, media reporters, and expert gurus. And there are our families—spouses and children—as well as our own internal voices of conscience. In short, a basic reality of the values horizon of healthcare ethics is that *multiple* legitimate expecters exist in the ethical dimension of our professional work, and their values tend to touch us—sometimes grab us—in very real expectations on our behavior. Indeed, from my own experience the words "values" and even "expectations" are much too soft to depict the reality: words like "pressures" and "demands" are much more accurate.

Specifically, in the daily routine of our healthcare work codes of ethics sometimes decorate the walls, but there are also: (a) our boss telling us to get this done and that out; (b) our patient asking over and over when he will be treated; (c) our spouse on the phone telling us the roof is leaking and a new roof costs $10,000; (d) our Joint Commission official requesting more documentation; (e) the union representative filing a grievance on behalf of our incompetent employee; and (f) our inner soul feeling the stress of it all. And what are these actors shouting at us? "Get the job done!" "Get *my* treatment done!" "Get a salary raise or we'll all get soaked!" "Get the job done by the book or I won't let you do the job!" "Don't expect any extra help from your employee in getting that job done!" And finally, "Take a vacation before you burn out!" All of these voices compete for our time and attention. Who, then, gets our ear and who gets it first? To whom *should* we listen first? And what do all of these urgent demands have to do with ethics and values?

Nature of the Values Reality

First is the question of *responsibility*. To whom are we responsible and for what? In a nutshell, healthcare professionals have multiple responsibilities for multiple values. That modifier—"multiple"—makes a major difference. If our responsibility were simply to get the job done, or to be pleasant, or to follow our personal values, doing ethics might not be so cumbersome. But, as a classic study of the professions found, professionals are held responsible for many things like being fair, competent, honest, *and* responsive.[1] Mary Guy identifies ten core values required for what she calls "high reliability management": caring, honesty, accountability, promise keeping, pursuit of excellence, loyalty, fairness, integrity, respect for others, and responsibility.[2] What do *we* find that we are held responsible for in the daily routine of our healthcare position? What do our bosses expect? Competence and productivity? But what about loyalty and obedience to their authority? What do our subordinates expect? Fairness in dealing with them? What about our peers? Do they expect a consistently high level of skill and expertise? And professional loyalty to them? And what do the patients expect? Besides valuing our expertise do they hold us responsible for responsiveness to their particular needs? And ourselves?

Do we expect honesty of ourselves and value our own sense of integrity? How about our families? Do they value our job security? Don't forget the Joint Commission on Accreditation of Healthcare Organizations. Does the Joint Commission hold us responsible for adherence to the rules and procedures?

When we focus on responsibility, a dizzying kaleidoscope of values emerges. In organizing this reality it may help to distinguish between the "big picture" values and what I call the "little picture" values. This is a practical translation of the ancient conceptual dichotomy of society versus the individual, of the value of the whole versus the value of the person. In the big picture we value our organization and profession, and under this rubric lie cherished and expected values: efficiency, expertise, legality, authority, rationality, organizational loyalty, and organizational survival. For the sake of the big picture are we not expected—especially by our superiors, peers, and the courts—to uphold those values? Are we not held responsible for them? But the little picture also comes into focus in our daily professional work. Here we are held responsible for individuals and relationships; under this rubric stand cherished values like caring, responsiveness to each individual patient, dignity, fairness to each employee, honesty to oneself, loyalty to the boss and one's immediate colleagues, and personal and familial survival and preservation. For the sake of this little picture are we not expected—especially by our patients, subordinates, superiors, selves, and families—to uphold these values? In my experience these are all real and salient pressures.

When we step back and contemplate all of this we see a major challenge here. While we mortal healthcare professionals may not be expected to be all things to all people, it does look like we are expected to be and are held responsible for being a lot of things to a lot of people. Undeniably, the values reality of healthcare is rich and complicated.

Second, what is the reality of our *consciousness* of the wealth of these expectations, of the plethora of values we are expected as professionals to uphold and cherish day in and day out? In the routine of our work are we fully aware of our responsibility to all of those expecters for all of those cherished goods? Is our behavior and our decision making affected by any awareness of the values involved, or are we more often guided by whomever exerts the most pressure at the time or by whatever expectation is most apparent in the situation? Does the level of our consciousness of values have anything to do with ethical maturity? Does it have anything to do with simple professionalism in contrast to amateurism?

The American Hospital Association has strongly suggested that we are not as conscious as we should be: "In the course of a normal day's activities. . . . Most of us do not take the time to articulate the ways in which our particular choices and actions mirror a certain system of values."[3] Health ethicist John Glaser is similarly convinced that our value preferences usually remain "below the threshold of our attention."[4] Reasons why such a lack of values consciousness might exist in our daily work were suggested some time ago in a brilliant reflection by Stephen Bailey. He observed that the plethora of values in public service results in a situation of "ambiguity" that can easily dull the conscious state.[5] Glaser's compatible explanation is that "the everyday nature" of the values reality conceals its presence.

In any case, ethical maturity may require a raising of our values consciousness. "What is most important," argues health ethicist Emily Friedman, is that healthcare professionals "make their choices consciously."[6] Central to ethical development, asserts the American Hospital Association, is "understanding what values are indeed being furthered by our behavior."[7] They are referring to the macro dimension of healthcare; in the micro dimension it is equally as true but probably more difficult to accomplish.

Third, once we gain consciousness of the multiplicity of expectations around us, it becomes starkly evident that *conflict* and competition among these values are rampant. In Cooper's words, "Conflicts of responsibility are the ways in which ethical dilemmas are typically experienced."[8] Friedman describes it as a conflict of "right" in all the meanings of the right thing to do, and she views this conflict as the "core of ethics."[9] Cleary eloquently articulates the reality as a matter of "conflicting responsibilities."[10] Being responsible even to clarified, conscious values can put us in the midst of conflict. Consider our professional responsibility to provide healthcare expertly and rationally; our social responsibility to provide it fairly and responsively; our organizational responsibility to do it efficiently and loyally; our legal responsibility to accomplish it procedurally and with due process; and our personal responsibility to do it honestly. Concurrently upholding all of these responsibilities can be a mighty task. The professional in the micro dimension may constantly face a competition among these diverse responsibilities.

Often, for example, it is inefficient to explain fairly the implications of a consent form to a not-so-bright patient. It takes time away from other patients needing healthcare. Frequently, it violates the professional claim of expertise to respond to a patient's request to cut through red tape procedures. Sometimes, loyally following a directive from above may compromise legal requirements as well as one's sense of honesty. And more than occasionally, ordering expensive, unreimbursable care for a patient can jeopardize the financial stability and eventual survival of our hospital, while not ordering the care jeopardizes an individual human life.

Values clarification in microethics puts us in the midst of conflict, and embracing conflict can be distasteful. It is easier to blithely ignore it and "make believe," or at least to minimalize the conflict reality. We can easily view ethics as just a matter of values when, in fact, it is a matter of *conflicting values* with that modifier making a major difference. Glaser, from his extensive healthcare experience, is convinced that we are hesitant in embracing this reality: "We have not taken sufficient note of this underlying values-in-conflict fabric of our ethical life."[11] Even revered ethicists seem to fall prey to the tendency to minimalize: witness Dr. Veatch, who states that values come into conflict only "upon occasion"[12], and Terry Cooper who, after articulating the reality of conflict, falls into the understatement, "There is a possibility of conflict among competing values."[13]

These issues of multiplicity, consciousness, and conflict can perhaps be better clarified through exercises and cases. Consider the following scenarios. After reflecting on each make a judgment of whether the behavior described is ethically acceptable or unacceptable, and explain your reasoning:

A. Paul steals $10 from Penelope's purse while she is walking by.
B. Paul is an administrator in the clinic billing office. He notices that Penelope has overpaid her account by $10 but that it is too late to stop the payment process. He is also sure that she does not realize the error. Realizing it will take a chunk of time to correct the error, that he is under heavy pressure in the office, and that it is a measly amount of money, Paul lets it ride.
C. Paul works for a medical center hospital. Last week he took $10 worth of excess office supplies home for his children to use in school. Everyone else in his unit also seems to take a few supplies home from time to time.
D. Paul works in a large state hospital and lives in a rural area some distance away. Last year he used his office phone to make about $10 worth of personal calls during work hours.
E. Paul is the administrator of a major long-term care complex. Yesterday he took about $10 worth of old painting materials from his facility and gave them to the youth director of a poor inner-city church to use for the children.

When I use exercises like this in workshops with healthcare professionals, inevitably the discussion begins one-dimensionally. The judgments are quick, the reasons are crisp: Of course it's unethical for Paul to steal from Penelope. It's her private property. It's against the law to steal. It's against the Fifth Commandment too. Paul in the billing office is also wrong, but I can understand the pressure he is under. Besides, the computer is probably programmed to show Penelope a credit. Hospital Paul is probably wrong but weren't they old supplies that would be thrown away anyway? And everyone does it. Matter of fact the pen I'm holding has my hospital's logo on it! Give me a break with phone-calling Paul. His facility has a regional calling plan so it doesn't cost any real dollars. What's he supposed to do? Run down to the public phone in the cafeteria while he could be getting work done at his desk? As for administrator Paul, his facility has a ton of painting supplies donated by local merchants. Maybe he shouldn't take them, but isn't it better that they be used by church kids who don't have anything?

What's interesting in doing these kinds of exercises is the consistency of the low level of awareness *pursuit*, even as the scenario described hits closer to home. Amazingly, no one ever asks why Paul steals the $10 from Penelope's purse. It seems there is no need to ask. Wrong is wrong. When I explain that Paul has lost his job and home and is living on the street with his two small children; that he stole the $10 to buy food for his hungry youngsters; that Penelope was wearing a mink coat and angrily walked by Paul when he approached to ask her for money, the usual response is that he should go to an agency or a church or a soup line. When I ask what values are involved, there is high consciousness of the sacred values of law, private property, and fairness to Penelope; there is little consciousness of the sacred values of human welfare (Paul's children), justice, or responsiveness, all of which might, at least, be at stake; and when I suggest that a conflict may exist here between rules and relationships, between law and life, the suggestion is usually not tolerated very well. Whatever possible conflict is acknowledged quickly dissipates amidst assertions of the sacredness of the moral code and the civil law. "Thou shalt not steal" easily prevails. And I am just about thrown out of the room when I suggest that *maybe* this is similar to the Milgram shocking experiments (discussed in the previous chapter.) Shocking an individual person was all right for most of the "teachers" because of the value of the greater good of society. So, then, is the continued hunger of Paul's individual children okay because of the greater value placed on the law, private property, and social order? And does this help explain why most people administered the Milgram shocks?

The fervor of the judgment mellows a bit as we consider billing office Paul. He is still judged unethical but there is some expressed awareness of the possible conflict between values of efficiency and fairness to Penelope. Actual experience seems to influence the level of consciousness and awareness of conflict. No one in the workshop has ever been in homeless

Paul's shoes, but most of us know something about the situation of billing office Paul. Fervor really begins to mellow when we reflect on hospital-based Paul. Our consciousness is pricked as we realize that we have done just that—taken a pen or a notebook home from the office. We were quick to condemn homeless Paul for taking a mere $10 to feed his children; it is not so easy to condemn hospital Paul for what we have all done. "After all, the hospital is loaded with pens and notebooks! They would go unused or wasted if I didn't put them to good use. I knew there was a good reason why I've done this!" Now the ethical judgment doesn't seem so crisp.

When we get to long-term care Paul, fervor really eases up. Here the suggestion is that stealing $10 is stealing $10 whether it is homeless Paul or me, but I have a job to do, and it's very hectic, and I have a family. You're going to tell me that it might be unethical to use the office phone for a personal call or two? I work many dedicated hours for my facility for which I am not paid extra. A phone call doesn't begin to address the value of fairness, for example.

As we proceed, the dynamic of reflection and discussion, of thought and emotion, of consciousness and awareness usually changes drastically. We begin with a bias of blindness to the values that homeless Paul sees and an extreme clarity to the values that we see. As we move along, the bias of blindness and the direction of clarity shift. In the ordinary routine of our healthcare work similar biases may well condition our awareness, understanding, and appreciation of multiple and conflicting values in our reality.

Two categories of values are, I believe, particularly prevalent and underrecognized in the micro dimension of healthcare. One is the **individual versus society conflict** alluded to previously. The daily routine of healthcare is rife with stress involving these two basic values. Our organizations, our systems, our procedures, our laws and standards are all established for the sake of the whole, so that society—the community in which we work—can be cared for. But at the same time we healthcare professionals are trained for and expected to be dedicated to the welfare and dignity of each individual patient. In our daily work there is an inherent tension between these two sacred, valued realities—the individual and the community. *One Flew Over the Cuckoo's Nest* dramatically contrasts the individual dignity focus of McMurphy with the community order focus of Nurse Ratched. For which focus are we ethically responsible? For both, of course, so how do we play out the conflict and tension that routinely emerges between these responsibilities? Are we like Ratched or McMurphy, or someone else? As administrators, for example, do we focus on the value of organizational survival when it comes to providing costly care that will not be reimbursed? Do we minimalize the value of the individual patient in these contexts? Or do we, as care providers, focus on the value of each individual patient and instead minimalize the value of the organization's financial stability?

The other underrecognized values category is the **survival-loyalty phenomenon.** In my experience and study the value of professional survival is, in reality if not in theory, tremendously operative. I place a high value on my professional work and on the opportunity to do it. My survival as a professional is instinctively important to me; it is very apparent on my values horizon. So, too, my own personal welfare and that of my family, including our economic welfare. To put it tersely, keeping my job and getting ahead are very valued expectations. This survival value is not only an intellectually vivid part of my outlook; it is a visceral presence. When push comes to shove, the importance of this value rises right to the surface and easily conditions my behavior. Failure to be conscious of this can doom my quest for ethical maturity. Am I, for example, as a healthcare professional in a medical complex, biased toward the value of organizational welfare, knowing that my salary increases will depend on financial performance? And am I consequently less attuned to the value of the underinsured patient seeking an expensive procedure?

In many ways ethical analysis can be reduced to the simple question of who survives in the daily routine of my professional work. Do I survive—emotionally, economically, psychologically, professionally? Is it ever ethical to jeopardize my own survival, my own ability to continue doing the wonderful things I do? Is it ethical for the sake of making a point like principle x? Does my patient survive (and I don't mean just physically)? Is it ever ethical to jeopardize my patient's dignity? Is it ethical for the sake of other patients' care? Do my subordinates, my peers, my boss survive? Is it ever ethical to undermine my superior and the authority she represents? Is it ever ethical not to? Do the law and procedure survive, or do I undermine them for the sake of some other survival? Does the individual survive, by virtue of what I do, or the organizational community, or both? And, by the way, ethically speaking, who *should* survive? Mitchell and Scott are challenging in their discourse about this, suggesting that the professional survival value is thriving to the detriment of community.[14]

Similarly, in my experience, the value of loyalty has a tremendous influence on our behavior. Unlike the value of survival it has been studied somewhat though not extensively. Marcia Bacon's little-recognized treatise is outstanding.[15] She enlightens us to the notion of loyalty's ethical goodness. Cooper, on the other hand, alerts us to the ethical badness of loyalty.[16] In any case organizational and professional loyalty is as strong and subtle a value as there is in the micro dimension of healthcare, yet it is little discussed or appreciated. The socialization process of professions and organizations nonetheless brings it right to the surface of professional behavior, albeit perhaps less than consciously. The value of loyalty to professional peers has more than once confronted head-on the value of patient well-being, and has won in a heartbeat. But, more than once, other values have confronted the value of organizational loyalty and have won, to the great detriment of good healthcare organizations. Failure to be conscious of these values and to reflect on the conflicts that emerge from them can impede the road to ethical maturity.

Dealing with Competing Values

Finally, there is the reality of values **conflict resolution**. It happens. It has to happen for us to function. But does it more often happen willy-nilly or blindly than reflectively, maturely, professionally? How do we in fact resolve the value conflicts in the daily routine of our healthcare work? Do we rely on instinct, that wonderful inner sense? Do we follow the squeaky wheel principle and favor the momentarily clearest value? Most writers seem to suggest that resolution should occur through a reasoned process of *prioritization*. Similar to the utilitarian approach of seeking the greatest good with the least harm, these ethicists lean toward sacrificing some values for the sake of others that seem more important in the particular situation. Glaser, for example, recognizing the reality of limited options in our daily routine, embraces the conflict resolution methodology of deciding which values deserve priority.[17] Cooper agrees: "The ethical process is the examining and *ranking* of our values, or principles, with respect to a particular decision."[18] This approach is often termed "values ascendancy," meaning that some values are deemed, in particular circumstances, to be more sacred than others.

I have a problem with this approach. For one thing it sets us up to surrender too easily, too quickly. For another thing I worry about the values that are thrown to the wind in such an approach. The Krafts are representative of this bent when they remark: "Resolution of such [values] conflicts ultimately depends on determining which needs ought to be met."[19] But isn't it true that all legitimate values ought to be honored and that we should at least *try* to salvage *all* values involved? We may not succeed always, but a little success is more professional than none. For example, with the benefit of prioritization reasoning I might serenely let one not-so-sick patient on my floor linger so that I can attend to three who are very sick. But, if I pause and reflect an instant without a prioritization mentality, I *might* find a way to have all patients attended to.

After all, isn't each individual of value? Furthermore, a values ascendancy approach can easily slip into begging the question. For example, if the profit margin of a healthcare facility conflicts with the provision of care to an uninsured patient, that is one thing. Profit, as opposed to organization *survival*, is not in the same values league as patient welfare. An ascendancy approach can help clarify that and resolve the competition. But organization survival *is* in the same values league as patient survival—they go hand-in-hand. In not distinguishing categories of sacred values from categories of less important values, ascendancy proponents tend to minimalize the competition *within* the league of sacred values.

With this in mind the notion of *balancing* can be helpful in the quest for conflict resolution. Ethicists like Lilla and Lebacqz suggest this approach as a way of opening the door to ethical reflection beyond simple ranking and prioritization. This avenue to values conflict resolution may not be as viscerally satisfying, as clear-cut, as prioritizing. With this approach, for example, we would attempt to attend to all patients, but probably none of them would receive our best effort. We would "satisfize" but not "optimize," to borrow Herbert Simon's economic terminology.[20] And we can then ask what the ethical thing to do is in the harried day-to-day activities of healthcare, to optimize or to satisfize?

Pursuing this line of reflection I find the concept of values **reconciliation** to be the most helpful and enlightening for the conflict resolution quandary. It is implied in statements like Griffith's: "Modern healthcare is a unique melding of charity and business, of compassion and attention to fiscal responsibility."[21] It is promoted by Susan Wakefield in her rigorous discourse on ethical responsibility.[22] It is described by Neil Brady as a matter of "knowing how" *and* "knowing that," of combining paradox with principles.[23] It is convincingly and realistically conveyed by Kress, Springer, and Cowden in their analysis of housing programs: "Prescriptive polemics offered in the literature," they observe, "do not recognize the degree to which values from both perspectives are actively pursued in practice." They find that mature professionals can and do, in fact, find ways for conflicting values to "co-exist" and "interact."[24] Figure 4.1 depicts the concept, pictorially contrasting it with other approaches to values conflict resolution. As we reflect on our professional experience do we, too, see this, or do we subscribe to the need to prioritize? Is the possibility of values reconciliation worth pursuing in the micro dimension of our work?

In any case, accomplishing reconciliation is not easy. The great management guru Chester Barnard, in arguing that a professional manager's job is to help resolve conflicts of values, claimed that creativity skills are critical in this task.[25] Bill Kuhn advises that dialogue is the key

Figure 4.1 Values Conflict Resolution

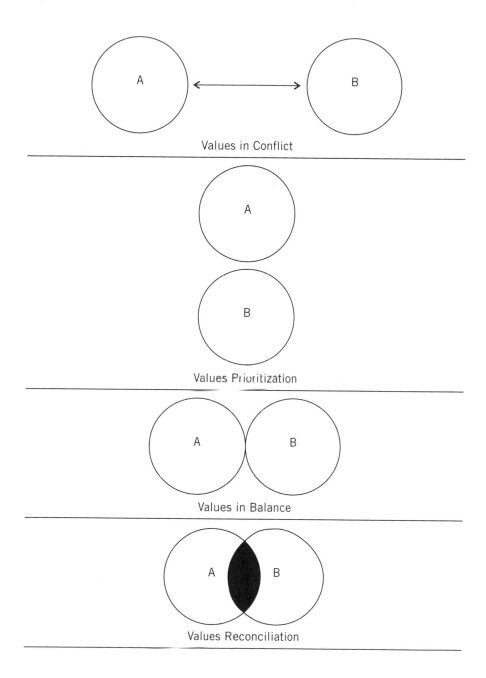

Values in Conflict

Values Prioritization

Values in Balance

Values Reconciliation

to reconciliation: "Conversations enable people to confront their opposites and to seek workable solutions within the midst of conflict, argument and tension."[26] And Marilyn Ray et al. similarly encourage "reflection in action"—sharing other's perceptions and developing reciprocal awareness—as a means toward reconciliation.[27]

But it can be very difficult. Consider cases like that involving Diane, the medical director at a big industrial complex in a small midwest community. Her staff informed her that environmental conditions within the plant were marginally healthy and probably in violation of government health and safety regulations. She reported this to senior management and was told that the matter was known and was being taken care of at higher levels in the organization. Several months later her staff reported no improvement in conditions. After discussing it with her immediate superior who brought it to the attention of top management, word came back to take no further action as the matter was still being attended to at the highest levels. As weeks passed Diane became more and more concerned. What should she do? What was her ethical responsibility?

She felt a real conflict between the expectations of legitimate authority in telling her to back off and her own professional expertise and concern for human welfare in telling her she must do something; between loyalty to her superiors and responsiveness to her staff and the firm's employees; between her own job survival and the requirements of law and regulation. If she deferred to her bosses, the values of organizational authority, of loyalty to superiors, and of her own career welfare would look good; but the values of employee health, of professional expertise, and of public law would appear to be in jeopardy. If instead she pursued the matter, the values of professional expertise, employee health, and public law would look good; but her own job survival, authority in the organization, and loyalty would clearly be in jeopardy. Her professional instincts were to "jump on the white horse and save the community"; her private instinct was to tremble over what that might mean for her and her two children for whom she was the sole support. She realized that she could threaten the hierarchy with exposure, that she could resign, and that she could leak word of the situation to the local press or state authorities. She could also, of course, defer to organizational authority, which always in the past had earned her respect. She thought at first in terms of ascendancy and prioritization. Which was more important: the health welfare of the employees or the security of her own family? Then, instead, she decided to begin a dialogue, first with her immediate supervisor with whom she shared a good, trusting relationship, then with a peer who was the medical director of a major firm in another state. Discussions with her boss clarified that their personal history with the organization supported the reputability of their superiors. They decided that they could and should push the issue and request higher-level dialogue.

Discussions with her out-of-state colleague raised the question of possible economic factors: he had experienced in his company fiscal difficulty with meeting environmental and safety regulations, which had resulted in political negotiations leading to tax abatements so that the company would not move to a different state. When this possibility was raised in the eventual higher-level meeting, the corporate CEO acknowledged that tax abatement negotiations were indeed under way, and that secrecy had to be maintained lest the negotiations fall apart. She then argued that remedial measures should at least begin. They all agreed.

Did Diane behave ethically? Did her behavior reconcile all of the values involved that had at first seemed impossibly in conflict? Had she jumped to expose the firm, as she initially had felt compelled to do, the company would likely have had to move, causing economic harm to the very employees she was presumably protecting. Had she caved in and simply deferred to superiors, chances are the unhealthy conditions would have lingered a lot longer. By opening dialogue before acting did she reconcile what had seemed in conflict? Was this dialogue and imagination the key to the outcome of reconciliation? For Diane, dealing with the situation and answering these questions was not easy. Her use, however, of the tool of open dialogue illustrates the relevance of Carter's conceptual approach.[28] It also limns the responsibility paradox of "agency *and* answerability" recently proffered by Harmon.[29]

Values are our guides in the ethical use of our professional power. Unfortunately, these guides are multiple and conflicting. The reality of microethics in healthcare is our routine position in the center of value conflicts that necessitate resolution. Developing skill at reconciling the value conflicts that go with the terrain is a key to growing in ethical maturity.

Notes

1. A. Carr-Saunders and P. Wilson, 1933, *The Professions* (Oxford: Clarendon Press), pp. 421–22.

2. M. Guy, 1991, "Using High Reliability Management To Promote Ethical Decision Making." In J. Bowman (ed.), *Ethical Frontiers in Public Management* (San Francisco: Jossey-Bass), p. 193.

3. American Hospital Association, Committee on Ethics, 1980, A Perspective on Teaching Medical Ethics (Chicago: AHA), p. 7.

4. J. Glaser, 1994, *Three Realms of Ethics* (Kansas City, MO: Sheed and Ward), p. 7.

5. S. Bailey, 1964, "Ethics and the Public Service." *Public Administration Review* 24, no. 4 (December): 234–43.

6. E. Friedman, 1987, "Searching for the Right." Health Management Quarterly 9, no. 3 (Third Quarter): 6.

7. AHA, Committee on Ethics, A Perspective on Teaching Medical Ethics, p. 8.

8. T. Cooper, 1982, *The Responsible Administrator* (Port Washington, NY: Kennikat), p. 62.

9. Friedman, "Searching for the Right," 3.

10. R. E. Cleary, 1980, "The Professional as Public Servant: The Decision-Making Dilemma." *International Journal of Public Administration* 2 (2): 151–60.

11. Glaser, *Three Realms of Ethics*, p. 3.

12. R. Veatch, 1981, *A Theory of Medical Ethics* (New York: Basic Books), p. 3.

13. Cooper, *The Responsible Administrator*, p. 116.

14. T. Mitchell and W. Scott, 1990, "America's Problems and Needed Reforms: Confronting the Ethic of Personal Advantage." *Academy of Management Executive* 4 (3): 23–35.

15. M. Bacon, 1984, *The Moral Status of Loyalty* (Dubuque, IA: Kendall/Hunt).

16. T. Cooper, 1987, "Hierarchy, Virtue and the Practice of Public Administration: A Perspective for Normative Ethics." *Public Administration Review* 47, no. 4 (July/August): 320–28.

17. Glaser, *Three Realms of Ethics*, p. 5.

18. Cooper, *The Responsible Administrator*, p. 52.

19. S. Kraft and A. Kraft, 1982, "Leadership Strategies and Values in Times of Scarcity." *Administration in Mental Health* 9, no. 3 (spring): 177.

20. H. Simon, 1947, *Administrative Behavior* (New York: Free Press).

21. J. R. Griffith, 1993, *The Moral Challenges of Health Care Management* (Ann Arbor, MI: Health Administration Press), p. xvi.

22. S. Wakefield, 1976, "Ethics and the Public Service: A Case for Individual Responsibility." *Public Administration Review* 36, no. 6 (November/December): 662.

23. F. N. Brady, 1986, "Aesthetic Components of Management Ethics." *Academy of Management Review* 11, no. 2 (April): 337–44.

24. G. Kress, J. Springer and A. Cowden, 1986, "Administrative Values in Conflict." *State and Local Government Review* (fall): 125–31.

25. C. Barnard, 1938, *The Functions of the Executive* (Cambridge, MA: Harvard University Press), pp. 278–83.

26. W. A. Kuhn, 1990, "Toward an Agenda for Business Ethics Research." *Academy of Management Review* 15, no. 2 (April): 315.

27. M. A. Ray, V. Didominic, P. Dittman, P. Hurst, J. Seaver, B. Sorbello, and M. Stankes-Ross, 1995, "The Edge of Chaos: Caring and the Bottom Line." *Nursing Management* 26, no. 9 (September): 48–50.

28. See S. L. Carter, 1996, *Integrity* (New York: Basic Books) for the suggestion that this sort of dialogue and quest for the right answer is the essence of true integrity.

29. M. M. Harmon, 1995, *Responsibility As Paradox* (Newbury Park, CA: Sage). See also his "Harmon Responds," in *Public Administration Review* 56, no. 6 (November/December): 604–10, for a crisp precis of his thesis.

READING

Jim Summers' 1984 article quickly became a classic in the field because he was among the first to recognize and attempt to deal with the practical conflict of values in healthcare management: doing good (people values) versus doing well (organization values). His discussion enhances this chapter in two major ways. First, it rigorously articulates the nature of the values conflict in healthcare administration; and second, in focusing mostly on the macro dimension it accentuates our insistence on attention to the micro dimension.

The article stresses the need for clarifying values and suggests some means of doing this. It is extremely helpful on these points. It is distinctly limited, however, in helping us bridge mental and verbal consciousness with behavioral consciousness—our high-level behavior with our ordinary, routine activity. For example, is concern for the dignity of people demonstrated more by promoting the one-time building of a hospice, or by the daily interaction of the healthcare professional in that hospice with his or her patients, subordinates, and visitors? Is my failure to say "good morning" to a janitor or colleague an indication of the level of my consciousness of personal dignity? A fundamental argument of this book is that it is very difficult to become skilled at doing well and good in the macro dimension, as Summers discusses, unless we first learn how to do it in the ordinary routine of our working day.

DOING GOOD AND DOING WELL:
ETHICS, PROFESSIONALISM, AND SUCCESS

James W. Summers

Health-services administrators face no shortage of pressures to ensure that their institutions are doing well. Indeed, with all the concern over cuts in reimbursement, prospective payment schemes, rate review, rate regulation, consumer-choice health plans, preferred provider organizations, competition and regulation, it is no wonder if we often see our roles in financial terms. Much of the literature on models for hospital organization or on the meaning of being a professional administrator exhort us to adopt business-like ways as the solutions to our problems.[1] Graduate training encourages us to see hospitals as analogous to manufacturing facilities where physicians are customers and patients the raw material. We have learned much from study and application of these business skills. We speak now of diversification, mergers, corporate restructuring, financial maximization strategies and marketing with considerable aplomb. Apparently, we have succeeded too well.

Robert Cunningham argues that a shift from patient care values to business values will lead to a loss of public confidence.[2] Recent chairpersons of the American Hospital Association (AHA) have stressed the need for retention of humanistic and charitable values. Stuart A. Wesbury, Jr., Ph.D., FACHA, President of the American College of Hospital Administrators (ACHA) [now the American College of Healthcare Executives, ACHE], argues that our leadership role forces a consideration of ethics.[3] Peters and Wacker say that hospital strategic planning must be rooted in values and ethics.[4] Echoing Cunningham, they note that the legitimacy of hospitals in the public eye is tied to perceiving hospitals as "sustenance organizations," with a charitable ethic instead of an exchange ethic. Failure to keep this in mind while considering diversification, divestment, nontraditional revenue sources and the like poses such a threat to public confidence that it may threaten their survival in the traditional forms. Harry Levinson, noted management consultant in organizational theory, motivation, and the management of change, shows that for the administrator to succeed he/she must build a values consensus with the board, the medical staff, and the other employees.[5]

This literature and the concern of our leaders, while overwhelmed by cost and operational issues, is noteworthy. It seems important to

James W. Summers, "Doing Good and Doing Well: Ethics, Professionalism, and Success," *Hospital and Health Services Administration* 29, no. 2 (March/April 1984): 84–99. Copyright 1984, the American College of Healthcare Executives. Reprinted by permission. James W. Summers was vice president of services for Inter-health Corporation.

achieve two goals relative to this sentiment. First, in terms of leadership as individuals and in terms of professional development as persons in the role of hospital administration, it seems we need to become clear on just what our values are. Part of this essay is devoted to doing that and along the way showing why such clarity is needed at this time in the history of our profession. Second, the article addresses techniques by which discussions about values and ethics can be useful in achieving success at leadership. Doing good and doing well are compatible. With these tasks in mind we may begin to question ourselves about our values, why we hold them, and the consequences on our long-term effectiveness.

Why Are We Here?

The quickest way to find out what your values are concerning hospitals is to ask yourself why you are in the field—why you chose it, why you remain. Most express the view that they are in health-services administration because they like the idea of involvement in a meaningful way with an organization that helps people when they seem to most need it, what Peters and Wacker called a "sustenance organization".[6] There is a value in "doing good" which tends to influence our actions, whether we are in the investor-owned or non-profit sector.[7] But unlike our colleagues in medicine, nursing, and other health-professions, or even non-professional employees, this ethical commitment to doing good seldom surfaces. In fact, our training and our ideas about professionalism in management make it appear that we deliberately distance ourselves from such "sentimentality" and "subjectiveness." However, this leads to a conflict.

Administrators face this conflict, not just as individuals with their own values, but as professionals and persons trying to understand or even redefine the hospital's mission. We see management and professionalism in terms of the bottom line results and pride ourselves on these successes. Our skills in translating problems and solutions into quantifiable terms, in being able to transcend management by crisis through planning and implementation of sound policy, are essential and should be matters of pride. Yet the results-oriented, no-nonsense approach is sometimes packaged in a suit of callousness, empire building, and ruthlessness, all of it then festooned with an aura of manipulation which we may believe is the attitude of objectivity. But this misguided management style leads to conflict with the values of the boards, the healthcare workers, and perhaps even the now-suppressed values of administrators. The emphasis on doing well, in terms of a purely business model, is limited by the public image of hospitals, an image enforced by the board.

The Trustee Image of the Hospital

As Johnson points out so well, trustees consider significant amounts of black ink on the bottom line to be taking advantage of the public.[8] Even if the hospital is owned by a for-profit chain, management is typically careful to present an image of public and social concern for the medical needs of the community, including the indigent. To fail in presenting this image usually means the community perceives the values of the institution as somehow suspect.

The trend toward investor-owned hospitals has probably saved many non-profits by helping to legitimize the need for a reasonable return on investment in the trustee community, thus avoiding bankruptcy, extreme deficits, or takeover by the same for-profits. While days of worry about excessive black-ink may be few and far between, this is still a profession where applying management skills prompts us to "do good" along with "doing well." These two values are not in conflict; "doing good" does not mean spilling red ink, although sometimes people outside of the healthcare field tend to impulsively act as if it does.

The public image of hospitals as not just another business, of having a "product" that is something besides a mere economic commodity, leads to problems not just with the board, but with the medical staff. These problems may not be solved unless we more deliberately see our own values commitment to doing good brought to the fore in our activities and in our professional identification. Why is this the solution?

The Medical View of Hospitals

Physicians and nurses embody, in their own minds and in the public's conception of them, a dedication to the relief of individual suffering. Their professional identity has been clear about this primary obligation for a long time, both clear to them and to the public. Failure to live up to this obligation to individual patients is not seen as a failure in the formulation of the professional role but as a failure among the practitioners. Trustees, the public, and typically both physicians and nurses see the hospital as a place for them to carry out this role. Johnson states the problem well.[9] This grouping of role players sees the purpose of the hospital in terms of a cause, not a business. They all identify the hospital as primarily a medical institution. Neither trustees, physicians, nor nurses typically see the hospital chief executive as the person who leads and inspires for the sake of this cause. Levinson puts the problem in a sociological perspective.[10]

Physicians and nurses are socialized to identify with their professional role and its obligations above all. These roles and obligations, in

Freudian terms, are super-ego oriented, resulting in conscience-driven or conscience-guided behavior. Further, this orientation is on person-to-person services; the goals of their activities take on strong moral overtones. The mission—the purpose of the institution—is experienced in terms of facilitating their meeting the ethical obligations of their cause.

Given such powerful needs to do good, there is a vast problem in living up to the professional role. Obviously a person who prevents them from providing "quality patient care" sets himself up as a target or scapegoat for ventilating a sense of inadequacy or perhaps even sin. Rules, budget constraints, quality assurance, DRGs, all these sorts of things pose a threat that doing good will be harder or that inadequacy in doing it will be verified and made public. Small wonder that we find ourselves subject to vociferous attacks on our motives, our values, our roles, and that what seem to be obviously beneficial policies or changes are resisted tooth and nail. The response seems to have been to suppress our own doing-good values behind a veil of business-like professionalism, much to our disadvantage.

Board Suspicions Verified

If hospitals are perceived primarily as value laden, cause oriented, ethically superior institutions . . . as places for the practice of skills which fulfill these values, then administrators should not be surprised to find themselves expendable when the medical professions begin to complain that administrator behavior prevents the organization from carrying out its mission. The seeming injustice and arbitrary nature in which boards carry out medical staff wishes stems not just from recognition that physicians control the revenue, but from sharing their views about the purpose of the hospital. Sensitivity to this mission by the board leads them to quickly side with the physicians against an administrator who appears to "stand in the way" of good medical care.[11] Cultivation of purely business values does little to let do-gooders feel inspired or motivated. If we are to be leaders, we must plug into the value system in a deliberate way instead of cultivating an image that places us outside it or even as an enemy of it.

Careful Redefinition of the Hospital

The current move into diversification and corporate restructuring carries great risks in terms of diluting the good will hospitals have enjoyed in the public eye and from the employees. Workers no longer accept low pay and poor working conditions as a just sacrifice to the cause. A variety of factors explain that, but one frequently overlooked is the loss of the ability to identify oneself with a cause through the institution. Self-sacrifice is not expected in a business. The more removed one's task is from the cause of alleviation of suffering and the more it seems bureaucracy, machinery, or bigness inhibits this work, the more likely one will be unwilling to endure unnecessary sacrifices. However, let's examine what we say in the mad dash toward diversification, corporate restructuring, and the business model.

Moving into non-traditional revenue sources[12] such as manufacturing of products, real estate, restaurants, hotels, health spas or even the new prevention and wellness services, requires a restatement of the hospital mission. Mergers, acquisitions, development of multi-hospital systems, and corporate restructuring, in general, create, for these superego people, a problem regarding the hospital's purpose and their relation to it.[13] To the extent management seems to become more powerful and more able to control their activities, they will be threatened, feel their ability to fulfill the cause is being undermined. The changes prospective reimbursement will require in administrator-physician relations is especially threatening for this reason. However, that topic requires a separate article.

If corporate restructuring is perceived as making medical professionals accountable to a chief executive, instead of to the standards of the role, it will be fiercely resisted, with the expectation of administrator demise or a curtailment of authority.[14] To the extent management is involved in the heady game of setting up non-traditional services, non-traditional revenue sources, or involved in the multi-hospital system game, he/she will be perceived as empire building, which is at least suspicious, and perceived as threatening if this may result in power to influence medical decisions. If these actions are justified in terms of institutional survival or progress and no clear and present danger is perceived by the medical staff or the employees, the games will still be seen as empire building or be seen indifferently. In any case, these activities will be seen as tangential or irrelevant to the cause and make it harder to identify the hospital with that cause, a loss of goodwill, conceived internally. But this need not be.

Redefinition Can Confirm Shared Values

The redefinition of the hospital presents a superb opportunity to gain respect, tie into the value system, and get the entire hospital organized psychologically and normatively around a mission that might help overcome resistance, fear of interference, and disparagement of the chief executive. The quickest way to begin is to emphasize how a hospital differs from a business in mission, values, types of employees, why they work there, and so on. MHA schools would do well to consider this. Quite frankly, the emphasis on the business model and quantitative methods seems popular because it is easier to teach. Values are somehow soft where bottom lines are hard. Relating to people is far more difficult to teach than management science, finance, marketing and the like.

When relating is taught in terms of negotiation or motivation or the management of change, it is frequently done in a context of manipulation, conceiving the other as an adversary to be overcome or the mere means to an end.[15] Learning to relate to people in a manipulative way is easily identified by cause-oriented persons who do not subscribe to that view of how to get along. Certainly it does nothing to inspire confidence as a leader to them, for a leader must share the values of the cause. We are being taught to squander the ingredients that make us leaders in more than title: a shared ethics with our colleagues in medicine, one which emphasizes how hospitals and health professions differ from businesses and business professions.[16]

Regaining Confidence

Being credible to suspicious or hostile physicians or nurses about the fact you share their commitment, their values, but from a different perspective begins with the self-analysis noted earlier and is worth emphasizing again. Why did you choose this field? If it was a second or third choice, what relationship did it have to those first choices that led you to select it? Why do you stay? Besides reasons such as prestige, fairly good money, having a position of power, I suspect most will agree we chose hospital work because there is a fundamental, gut-level congruence of the work with our values. We want a role in helping people and that is what hospitals do. Probe the psyche of a dedicated hospital worker, or even a burned-out one, and you find a do-gooder. Why should we hide it behind some sort of model of ourselves as business people? Sure we are in business, but it is what is special about this business that made us choose it. Let us emphasize that specialness and find a way to join hands with doctors and nurses because of it, instead of crossing swords. Our professional identity should build on the value in helping those who need it, as should our hospital mission and any redefinition it may get.[17]

Tremendous opportunities emerge from the decision to flaunt your specialness and your values, opportunities physicians and nurses have used to distance themselves from us. The project of clarifying the hospital's mission should be one which involves all employees, beginning at orientation. Learning what a place is, what it stands for, why it is there, and continually showing it, serves as a tremendous motivation to get people to pull together, put up with adversity, and even to define their role—perhaps even themselves—in terms of that mission.

Diversifications, mergers, corporate restructuring, new services—all of these projects present an opportunity to inquire again into the mission, inquire with the employees and the medical staff in a way which reaffirms the congruence of these changes with the mission and shows that the mission statement is a living document. In a certain sense, this is like zero-based budgeting, but on a value level—why are we here, what are we doing, should it continue, and how much of it? Now, this may be valuable in becoming worthy of leadership in the eyes of medical workers but it will become more powerful if the role of hospital leadership is seen as part of the proper role of a health-services administrator *per se* and not just as a quality found in a particular administrator. This means doing some hard thinking about professional identity, what it says to the outsider, and what we have to do to get it accepted such that the failure to be a leader is seen as a failure in fulfilling the professional role instead of something which was never expected anyway.

Leadership Is More Than Administration

An extremely important reason the administrator must not only take, but earn, the right to a leadership role is because external pressures are forcing the hospital into a reconsideration of its mission in order to survive. There is no need to belabor this point or the reasons for it.[18] The point is that physicians no longer embody the mission of the new hospital and it falls to the chief executive officer to rise to the occasion. Prospective reimbursement will add force to this shift upward in status. And *rise* it must be, for if this analysis is correct we are seen neither by the public, by the medical staff, nor by professional or non-professional employees as embodying this new mission, which is itself not yet clear. To achieve a consensus on the mission of a health services facility, to seek to exemplify the ethical ideals of that mission in personal conduct, to belong to a profession which encourages and supports these two goals . . . that is professional development in a sense which properly transcends the mere emphasis on competency at business skills. And this is necessary to become a leader and be followed, or to get beyond the problems of a role-oriented organization in which we are obstacles or enemies and begin molding a task-oriented organization which is characterized by shared values, trust, and role flexibility so that success for the nurses, for example, is not understood as a victory over physicians and administrators.[19] How does one do this? There are three levels of inquiry: What are my reasons for doing hospital work? What does my profession seem to expect of me? What really is the mission of my hospital, or even hospitals in general, and what can I do to get it to meet that function? When these are reasonably clear, then the ongoing effort at achieving consensus and being recognized as the leader may begin.

Building a Values Consensus

The first level, the individual inquiry into values, has already been mentioned. Openness, instead of manipulation, seems to be highly valued as an ingredient in building the confidence base for recognition as a leader.[20] Second level inquiries lead to the profession itself. What do we expect of ourselves as administrators? What are our yardsticks of success? Our values? Our obligations?

The superficial answer is that professional success is evidenced by promotions, increasing responsibility, higher pay, advancement in the American College of Hospital Administrators, holding office in various hospital associations, etc. Success for a hospital, in our eyes, is an extension of those things by which we measure our professional success: strong financial position, latest equipment, good consensus, competent and loyal workforce and medical staff, expansion of services, perhaps corporate restructuring, the institution being the flag ship in a multi-hospital system, recognition and respect from colleagues that it is a good hospital, as evidenced by referral patterns, and so on. But lacking in any of these indicators of success for the administrator or the hospital is any evidence of dedication to values, to the cause that motivates other health-care workers. Does the professional organization for healthcare administrators provide that sense of identity, mission, obligation?

Essentially, the American College of Hospital Administrators[21] (ACHA) is the only organization claiming to represent administration in general. It states the goals of the profession in its seven objectives,[22] eight obligations of individual practitioners,[23] and provides a fairly detailed *Code of Ethics*. The ACHA, now in its 50th year, claims to have had as a goal creating a profession where there was none.[24] Our fellow professionals in the cause do not have the problem of creating a professional identity.

Physicians, who could be said to embody the ethical values of individual medical care, at least in an ideal sense, have a well-recognized ethical tradition which has endured thousands of years. Nurses have a much briefer history as a profession, but can look to Florence Nightingale as the model of devotion, care, and self-sacrifice. Nurses can even point to their key role as care-givers since the origin of hospitals as pest houses, places people went to die, or places for the impoverished. Again, there is an ethical ideal which nurses are to strive for. Is there such an ethical ideal available [to the] administrator?

What the American College of Hospital Administrators Says

The ACHA publications describe our obligation as to the institution.[25] We are urged to identify ourselves with this role of dedication to the institution. It becomes appropriate to then question the function of the institution. The ACHA refers us to the American Hospital Association's (AHA) Hospital Code of Ethics. There we recognize multiple responsibilities—patient care, the community, the employees, the medical staff, and so on. This multiplicity of responsibilities, this conflicting constituency[26] includes all the above but also creditors, suppliers, regulatory agencies, third party payors of all kinds, perhaps the other elements in our multihospital system, the various associations, and even shared service organizations. It is this incredible diversity of conflicting responsibilities which puts the chief executive in a position of authority to be a leader, to pull together a values consensus on how the institution shall represent itself externally and internally to these constituencies. But while the board, physicians, nurses, and other employees may recognize the difficulty of this task, it is not likely that stating it in this way will result in them sensing many shared values with us. Nor is it likely to give rise to such sharing if we appear to be deliberately adopting business values and attitudes, attitudes that will seem less than pure at their best.[27]

Perhaps some self-analysis is again useful here. Did we get into hospitals primarily because we like the management of complex organizations or did we get into hospital management because we wanted to help people through management? Use of power—use of management skills to help people in the aggregate—seems no less laudable than direct patient care. Surely we can point, if only statistically, to patients saved, patients getting well quicker, patients avoiding iatrogenic infections, people served better by new services and new equipment, employee or patient or family benefits resulting from shared services, diversification, multi-hospital systems, and the like. Since the belief is that power corrupts, we must show how we have used it to help, in terms they understand—benefits to individuals. Our work may benefit large numbers of people we will never see, but that is no reason for hands-on care providers to consider us as having non-caring, nonhumanistic values.

Indeed, business today is moving to try to show that good business is compatible with such values, not greed, exploitation, empire building, and ruthless achievement of profits at any moral, human, or environmental cost. Yet we foolishly squander our possibilities for being viewed as leaders by cultivating a business image, an image crusading do-gooders will see in the worst possible light because we often have to control their spare-no-expense approach. It will be tough winning their confidence, but getting them to think about the hospital mission and seeing how your values as a professional mesh with theirs, even if the perspectives differ significantly, is a start. In other words, the professional obligation of the healthcare administrator is helping people, not just patients, and helping them through the skillful use of management techniques. It gives a point of leverage. Now, how does one go about building this consensus?

Specific Techniques—Professional Development

Administrators are experts at achieving results and discovering things by indirect methods. The following ideas should show that developing a hospital mission which helps us to achieve a sharing of values, a task orientation, is not too different from launching other touchy projects.

A good place to begin to find a commonality of values is with your subordinates or with other administrators over lunch or drinks. One need not appear foolish by asking why someone chose hospital work when other work might have been less stressful and more lucrative. If most of us are closet crusaders, getting that confession out into the open serves as an important basis for values consensus. Probe their thoughts and your own about what it is about hospitals that is special and inspires a bit of dedication. Discuss the value conflicts Levinson and Johnson point out among administration and both the board and the medical staff, not to even speak of most of the employees. Note reasons for the conflicts and note places you really share values. Shared values can be a powerful force and savvy managers will discover them or create them and do their best to make them meaningful. Such a source of goodwill should be looked on as a valuable resource not to be squandered. In terms of management, this phase could be considered professional development. The next stage in getting you in the leadership role is organizational development.[28]

Organizational Development

Organizational development must begin indirectly to properly build a credibility base. At appropriately informal times, created if need be, the administrator might begin asking physicians, department heads, key nurses, long-term employees, etc., why they are in medical or hospital work. Assuming patient-care values are the typical response, the very fact you showed concern about values should be a step toward confidence building.

Of course, if the context of the hospital's administrative style is one of reciprocal manipulations, such questions will be suspicious, threatening, leading to second guessing about motives. Consensus building in this area is not like putting together a coalition of self-interested groups for a specific purpose; it is instead the creation of a group by establishing common values.

For these questions to be confidence builders, there must have been a tradition of openness already. Discussion can then lead into comparisons of views about the purpose of hospitals, especially in the changed environment of today. An administrator must be sensitive enough to the professional and ethical obligations of direct-care professionals not to become agitated if his role is described in support function terms. Being in a support position does not mean being a lackey. Our goal is to help people through the management of a complex organization dedicated itself to helping people.

As confidence builds and these discussions continue, the administrator may discover an awareness of apparent value conflicts between the roles and then find ways to prove the essential convergence of his/hers with theirs. At the same time, the administration may find out the length of the row that must be hoed before these value conflicts are overcome sufficiently enough for him to be the leader. It is important here to be sensitive to the fact that they may suspect your values because of the strong business coloring. Further, their values have a much longer tradition and a profoundly greater degree of public respect. It is your values which must be seen as meshing with theirs. Perhaps opportunities will arise to point out how your perspective has long range usefulness in helping them fulfill their obligations.

After these discussions have been going on for awhile, perhaps even with board members, depending on the situation, some will suggest following up on these questions about values, role conflicts, shared goals, and the hospital mission at staff meetings. These issues will interest them, as indeed they should, if the seeds planted on that row have been tended well.

The progression from staff meetings to departmental meetings should follow, with the administrative staff helping to explore the questions. If the process works, there should be less fighting over turf and more task-oriented behavior. Causing this to happen means breaking down suspicions and encouraging a sense of common goals, resting on a foundation of common values. It means breaking out of the zero-sum game mentality where every department in the hospital tries to maximize their position at the expense of the others. This process will be ongoing, but opportunities to find and use common values will be frequent as hospitals try to find their way in a rapidly changing and often hostile environment.

Merging Ethics and Management

Dr. Wesbury notes that if we are to fill this new leadership role which circumstance has cast upon us, "our personal values and those of our institutions must rise to the surface and become a part of the decisions that we must make."[29] This involves testing oneself and one's institution, not just developing slogans or developing mission statements which are filed away. As Dr. Wesbury says, "stimulate in your own mind problem situations. Think through what your role might be in these situations and the possible outcomes."[30] "Discuss ethical situations openly with a variety of people on a frequent basis."[31] Discussions of cases at staff meetings or with different departments can bring role conflicts to the surface and present opportunities for everyone to emerge with a sense of a bigger picture. Some examples illustrate the point.

Medical professionals are presumably committed to the ideals of informed consent and protection of individual autonomy. Present a case which shows a conflict between doing good, from their point of view, at the cost of informed consent and autonomy. After a discussion of the medical uses of information point out your own commitment to openness and accuracy in dealings with them, how that ties in with their values and repudiates the view that management, like some paternalistic medical professionals, will be manipulative about information, seeing it as a tool to their own ends. Most medical professionals have probably never thought about how the values of informed consent apply to management. Having reviewed the Codes of Ethics of the professionals with whom you are speaking will bolster your prestige and keep them honest. Most professionals know as little about their Code as you probably do about the ACHA code. Of course, these Codes are not laws from on high, but subject to interpretation or perhaps even rejection. Or maybe the Code does not go far enough. Working these problems through in a group is an effort to reach a consensus on values that transcends mere role identity and is a major element in gaining the consensus you will need to function as a leader.

Discussions about the right to refuse treatment, death with dignity, and euthanasia may get some consensus going about the possibilities of more humane care, respect for persons, and the like. This could be channeled into a desire to open a hospice. Your homework should be done ahead of discussions that might lead to the suggestion of a hospice. If the numbers will not allow it to contribute, be ready to explain it. Many discussions about values may lead to discussion of specific services. This presents an excellent opportunity to bring up questions about resource allocations and the obligations of the professions and the institution, and so on.

Choosing the Right Cases To Discuss

Dilemmas about resource allocations are generally understood by medical people as agonizing over which patient gets the life-saving equipment when there is too little of it. This sets up the situation with you being the fall guy for why they cannot do their job, or leads to talk about rights, government stinginess, the "real world," and so on. Instead of letting this happen, guide discussion to allocation cases which pertain to decisions about opening entirely new services. Here the patients are in the abstract and you can get the direct-care people to think more in terms to which you are accustomed.

Use the new service case—perhaps a burn unit, or a pediatric intensive care unit—as an opportunity to discuss the realities of third party reimbursement and the ideal of highest quality, state of the art, patient care. The impact of giving the medical practitioner a virtual blank check to use for the benefit of his patients may have been great for their crusading superegos and their patients, but certainly turns its back on social responsibility. Getting them to recognize a social responsibility and then to *feel* the moral dilemmas of a value conflict in *their* professions may do wonders when you point out your own value conflicts and how they are no less troubling in the administrator's office. Particularly good cases are those which show how extreme emphasis on doing good for an individual patient or perhaps even specific types of patients consumes so much resources that it renders problematic the ability to handle other patients in the future. The issue of inequity will trouble crusaders and certainly you can show how your job requires balancing and weighing these equity issues in a way which may be *more responsible* than what they have been doing. Some good things can result from discussion of resource allocations which are a step removed from their ordinary specific patient concerns.

Cases Which Support Management Goals

Something as simple as the need to be more reasonable in cooperating with a shared service organization or even group purchasing may suddenly be perceived as having the moral overtones of social responsibility. Representatives of multi-hospital systems can explain why these forms of organization reflect an effort to be socially responsible in the sense that effectiveness and efficiency help the community and the nation, and assist the direct care giver by enhancing institutional viability. Making all these points may take a series of discussions, but it will be interesting to these crusaders if you *continually* relate what you are doing back to values they recognize and acknowledge. Diversification into nontraditional revenue sources must be handled the same way.

A hotel can be seen as showing a real interest in the families of the patients. Apartments and real estate firms can show an interest in the employees. Manufacturing can be justified not only in cost terms (if it can be this must be demonstrable) but in terms of quality control. Profits can be seen as not evil but as used *to* help them help patients. Here openness about how money moves is important.

It can be surprising to discover how little direct-care professionals know about the financial side of hospitals. Remember, concern with money is a pejorative in their eyes. Even if it has been previously explained, they may have tuned it out. Relate it to value issues which help them do good by seeing why what you are doing is coherent with those concerns. Explain third-party reimbursement, cross subsidization, costs versus charges, the different sorts of third-party payors and what they pay. Just remember their common denominator is not the bottom-line, but values, the cause. You cannot go back to values enough.

If you succeed, your difficult job will be respected as one which has values like theirs. Get *them* to emphasize how a hospital is different from a business. Get *them* to recognize that hospitals must change to survive. And get *them* to see how what you must do does not violate that specialness. They may well suggest and then support new services you want. Those who see how to fulfill their values through specific projects can become very enthusiastic crusaders. If their suggestions are financially or politically ill advised, be prepared to explain it to them in value terms.

Retreats, continuing education, seminars, consultants, all the usual educational tools for the management of change are likely to be employed as the process gets rolling, especially at larger institutions or multi-hospital systems. Bringing out the values involved and their congruence may require the help of people skilled in values analysis. They can serve as coaches to the administrator, help facilitate discussion, provide feedback on how well the discussions met the needs of the administrator and keep the discussions on track. But it is discussion, not *lecture*, which is needed.

Success in this project occurs when the administrator is recognized as the leader, the one who inspires, who embodies the ethical ideals, the obligations of the whole institution, a person "of unimpeachable character . . . that will make integrity his way of life.[32] A tall order indeed, but crusaders require goodness in their leaders, and it will take people who are willing to fill tall orders to keep hospitals on track in the days ahead. Levinson describes the administrator-leader as therapist for the whole institution, whose tools are the abilities to reach consensus on values and effectively use management skills from that base.[33] Presenting the administrator as a value therapist is likely to help him/her achieve recognition as a leader, far more than merely presenting himself/herself as a businessperson—and the institution as merely a business.

Notes

1. For representative articles see H. L. Hirsch "Health-Care Is A Business!," *Medical Trial Technique* Quarterly 25, no. 1 (Summer 1978): 77–83; Richard McQueen, "Hospitals Need Business Instincts Too," *Health Care* 4, no. 10 (October 1979): 58; Alan L. Applebaum, "Hospitals Must Be Businesslike," *Hospitals* 53, no. 21 (November 1, 1979): 107–108, 111–112; Richard L. Johnson, "The Wobbly Three Legged Stool," *Trustee* (May 1976): 9–14.

2. For a very good short piece on this theme see Robert M. Cunningham, Jr., "More Than a Business: Are Hospitals Forgetting Their Basic Mission?" *Hospitals* 57, no. 2 (January 16, 1983): 88–90. See also a collection of his articles in *The Healing Mission and the Business Ethic* (Chicago: Pluribus Press, 1982). Cunningham, a contributing editor to *Hospitals* could be likened to our conscience, a role also being taken on by Emily Friedman, a field editor to *Hospitals.*

3. Stuart A. Wesbury, President of the American College of Hospital Administrators, in a very excellent speech, "Ethics in Health Services Administration: A Case for Constant Reevaluation," the Eighth Annual Reverend J. Flanagan, S.J. Lecture in Hospital Administration to the St. Louis University Alumni Association (March 19, 1980), argues that technological changes, social changes, and the involvement of third parties has changed the health-care system such that administrators are the logical leaders. And leadership involves a clarity about values and mission we seem to have lost in our concerns over the problems management itself presents, a problem he wishes to redress.

4. Joseph P. Peters and Ronald C. Wacker, "Strategic Planning: Hospital Strategic Planning Must Be Rooted in Values and Ethics," *Hospitals* 56, no. 11 (June 16,1982): 90–98.

5. Harry Levinson,"The Changing Role of the Hospital Administrator," *Health Care Management Review* 1, no. 1 (Winter 1979): 79–89. This article should be obligatory reading; it points out the root causes of many of our frustrations in a very clear way.

6. Peters and Wacker, "Strategic Planning," p. 91.

7. Cunningham, *Healing Missions and Business Ethic*, p. 13 notes that twenty years ago the difference in values between these two sorts of ownership belied an underlying philosophic difference. This opinion still breaks out, which perhaps because of the emergence of the Federation documents, in spite of counsels to the effect that the phrase "not-for-profit" is a mere technical legal term. See Hugh W. Long, "Valuation as a Criterion in Not-For-Profit Decision-Making," *Health Care Management Review* 1, no. 3 (Summer 1976): 34.

8. Richard L. Johnson, "Revisiting The Wobbly Three Legged Stool," *Health Care Management Review* 4, no. 3 (Summer 1979): 17. Long, "Valuation as a Criterion," recognizes this same set of beliefs and urges they be transcended because of the real needs for substantial return on investment in order to survive.

9. Johnson, "Revisiting," 17–20.

10. Levinson, "Changing Role of the Hospital Administrator," 79–89.

11. Johnson, "Revisiting," 17–20.

12. Jeff Goldsmith, "Diversification", *Hospitals* 56, no. 23 (December 1, 1982): 68–73 and Salvinija G. Kernaghan, "Nontraditional Revenue," *Hospitals* 56, no. 23 (December 1, 1982): 75–81 point out some of the sorts of diversifications and the issues to be considered. While both mention the need to be consistent with the hospital mission the emphasis is on how to do it and make money, requiring administrators to "expand the limits of their vision beyond the traditional hospital role of patient caregiver" (p. 75). As noted, such expansion should not risk losing good will.

13. Cunningham, "More Than a Business," 89.

14. Johnson, "Revisiting," 21–22, and Cunningham, "More Than a Business," 89.

15. That this is often the way it is does not excuse us for letting it continue or for seminars or other training to try to legitimize it. Richard L. Johnson, "The Power Broker—Prototype of the Hospital Chief Executive," *Health Care Management Review* 3, no. 4 (Fall 1978): 67–73 exemplifies to the extreme the values, or manipulation, prompting in the "letters to the editor" criticisms by a physician—Summer 1979—and approval of its accuracy by an administrator—Winter 1979. While I totally agree with its accuracy, the long range consequences will only further alienate us from our values and prevent any likelihood of becoming a leader in the eyes of medical workers. As the sociologists Peter L. Berger and Thomas Luckmann, *The Social Construction of Reality* (New York: Doubleday, 1967), pp. 172–173 point out, "If this phenomenon becomes widely distributed, the institutional order as a whole begins to take on the character of a network of reciprocal manipulations." The ensuing distrust, suspicion, second guessing, and cynicism do little to enhance an environment conducive to leadership or patient care. The accuracy of Johnson's article should be a matter of major concern, not applause. It is also noteworthy that the very good article of his—"Revisiting"—points out that many administrators "say that the fun has been taken out of their profession" (p. 21). Certainly in a network of reciprocal manipulations the sense of working together in a common cause would seem to end. Perhaps it is not just fun we have lost, but a sense of values.

16. Cunningham, "More Than a Business," 89, argues that the only difference in the hospital and physician ethic is one of application. Hospitals have collective obligations; physicians have individual obligations. Peters and Wackers, "Strategic Planning," 97, describe this collective obligation as to the community. Long, "Valuation as a Criterion," 36, makes a similar point for non-profit hospitals.

17. The redefinition of the hospital in terms of these values is what Cunningham and Peters and Wacker advocate.

18. See footnote no.3.

19. Levinson, "Changing Roles of the Hospital Administrator," 84–89 discusses the task-oriented hospital and what must be done to achieve it.

20. John T. Foster, "A Letter to a Young CEO," *Hospital and Health Services Administration* 27, no. 3 (May/June 1982): 57–64, esp. 62; Wesbury, "Ethics in Health Services Administration," 11–13; William C. Parrish, "Is Fear a Part of Your Management Style?" *Health Care Management Review* 2, no. 3 (Summer 1977): 17–24, esp. 23–33, all make this point. Levinson, "Changing Role of the Hospital Administrator," 88, is emphatic that administrators must understand their own values and their conflicts and assess their fitness for the leadership role in terms of the values it requires.

21. The organization was unsuccessful in its 1981 effort to change the name to the American College of Health-Care Administrators, perhaps noteworthy of our own ambivalence about the changes in the mission of the hospital and our role in it.

22. The seven objects focus primarily on competency and education.

23. The eight personal obligations stress integrity and dutifulness along with helping to advance the profession *per se*.

24. American College of Hospital Administrators, *A Brief Description* (Chicago: ACHA, 1982), p. 1.

25. See esp. American College of Hospital Administrators, *Code of Ethics* (Chicago: ACHA, 1976).

26. Daniel Bell, "The Revolution in Rising Entitlements," *Fortune* (April 1975): 99.

27. Levinson, "Changing Role of the Administrator," 86, notes that direct-care medical professionals pride themselves on not dirtying their hands with business and politics, activities a leader must not only do well, but take pride in. My own recent experiences bear out that academics are even more extreme than medical professionals. It is interesting that to those in business, being accused of having dirty hands is a major insult, whereas to these more or less outsiders any activities undertaken primarily for personal or institutional gain are somehow suspect. Levinson points out that recognition of these value differences is a major step toward directing them into a shared set of institutional values, operating under a transcendent but meaningful mission.

28. John R. Schermerhorn, Jr., "The Health Care Manager's Role in Promoting Change," *Health Care Management Review* 4, no. 1 (Winter 1979): 71–84 uses these terms and provides a check-list for effective change. His analysis is not targeted to values, which presents some different problems in terms of top management commitment.

29. Wesbury, "Ethics in Health Services Administration," 8.

30. Ibid., 14.

31. Ibid., 13.

32. Foster, "Letter to a Young CEO," 62, 64.

33. Levinson, "Changing Role of the Hospital Administrator," 88–89.

CASE D

THE PATIENT OR THE INSTITUTION

The director of a radiology unit at a large hospital is faced daily with making administrative decisions that pit institutional efficiency against responsive patient care. As director he has the authority to delegate, to hire and fire staff, to budget, and so forth. When dealing with staff he has the power to inform them of hospital policy and the need for efficiency, and he can choose to stress it or not. He can guide them in an unbiased fashion, expressing to them the hospital's needs and goals as well as what he may feel is right or wrong for the patients. He can also pressure them by selective commendation when they are acting in a way that agrees with his personal feelings. Finally, in dealing with those in his work environment he wields power over the patients who need the services rendered by his section. Patients can be made to relax or have their anxiety levels increase. This depends on how the technologist is instructed to use his or her own time—to be courteous or abrupt, to be prompt or let them wait, to show responsiveness or just get the job done.

Within the past several years this radiology unit has experienced a fiscal shift. Before the advent of prospective reimbursement policies, services of the radiology department were reimbursed retrospectively at cost per service. Thus, every radiologic procedure performed netted the hospital a fee. The more procedures, the more the patient's itemized bill, and responding to individual patients as people was all right.

The new reimbursement policies bill patients prospectively according to their diagnosis. They pay the same amount for a diagnosis of cholecystitis with two radiologic procedures as one with eight radiologic procedures. Thus, the more procedures performed on a patient, the more that particular service becomes a financial "disincentive" to the hospital. Consequently, the radiology department is under scrutiny to cut costs wherever and whenever possible. In this vein, the hospital has hired outside consultants to probe various professional services departments, including all sections of the radiology department, and to conduct efficiency evaluations. These "efficiency experts" have been collecting data on the number of procedures per day, the time factor for each type of procedure, how time is spent when not performing procedures on patients, and the number of technologists required. Responding to patients as people has now become not as all right.

Yet patients are usually people who are ill, frightened, hopeful, depressed, and so forth. The radiology technologist tries to be responsive, to consider their wants and to ease their worries, to be fair to each of the patients by not devoting too much time to one and neglecting or delaying another. And he tries to be honest. But when a patient asks, "Did you see anything wrong with me?" after the film shows a large mass, he is professionally and legally not at liberty to divulge the information. He considers himself compassionate and tries, for example, to be courteous even to a bitter, nervous, angry patient. He is, in short, a good person and a good professional.

But, in his role as unit director, he also tries to be efficient and loyal to the hospital. For the hospital to survive in today's financial crunch, efficiency is constantly stressed by the administration. The radiology director knows that if efficiency is not achieved, the hospital's future will be in jeopardy. He believes that loyalty to the organization is important for survival, not only the hospital's survival but also the survival of his own job, of the staff and even of the patient community.

In this context he utilizes three examination rooms each day with a set schedule of inpatients and outpatients. He must also allow time for emergency "add-ons." Frequently, an outpatient shows up late. He must then decide whether to cancel that patient for the sake of fairness and responsiveness to other scheduled patients, or to instruct the technologists to understand the late patient's situation and squeeze him in, thus keeping on-time patients waiting and delaying emergencies. This situation often leads to lower-quality exams for all involved. Is that ethical? He wonders.

With regularity his superior directs him to stress efficiency to the staff. He knows that quality suffers in most cases of forcing the most exams per time unit/per technologist/per day for the sake of producing high patient volume. Efficiency for hospital survival seems to conflict with compassion, fairness, and quality care.

As a professional, it troubles him to be the one who places restrictions on patient care. He also worries that businesslike efficiency may not be profitable for the hospital in the long run. He believes that overshadowing courtesy and responsiveness to patient needs with efficiency has a detrimental effect on hospital survival. As a result, on some days he presses the staff to produce, and on other days he yells at them for not spending more time explaining procedures to patients. Yesterday he ordered a technologist to fit in a patient who is related to a close friend.

Questions for Discussion

1. Evaluate the ethical maturity of the radiology unit director. Is he sufficiently conscious of all the values involved?
2. What is the ethical way to deal with pressures to increase health delivery efficiency?
3. How could the unit director reconcile the competing pressures he feels?
4. Analyze this case in terms of who survives.
5. Distinguish the macro dimension involved in this case from the micro dimension confronting the unit director.

Annotated Bibliography

Bacon, M. *The Moral Status of Loyalty*. Dubuque, IA: Kendall/Hunt, 1984. A rare and perceptive discourse on the ethical impact of the value of loyalty.

Bayles, M. *Professional Ethics*. Belmont, CA: Wadsworth, 1981. A sound exploration of the conflicts among a professional's obligations.

Carter, S. L. *Integrity*. New York: Basic Books, 1996. A superb discourse on the nature of integrity as serious reflection drawing from dialogue.

Cleary, R. "The Professional As Public Servant: The Decision-Making Dilemma." *International Journal of Public Administration* 2, no. 2 (1980): 151–60. An articulate exploration of the conflicting roles of public service professionals.

Friedman, E. "Searching For Right." *Health Management Quarterly* 9, no. 3 (third quarter, 1987): 3–6. A brief and well-written probe of conflicting rights in healthcare.

Glaser, J. *Three Realms of Ethics*. Kansas City, MO: Sheed and Ward, 1994. An outstanding presentation of approaches to healthcare values conflict with structured cases.

Harran, F., J. Burnside, and T. Beauchamp. *Health and Human Values*. New Haven: Yale University Press, 1983. Written for macro level analysis this offers a clear presentation of the values horizon of healthcare.

Kress, G., J. Springer, and A. Cowden. "Administrative Values in Conflict." *State and Local Government Review* 3 (Fall 1986), 125–31. One of the few pieces that empirically explores values reconciliation in public service.

Lande, N., and A. Slade. *Stages*. New York: Harper and Row, 1979. A simple but enlightening presentation of Kohlberg's moral development theory that brings out bases of values conflict.

Okun, A. *Equality and Efficiency*. Washington, DC: Brookings Institution, 1975. A brilliant essay on the nature of the underlying values conflict in the economics of healthcare.

Ray, M., V. Didominic, P. Dittman, P. Hurst, J. Seaver, B. Sorbello, and M. Stankes-Ross. "The Edge of Chaos: Caring and the Bottom Line." *Nursing Management* 26, no. 9 (September 1995): 48–50. A good though brief analysis of a covenantal approach to reconciling value conflicts in healthcare.

Wakefield, S. "Ethics and the Public Service." *Public Administration Review* 36, no. 6 (November/December 1976): 661–66. A lucid presentation of the case for individual responsibility as the basis of public service ethics.

Whorton, J., and J. Worthley. "A Perspective on the Challenge of Public Management." *Academy of Management Review* 6, no. 3 (September 1981), 357–361. Distinguishes the values environment of profit versus nonprofit organizations.

ETHICS AND ACCOUNTABILITY: DEALING WITH CONTROLS

T HE THIRD lens of the ethics reality prism focuses our gaze on the mechanisms of accountability or control over the use of professional power. What are those mechanisms and controls? How are they manifest at the micro level? What are they intended to do? What do they actually do? What is our reaction to them? And what does it all have to do with ethics?

The Nature of Accountability

In the theoretical realm there is a rich tradition concerning the concept of accountability in public service professions.[1] An article by Charles Gilbert, reprinted in part to accompany this chapter, provides a fairly comprehensive familiarity with this. In the practical realm the concept has received energetic attention through professional development of codes of ethics. Both the American Hospital Association and the American College of Healthcare Executives, for example, have spent extensive resources on developing codes for professional accountability.[2] Not surprisingly, in both theory and practice, the emphasis has been on the macro dimension.

At both the macro and micro levels we can give specificity to the notion of accountability by posing some basic questions: As healthcare professionals to *whom* are we accountable? For *what* are we accountable? *How* are we held accountable? *Why* are we held accountable? And *what results* from all of this? Theoretically, we are accountable to our superiors, to our clients, to our profession, and to the law. And through unions and contracts we are accountable to our subordinates. We have *multiple* accountabilities, and in theory, they hold us accountable for many things: for our honesty; for our competence, efficiency, and productivity; for our adherence to rules and our fairness; and for our responsiveness. Does this sound familiar? To get this accountability from us they use a *maze of mechanisms* from articulated policies to budgetary controls to extensive reporting requirements. This is all because of the power we wield: to get us to use that power well and to keep us from using it harmfully. Theoretically, the results come together in a formalization process of (1) *confining* professional power by fixing its boundaries; (2) *structuring* professional power by regularizing and organizing it; and (3) *checking* professional power by monitoring its use.[3] Practically, what results? A royal pain in the proverbial pancreas! But that's just in theory. Let's ask the same questions in the practical micro dimension of our healthcare work.

To whom are we accountable in that dimension? The self-absorbed medical director, the obnoxious patient, the overbearing union representative, the nitpicking peer review team. What do they expect? Obedience, loyalty, and competence. Respect and responsiveness. Fairness and respect. Conformity and competence. How do they demand these things? Through authoritative orders and directions, through facial expressions and unstated threats of dismissal, through comments on performance and written evaluations. Through pestering phone calls, shouts for attention, patient advocates, and lawsuit innuendo. Through union contracts and grievance procedures. Through written accreditation standards and periodic inspections. Why? So that their view of what should be done prevails instead of our mere professional view. What results? That same royal pain in the proverbial pancreas—and some other things, too. We have ways of undermining that medical director behind her back, don't we? And when she is not around we can do things our way anyway. As for obnoxious patients, we can easily delay in getting to them, or pump the blood pressure cuff a bit tighter. As for my annoying subordinate, see if I approve his vacation dates. And those inspectors? We'll play their silly game: the day they arrive won't even resemble every other day of the year! They'll love what they see. I wonder if all of that's ethical.

Formal and Informal Realities

We can take a more disciplined look at this with the help of a matrix modified from that used by Gilbert in the reading that follows. This matrix (Figure 5.1) might help us conceptualize and organize the reality of controls in the daily routine of our healthcare work.

Figure 5.1 Mechanisms of Accountability

	(Controls Over Professional Power)	
	Internal	External
Formal		
Informal		

The *formal internal* reality refers to those official mechanisms within the organization or profession designed to direct or control what we do on the job. They are things like the chain of command, written policies, standard operating procedures, job descriptions, union contracts, standard reporting forms, performance assessment instruments, and codes of ethics. More specifically, they are our ornery-stickler or laissez-faire boss; the policy statement requiring us to inform the patient of the pending treatment and to secure his signature on a standard consent form; the written procedure specifying how we are to conduct triage; the sentence in our job description about preparing an annual budget; the clause in our employees' union contract establishing a formal grievance right for them; the expense form we must complete and submit before being reimbursed for our job travel to another state; the time clock we must punch every day; the awkward interview with our boss at performance evaluation time; and that clause in our professional code of ethics that says we cannot accept a birthday present from the vendor if its value exceeds $25 but that we can accept it if it costs only $24.95.

The *formal external* reality refers to those official mechanisms outside the organization and profession that attempt to direct and control what we do in our work. They are realities like the Joint Commission accreditation standards, the federal government's Medicare regulations, the state's malpractice statutes, the governor's healthcare delivery task force. More specifically, they are those inspection team members who come to our facility, those particular regulations that take up so much of our time and paper, that gadfly lawyer who hangs around our emergency room, and the 23-year-old staff assistant to the state senator who chairs the legislature's health committee.

The *informal internal* reality refers to those unofficial mechanisms within the organization and profession that try to direct and control our actual behavior at work. They are things like organization culture, peer pressure, one's own moral code, and workplace "climate"—often subtle permissions, prescriptions, and proscriptions.[4] More specifically, they are things like the practice of calling patients by their first name or their last name, like the norm of dressing casually or more formally, like the ritual of the white jacket uniform and the unwritten code of covering up our peer's mistakes.[5] These mechanisms of control tend to be subtle but very strong.

Finally, there is the *informal external* reality, those unofficial mechanisms outside the organization and profession that nonetheless influence what we professionals do and how we do it. In general, they are things like interest groups and media; in particular they are that patients' rights activist and the investigative reporter. Sometimes they are the Geraldo Riveras who really can affect our work. Other times they are just annoying inquiries from a faceless cub reporter or a vociferous patient advocate or an aggressive television cameraman. And they are all trying to exert some control over our professional work. Don't we love it? Or, do we really hate it all? What are our *feelings* about such controls and what do such feelings have to do with ethics?

To pursue this line of inquiry let's begin by asking some other questions. First, why all these mechanisms of control? Two general theoretical reasons and numerous specific ones can be linked to the reality of professional power examined in chapter 3. One general reason is the promotion of sound exercise of professional power. The great organizational theorist, Max Weber, argued that controls are indispensable for an *effective* bureaucracy.[6] The other general reason is to protect against inappropriate use of professional power. Herman Finer is representative of this latter reasoning: "The political and administrative history of all ages demonstrates beyond a shadow of doubt that there is abuse of power when external controls are lacking."[7] So the general theoretical reasons for all of these controls are to further effective and responsible professional behavior. Sound good?

The specific reasons for mechanisms of accountability stem directly from the preceding chapter: the promotion and maintenance of the sacred values of healthcare—competence, responsiveness, fairness, honesty, legitimacy, survival and so forth. Why the standard operating procedures? To promote competence and fairness. Why the Joint Commission standards and inspections? To promote competence and expertise. Why the peer pressure? To promote survival and loyalty. Why the grievance procedures? To promote fairness. Why patient's rights? To promote responsiveness. Why the travel reimbursement forms? To promote honesty. And on and on. Behind every specific control is a purpose to protect and promote some important value.

A second question is: what actually *results* from the exercise of these controls? Does protection of the intended value result? Do other things result? Without doubt values are protected and promoted by these mechanisms of accountability. Those Joint Commission standards certainly help keep clinical competence high and consent forms and patient advocates help keep us responsive to clients; and grievance procedures, lawyers, and codes undoubtedly help keep us fair, honest and legally sound. But what else results? For one thing, we spend a considerable amount of time and money on these controls. Let's reflect on the nature of a typical workday. How much time do we spend completing reports, answering questions, following procedures that are all related not as much to getting our job done as to complying with control and accountability mechanisms? Aren't complaints about the amount of paperwork health-care professionals must complete indicative of a time burden?

For another thing don't those same controls that promote some values actually undermine other important values? Don't those procedures and Joint Commission standards that promote competence also sometimes—perhaps often—result in a by-the-book undermining of efficiency and responsiveness to individual patients? And don't those grievance procedures sometimes—perhaps often—undermine legitimate authority and employee competence? Don't some legal reimbursement requirements sometimes—perhaps often—promote "white lies" or outright dishonesty? Is it not often the case that a direct result of accountability mechanisms is accentuated conflict and competition among values?

Behavioral Reactions

A third question gets at what I call the visceral reality. How, in fact, do we *feel* about controls? What is the result deep down? I suggest that sometimes—perhaps often—our feelings are not exactly positive. I suggest that often we are more aware of the values threatened and less aware of the values promoted, and that this negative awareness tends to condition our reaction. Indeed, in my own experience, I can attest that I don't like controls at all and that my visceral reaction is usually negative. As an experienced professional of high integrity I know well what to do and how to do it well. I don't like government telling me what to do in my professional work. I don't like people looking over my shoulder checking up on me, whether they are Joint Commission officials or union representatives. I can't stand it when incompetent employees threaten a grievance against me for trying to get them to work better. And when I hear about a doctor being sued for malpractice when he just tried to save a life and did his best, well it gets me going. Robert Miewald is probably on target in describing many of us when he observes that we professionals are inclined to be diametrically opposed to controls over our professional activity: "Being professionals they need not engage in a dialogue with anyone and least of all with misguided politicians. . . . There is no need for the hassle of politics which can only obscure the general interest. After all, if the professionals did not know what the general interest looked like, they would not be professionals."[8] While I am not particularly conscious of having this attitude, it may be more present than I'd like to admit.

At any rate, my visceral reaction usually leads to a fourth result. I am not stupid and I don't have to take absurd interference with my professional work. There are ways to keep those controls within reason, aren't there? As an experienced and savvy professional, aware of the danger of some controls and of the harm they can cause, I know how to play their "control" game and still protect the values that are being threatened. I know how to manipulate the controls so that not too much harm is done. I have behavioral reactions.

For example, I can and often do "bend the rules," as they say. When an immediate response is needed and the procedures obstruct it, I know how to get the job done despite the red tape. For example, when the inspectors visit to check on our conformity with standards, we "go by the book." When they leave we get back to doing things our way, which is the only way to get the job done in the real world. For example, I can make life miserable for my lax employee without technically qualifying for a grievance: I submit the required reports, but there are different ways of phrasing things. I find that from this reaction follows an intellectual result. In my mind I often think that I *must* manipulate the damaging controls. I have a responsibility to protect against the harm that otherwise would occur, harm such as unserved patients, wasted time and money, and unfairly treated peers.

Of course, it is sometimes useful to comply with controls that undermine important values. To put an obnoxious patient in her place I sometimes like to enforce standard procedures instead of responding as I could. To protect myself from malpractice suits I often call on by-the-book procedures even though I doubt their efficacy and know the expense involved. And I know well how to use good old peer pressure to protect a good colleague who has made one mistake.

To illustrate behavioral reactions to mechanisms of accountability let's look at two outstanding healthcare professionals, careful Carol and loyal Luke, both of whom you probably know. Carol's job as an administrator for a large medical center entails regular travel. Her organization's reimbursement policies limit hotel and meal reimbursements to a maximum that sometimes does not cover Carol's actual out-of-pocket expenses. This occurs only occasionally, when she travels to a large city and chooses to stay at a more expensive hotel for personal security reasons. A year ago she was mugged while staying at a cheaper hotel. So on these trips Carol pads her expense reimbursement report with small taxicab items that do not require a receipt. She is meticulously careful in ensuring that her total reimbursement claim, padded in this manner, never exceeds her actual total expenses—it just covers the difference between the maximum hotel reimbursement and the actual hotel charge. It is not a lot of money and Carol does this only as a temporary measure until the reimbursement maximums are raised, an action that the organization is planning.

Notice what is happening here. Accountability and control mechanisms—namely travel expense policy, reimbursement forms and review procedures—are in place to structure Carol's discretion so that travel is done efficiently. Receipts are required to promote honesty in claims, and reimbursement forms are used to promote legal compliance with authoritative travel policy. These mechanisms have developed over time partially as a result of submittal of exorbitant travel claims and partially as a result of external pressures to contain costs. And securing receipts and completing travel forms now take time and energy away from productive work.

Further, this whole scenario is happening because travel is a condition of Carol's work, not something she chooses to do. She is as conscientious a healthcare professional as one could meet. She works hard, takes pride in her productivity, and is an upstanding single parent putting two children through college. Largely because she is so conscientious, the travel reimbursement nonsense has always irritated her. "Don't they trust me to use good sense?" she wonders. When she worked in the private sector it was so much simpler.

After she was mugged she really became irritated at the system. "It's not fair that I should foot the bill when I am directed to work in the city and am trying to be productive," she told me. "It's not safe at those hotels that are within the reimbursement rate and my anxiety there shuts down my productivity." Carol clearly has very real *feelings* about the reimbursement issue, and these visceral reactions have led her to cleverly undermine the honesty and legitimacy that the controls are designed to promote. But Carol does not see it as dishonesty. Meticulously ensuring that she claims no more than her actual "reasonable" expenses by using a reimbursement loophole, she sees it as an honest way to safeguard the cherished values of fairness, physical safety, and, by the way, work productivity. To hear her tell it, she has an ethical responsibility to protect fairness, safety, and efficiency.

Is Carol on the proverbial slippery slope of sin? Or is she merely showing good managerial ingenuity by maintaining common sense despite systems that sometimes appear to get in the way? After all, the amount of money involved is only a few hundred dollars; and to Carol it is not so much the money, anyway, it's the principle! Or is she rather justifying unethical behavior by focusing on some values and blindly dismissing the values that prompted the mechanisms she manipulates? Has she been led to this place by real visceral feelings instead of by professional ethical reasoning? Is it ethical for Carol to do this? Would it be ethical for her not to do it and instead to be less productive, less safe, and less fairly treated? Is it sometimes our ethical responsibility to manipulate controls, or is it never ethical to do such a thing?

Carol never got caught, by the way, and it is unlikely that, in things like this, many of us will. Besides, isn't this kind of "getting around" controls more or less common practice precisely for the reasons Carol articulates? But, again, is it ethical when an internal, informal control—Carol's moral outrage—overrides a formal mechanism of accountability?

Then there's my golfing buddy, loyal Luke, as fine a guy as you will ever meet despite his ten handicap. Luke is a unit director at a major Blue Cross/Blue Shield. His friend, charming Charley is director of a different unit at the same Blue Cross organization. They both joined Blue Cross about 12 years ago and have socialized ever since. Their families vacation together and their children are friends, too. Over a period of several months Luke has noticed a change in Charley's behavior and strongly suspects that his friend is in the midst of a drug problem.

Because of numerous drug-related incidents in recent years as well as other ethics matters, Blue Cross formed a committee last year to develop an organizational response. Luke was on this committee and it produced a "Standards of Integrity" document that after months of review and revision was formally adopted, with every employee required to sign a pledge to abide by the standards. One of the standards specifies that being under the influence of drugs or alcohol is unacceptable and that employees are "responsible for bringing to the attention of their immediate superior any situation that appears in violation of these Standards of Integrity."

When Luke finally confronts Charley with his suspicions, Charley at first denies any problem then assures Luke that he is getting help. Charley begs Luke not to report him lest his career be jeopardized. "You know how these supposedly confidential matters somehow get known. I'll be blackballed and you know it. Work with me. I promise I'll get clean, but please, Luke, don't report me."

Should Luke focus on the values of loyalty to his friend and his friend's economic welfare, and ignore the official standard of integrity that requires him to report the situation to his superior? Or should he honor the standard and report Luke, telling him it is "for your own good" or something like that? The organization has spent significant time and money developing this mechanism of accountability because some terrible things have happened. But Charley is a good guy as well as Luke's pleading friend.

Consider the situation. Luke is *feeling* deeply the cry of his friend for loyalty and safe-being. He knows in his mind the sacred importance of that standard of integrity, but it seems to be mere ink on paper. Charley is flesh and blood. So Luke violates the standard requiring him to report the situation to his superior. Instead, he goes with Charley to a rehab program and monitors his friend's recovery. No one in the Blue Cross hierarchy finds out, and Charley is still clean a year later.

Did Luke behave ethically? Was it ethically responsible to violate the very standard he had helped develop so that his friend would be economically safe? Or was his ethical responsibility rather to violate loyalty to his friend and jeopardize Charley's career so that a sacred standard would be honored? His visceral feelings led him to do the former. In effect, the informal control of peer loyalty, conflicting with the formal control of official policy, won out. To whom was Luke accountable and for what? In undermining a mechanism of accountability did he behave ethically? Did he have an ethical responsibility to undermine it? What about the factor of friendship? If Luke had not been Charley's friend, he undoubtedly would not have had the same visceral feelings. Should that make any ethical difference? Would it likely have made a behavioral difference?

Summary: Whose Judgment?

In the end the cases of careful Carol and loyal Luke—and indeed the whole subject of accountability and controls—come down to one basic question: Whose judgment should prevail? In fact, the whole subject of professional healthcare ethics could focus on that one issue. Whose judgment of what is ethical *does* prevail, and whose judgment *should* prevail? Mine or my superior's? The patient's or the doctor's judgment? The court's judgment or the profession's? In the case of Carol, legitimate authority had judged what travel policy should be. Carol's judgment disagreed with it, and she found a way for her judgment to prevail over that of the authorities. Since she is the professional on the scene, should her judgment prevail or should that of the legitimate authority? In the case of loyal Luke, the organization had decided that any appearance of drug influence should be reported. Luke apparently disagreed and his judgment prevailed. But, ethically, whose judgment should have prevailed? Maybe the organization's judgment is faulty, but who should judge that? Should we professionals take it upon ourselves to be the final arbiters of what is ethical and, whenever necessary, override the judgment of whoever else is involved? Just to whom are we accountable and for what? When push comes to shove we can often—like Carol and Luke—neutralize the notion of accountability and turn it into accountability to ourselves for what we determine.

Another way of reflecting on these questions is to consider whether healthcare ethics is more a matter of *daring* or of *deference*. Is it a matter of daring to stand up for what we believe is right and to manipulate obstructive mechanisms of accountability, or is it rather a matter of deferring our judgment to that of others? Remember the case of Diane in the previous chapter? She deferred her judgment to that of her bosses. Remember the Milgram experiments described in chapter 3? The teachers there deferred their judgment to that of the experimenter. Remember the story of *One Flew Over the Cuckoo's Nest*? McMurphy dared to have his judgment prevail and Nurse Ratched wasn't about to defer to his judgment on anything! From these examples, then, is ethics a matter of daring to make the judgment or of deferring personal judgment to the judgment of someone else?

Thus, when we focus that reality prism on mechanisms of accountability, we see an ethically richer picture than is apparent on the surface. Controls over our professional behavior, and our reaction to these controls, are key elements of the microethics of healthcare.

Notes

1. See, for example, the work of K. C. Davis, 1977, *Administrative Law Treatise* (St. Paul, MN: West Publishing), and 1969, *Discretionary Justice: A Preliminary Inquiry* (Urbana: University of Illinois Press); and H. Finer, 1941, "Administrative Responsibility in Democratic Government." *Public Administration Review* 1, no. 4 (December): 335–50.

2. See Appendix A and Appendix B for copies of these *Codes*.

3. H. K. Hibbein and D. H. Shumavon, 1983, "Methods for Structuring Administrative Discretion." *State and Local Government Review* (fall): 124–29.

4. See B. Victor and J. Cullen, 1988, "The Organizational Bases of Ethical Work Climates." *Administrative Science Quarterly* 33, no. 1 (March): 101–104 for insight on this point. This article is reprinted in part as a reading in chapter 6.

5. For a sophisticated analysis of this control, see L. Trevino and B. Victor, 1992, "Peer Reporting of Unethical Behavior." *Academy of Management Journal* 35, no. 1 (March): 38–64.

6. M. Weber, 1947, *The Theory of Social and Economic Organizations*, trans. by A. Henderson and T. Parsons (London: Oxford).

7. H. Finer, 1941, "Administrative Responsibility in Democratic Government." *Public Administration Review* 1, no. 4 (December): 336.

8. R. Miewald, 1978, *Public Administration: A Critical Perspective* (New York: McGraw-Hill), pp. 52–54, 68–70.

READING

Controls on government power have spilled over to healthcare and have been mimicked there. Government regulation, hospital procedures, the Joint Commission, are well known to healthcare professionals. Systematic analysis of controls in healthcare has, however, been meager. We therefore turn to more generic analyses to enlighten our discussion. The following seasoned piece by Charles Gilbert is among the most conceptually sound reflections that have appeared, and it is easily applied to our healthcare focus.

By probing the concept of "administrative responsibility" Gilbert classifies means of achieving it, means that are germane to healthcare and that can help us identify specific controls in the micro dimension. He begins with a discussion of basic values that controls are geared to uphold, a discussion that builds on our previous chapter. Using the simple four categories of control employed in this chapter—formal internal, formal external, informal internal, and informal external—he then deftly illuminates the nature of controls. Of course, Gilbert's interest is uniformly macro and governmental making it necessary for the reader to think and translate in order to apply the concepts to the micro dimension of healthcare. In his discussion of "representative" administration, for example, as an internal, informal control over behavior, we could well reflect on the way we interact with patients of our own socioeconomic-ethnic background versus those of another background. In his discussion of judicial controls we could profitably reflect on whether fear of legal sanctions influences our daily interaction with subordinates and patients. And his discussion of external, informal controls might well trigger reflection of how we react to the influences of labor unions and patient rights groups in our daily work.

In the end, Gilbert poses a key question for improving our ethical skills in the micro dimension of healthcare: What will the probable results on our basic healthcare values be as we reflect on control mechanisms and tinker with those that impinge on our daily routine?

THE FRAMEWORK OF ADMINISTRATIVE RESPONSIBILITY

Charles E. Gilbert

In this paper an attempt will be made to restate the problem of "administrative responsibility." Our literature has so far not come to much agreement—at least, explicitly—upon conceptualization of the problem, though the past quarter century has seen a number of penetrating institutional studies of it.[1] This study is limited to American experience and to the federal government; most of the literature discussed here does likewise. If, however, a workable framework for discussion and analysis emerges it should have a more general application. The two aspects of the problem . . . will be examined in what follows. This involves, first, an analysis of the term "responsibility," and second, a classification of the institutional means of its achievement. The resulting framework of analysis will then be applied to some of our main schools of thought on the problem of administrative responsibility.

I

Governmental administration in a society such as our own operates amidst a complex of presumptively popular values which are further presumed to guide the making and administration of public policy. Every teacher and every textwriter has his own method of signalizing these values or guidelines for public policy. These values and their relative emphases change, however, and the words that we use for them stand, in turn, for complexes of words or values.

The term "responsibility" as it is used in the literature of public administration seems nearly always to stand for such a complex of values.[2] It is not, and perhaps cannot be, employed with complete consistency from one situation to another. Probably it cannot be "defined" in any strict sense; rather, the term broadly bounds a set of values or concerns generally linked together in the administrative process. An attempt will be made to list and distinguish the chief of these values, without claiming that the list is either definitive or exhaustive. Nor does the author claim that the meanings here provided for twelve values more aptly summarize our constitutional theory, political folklore or academic writing than would other formulations. What is intended is a fair examination of the

Charles E. Gilbert, "The Framework of Administrative Responsibility." *Journal of Politics* 21, no. 3 (August 1959): 373–407. Reprinted by permission of the author and the University of Texas Press. The article is abridged. Charles E. Gilbert was political science professor at Swarthmore College.

term "responsibility" as it has been used in our literature, and the first step in this project is to discuss the values most frequently implied when the term is used.

1. *Responsiveness.* Prompt acquiescence by government (whichever part of government is under discussion) in popular demands for policy change (usually though not necessarily, voiced at the polls). The breadth and/or intensity to be required of "authentic" public demands are difficult to define, especially as regards demands not expressed through voting. A synonym which conveys the same notion is "popularness."[3]

2. *Flexibility.* Discrimination (not in an invidious sense) in the making and especially the administration of policy so as not to ignore individual group, or local concerns or situational differences relevant to effective achievement of policy goals. Such flexibility may be "responsive" to segmental popular demands, or it may result from executive or administrative leadership.[4]

3. *Consistency.* This is perhaps the most ambiguous word in the list. A common, equally ambiguous, synonym is "rationality", another and perhaps better synonym is integrity" in the literal sense of the word The idea is that governmental policy—as a whole, or within any "area" of policy, e.g., fiscal policy—shows as much freedom as possible from internal contradictions. The usual administrative term is, of course "co-ordination." Most writers seem to feel that this value has low popular ranking in our society.[5]

4. *Stability.* Public policy and its administration should be consistent over time, should be predictable where there is no evident public demand for change, and should forsake continuity only when public demand is authentic. This quality of policy and administration presumably has value for the whole society, but perhaps most—a point frequently made—for business and commercial interests. It also has obvious value in areas particularly subject to governmental "planning" i.e., centralized decision-making. As defined here, it is not necessarily at odds with responsiveness, but some would construe it in stronger terms than these and define "authentic" public demand as considered and long-term demand; not fluctuating and short term changes in opinion.[6]

5. *Leadership.* The demand—perhaps it is particularly a modern twentieth-century demand—that government do more than respond to public or publics, that it take initiatives in the proposal of solutions for problems and even in the definition of problems, subject, of course, to popular ratification.[7]

6. *Probity.* This appears to be a meaning frequently implied when we speak of a "responsible man" and, perhaps, a responsible institution. Three synonyms are honesty, integrity, trustworthiness. Inclusion of this concern brings the ethics-in-government problem within the meaning of "responsibility." Although the hems here employed cannot be clearly applied in all situations, all institutional approaches to administrative responsibility agree on the importance of the concern, and some take it for granted. There is disagreement as to whether it is best enforced by formal or informal, administrative or extra-administrative means.[8]

7. *Candor.* The policy-making and -administering process should be open to public scrutiny, leaving aside the question of at what stages open to scrutiny. Moreover, the political and governmental system in general should reach and deduce the merits of issues rather than obscure them through personal or procedural obfuscation. A further requirement might include that of reasoned justification of governmental decisions. Though logically three separate notions, they are lumped together here since they all have presumed value for public discussion, education and the sense of individual "responsibility" for public policy. Some theorists have not valued candor highly (save in the sense of the first requirement), fearing a tendency toward divisive or doctrinaire politics. Not everyone will agree upon which aspects of a complex issue constitute its "merits."[9]

8. *Competence.* The making and administration of policy should be guided by recognized objective or disciplinary standards where they are available, and appropriate expertise and specializations should be valued in administration. The perennial problems here concern the segregation of means (appropriate for decision by experts) from ends (which are presumably not meet for expert decision even though amenable to expert advice), and whether "objective standards" in fact exist in many controversial policy areas.[10]

9. *Efficacy.* Governmental performance of particular activities should be efficient, and governmental administration in general should be timely, thorough and conservatively priced. The term employed here is broader than the term "efficiency" because, where many ends or values are involved in governmental activity, the denominator of the efficiency ratio becomes practically inexpressible. Similarly, where differences between administrations are differences largely in energy or drive, the numerator of the efficiency ratio is also practically inexpressible. Not everyone will accept as realistic the conception of administrative organization and behavior upon which the technical notion of "efficiency" is based. "Efficacy" as used here means not only the performance in fact of programs undertaken, but the effectiveness or (in a loose sense) efficiency of the performance, given scarce resources.[11]

10. *Prudence.* Administrative action, in the normal case, should be deliberate rather than precipitate, informed rather than ignorant, and should display a care for consequences rather than negligence. This is the sense in which the terms "responsible man" and "prudent man" are generally taken in both lay and legal usage. Acceptance of this value, of course, implies acceptance of sufficient administrative discretion for its exercise. This is certainly not an unrealistic assumption, begging the question of the limits of discretion.[12]

11. *Due process.* It may not seem useful to distinguish this value; doubtless many would feel that it is comprehended under responsiveness, probity, candor, prudence. To the lawyer, however, it appears to connote something sufficiently special that it cannot properly be exhausted in these values though it does overlap them. The minimum procedural addition to these four values is the notion of non-arbitrariness as evidenced by procedure roughly similar to those of courts, though there is disagreement about how roughly and regarding what types of cases. Two frequent, more substantive, additions come under the heading of "justice": (a) proportionality in the sense that, where situations differ relevantly, they will have outcomes proportionate to their differences; and (b) equality, or equal opportunity at influence in the making of policy and equal treatment in its administration. Several separate concerns are thus included in the term due process (a lawyer's equivalent of our problem of "responsibility"), but in this paper this more general rubric has been retained. The term illustrates the difficulty of distinguishing between verbal statements of principles and institutional processes, for it seems to shift between the two in the language of courts. Of course, it also illustrates the difficulty, at the margin, of distinguishing between procedural and substantive values.[13]

12. *Accountability.* The relationship implied in this term is essentially one of agency; the concerns of the principal seem best expressed in Charles S. Hyneman's terms, "direction and control," and involve the demonstrability and regularity of the relationship. A good synonym is "answerability." The key question here is: accountability to whom or to what? Different sources and/or avenues of accountability will have different results in terms of emphasis or de-emphasis of various of the eleven other values just discussed.[14]

Several points will at once occur to readers of this list. First some of the twelve values as stated pose a complex set of dilemmas, or a complicated exercise in adjusting margins. Few of them can be pressed very far without infringing upon one or more of the others. Probably the chief controversies over American political institutions have involved various blends of the first five values listed here. On the other hand, other values are complementary; both consistency and candor may, for example, further accountability; accountability may further candor, though it will not necessarily further consistency.

Second, it is difficult to say much about the interrelationship of these values apart from their specific institutional context or embodiment—lacking these data, they are abstractions and guidelines, though nonetheless necessary or useful. I think one can say, however, that debate about their relative role in a governmental system is a matter of more or less. All of these ends must probably be met in some degree if a modern governmental system is to function.

Third, these values may be applied to administration per se, to other branches of government, or to the governmental system as a whole. Much debate about our governmental institutions concerns the particular institutions in which particular values are to be located or emphasized. The discussion that follows deals primarily (though not exclusively) with the realization of these values in administration.

Fourth, the weight that people will accord to various of these values will depend, in part, at least, upon the substantive area of public policy under discussion, though presumably men also make up their minds upon a balance as applied to governmental activity as a whole.

Fifth, the definitions are not very precise. I have tried to write of discrete concerns but, language being what it is, some will feel either that the twelve concerns overlap or that more categories are required. I will agree, but note the contrary peril of seeming precision that may exclude or torture both popular and academic thinking. The political scientist who undertakes to write of "operative ideals" and the jurist who writes of "due process" share the same problems whenever they leave description of existing institutions. An analysis of institutional patterns for the "values" they yield has generally to be couched in rather imprecise language.

Finally, all of the twelve words listed above, and the meanings there associated with them, have been comprehended by various writers under the rubric "responsibility."[15] The intention here has been to dissect this term for purposes of the subsequent discussion, and henceforth the word "responsibility" will be used only as a collective term for the twelve values discussed. Dissection, rather than definition, seems the only feasible approach to a term which, as noted above, simply bounds a group of concerns.[16] Much of our literature on administrative responsibility has not paused long over definition or analysis of the term "responsibility" but has focused instead upon analysis and prescription of institutional means for achieving something thus loosely described. Where analysis of institutions has differed it is likely, then, that the difference has stemmed from differentially including or weighting in the term "responsibility" some or all of the twelve values listed here, though differences as to premises may not have been explicit.

An earlier analysis of the term "responsibility" by J. Roland Pennock has served as a starting-point for this analysis.[17] Professor Pennock distinguishes two meanings of the term as essentially (1) accountability or answerability (including, by extension, the notions of identifiability and effective causation), and (2) susceptibility of rational explanation. While the first of these meanings is fairly explicit (save, perhaps, for its implications or extensions), the second—and especially the word "rational"—is much broader. The analysis above (focusing on the term "responsibility" as employed in the administrative literature) simply involves some further distinctions. "Accountability" is the same in both discussions. The further concerns with identifiability and effective causation are here expressed as "candor," "leadership," and "efficacy," though these values are also, I believe, implicit in arguments that (explicitly or otherwise) employ the term "responsibility" in Professor Pennock's second sense. The other concerns discussed above fall within the second usage of the term—a usage as broad as the word "rational" often is, which (in many arguments) can thus reflect such concerns as flexibility, consistency, stability, competence, prudence, probity, and due process. One of the chief points of Professor Pennock's discussion is to distinguish between the terms "responsiveness" and "responsibility." This analysis is in full agreement on this point, maintaining only (as does Professor Pennock) that the distinction is not always observed in discussions of responsibility.

Some may be inclined to recommend that we refrain from using the word "responsibility," in view of its breadth of meaning, or else use it solely as a synonym for accountability. But accountability, as Professor Pennock's analysis shows, has some logical extensions of meaning that are difficult to distinguish from his "rationality" dimension of responsibility. Moreover, we cannot simply scrap a word by fiat, and the word is probably a useful one if we are clear about its vaguely indicative nature. . . .

II

For the most part the literature on administrative responsibility and the issues in that literature have concerned institutional patterns rather than linguistic analysis of the term itself. Five traditions within this literature in terms of the emphasis they place upon certain avenues of "responsibility" will be discussed. As a simple framework for discussion, administrative relationships are divided into four main categories: *internal formal; internal informal; external formal; and external informal.* No writers advocate exclusive reliance upon any one of these four relationships. Moreover, the chief differences of emphasis occur not so much between the four types as between either of the two broader types: formal v. informal, or internal v. external. There is, then, no school of thought to be found entirely within any one of the boxes in the diagram, or in either the vertical or the horizontal column:

Internal Formal	External Formal
Internal Informal	External Informal

But there are decided differences in emphasis, and these have been at the center of modern discussions of our subject.

This fourfold classification is intended to include all relationships of administrative responsibility (as a collective term for the values discussed above), and to point to features of them that are important for those values. The same terms will be used, however, in describing five major approaches to responsibility which occur in the literature, recognizing that still other positions are possible within the above classification.

The five positions will here be termed the internal formal, the internal informal, the Congressional, the judicial, and the external informal. By the internal formal position is meant those approaches stressing direction and control by the President and via such hierarchical methods as budgeting, personnel management, standards and rules of procedure, and the structuring and restructuring of formal organization to the extent that this may be within the power or legal authority of the President (all these in addition to some personal suasion and intervention).[18] The internal informal position refers to those approaches emphasizing the moral, representative and professional aspects of public service as sources of "responsibility." The Congressional position places primary reliance upon external formal direction and control, though generally recognizing that Congressional-administrative relations often exhibit marked informal characteristics as well.[19] The judicial position comprises those emphasizing control by courts (external formal) and through "judicialization" of the administrative process (internal formal)— this position thus stresses formality and cuts across the descriptive categories of internal and external. Finally, in the external informal position are included those theorists who have urged and applauded experiments in interest-group representation, citizen participation, and "grass roots democracy," or the less planned interplay of organized groups and administrative agencies[20]. . . .

At the end of the preceding section some difficulties in using the classification of values set forth there were pointed out. A further difficulty in using the institutional classification just set forth exists. The difficulty concerns accountability; for while accountability to tome institutions or principals may be more demonstrable than to others, accountability in any direction at all is generally difficult to demonstrate. This difficulty is increased if the principal or source of accountability is not clearly defined. The following extended quotation aptly describes the problem:

> There is a tendency, in the literature relating to public administration to treat the decisions and instructions that make up direction and control of the bureaucracy as falling under one or another of three heads—political, legal, and administrative. To those three heads, some writers add two more—moral and popular. These titles [political, legal, administrative, moral and popular] suggest that the basis for the classification is the source of direction and control—that the type of direction and control is determined by the point in the governmental system at which the decision is made and the instructions are issued. . . . The truth is, however, that neither writers about public administration nor individuals who are caught up in practical situations adhere to any consistent basis in using these terms. Three of these terms at least—political, legal, and administrative—are used to describe the characteristics or the nature of the decisions and instructions that are involved, as well as to indicate where they originate. . . .
>
> I think we will best understand the relationships that are crucial to [our] purposes . . . if we organize our analysis about two considerations. One, what are the questions that must be decided and concerning which instructions must be issued . . . ? And two, who is to make these crucial decisions and issue the necessary instructions?[21]

This stricture is sound. In trying to handle "accountability" the only safe course is to define and designate as clearly as possible the institution (or other source) toward which accountability is presumed to lie. But the fourfold classification employed here (and the dimensions formal-informal, and internal-external) are justified on the ground that they manageably group together institutional patterns that have characteristic results for most of our twelve values and that are characteristically emphasized by both organization theory and political theory. The discussion to follow deals principally with the value "accountability." The formal-informal distinction relates to that value by the definition of accountability and has long been related to it in the literature of political science. Moreover (as already noted) this dimension draws on a conceptual distinction central in current theoretical approaches to organization. The internal-external dimension relates to concerns central in our constitutional and political tradition, including the putative politics-administration distinction. If these things are true, then the classification will be useful even though, as the quotation above suggests, it should be used cautiously and only to indicate probable tendencies of institutions; not to direct specific conclusions without more detailed and situational analysis.

III

Five broad positions regarding the institutionalization of administrative responsibility have been defined. In this section I shall deal briefly with each position within the framework just set forth. The analysis concentrates primarily upon the implications of each position for accountability, and secondarily upon the implications for the other eleven values. Each position is stated in a thoroughgoing version the better to illuminate major premises. I do not think, however, that I shall be discussing straw men, though I shall (somewhat artificially) be dealing with each position in isolation. It has already been emphasized that no one proposes to rely exclusively upon any one type of institutional arrangement.

A. The *internal formal* position.[22] This position, with its stress upon Presidential direction and control, appears to rest upon two lines of theory. One is a set of political values, assumptions and readings of evidence which has been called the "theory of executive leadership" and which aims at Presidential paramountcy in our political and governmental systems. The other is an assumption (and to some extent a reading of evidence) about the effectiveness of formal organization in instilling and organizing purposes and activities in large bureaucracies. Not all proponents of the theory of executive leadership will accept the second (administrative) assumption;[23] they will instead emphasize the role of a "representative bureaucracy" (discussed below) or such "informal" aspects of administrative behavior as loyalty to or identification with executive leadership. Where loyalty and identification are concerned it seems most difficult to distinguish between formal and informal organization as these terms have been employed in the literature, and debate about which most effectively supports Presidential leadership is likely to become bogged down in definitional controversy. While I shall not argue here that an optimistic assumption about the efficacy of formal organization in direction and control of large bureaucracies is an essential companion to the theory of executive leadership, the theory does seem to be more compelling with that corollary. Of course, advocates of more thoroughgoing Presidential leadership hope through political revision to relieve strains to which formal administrative organization is now subject at the federal level.

B. The *internal informal* position. This position includes and emphasizes (a) the "moral" factors of morale, identification, loyalty, and responses to leadership which have been stressed by many writers, (b) claims for "representative bureaucracy," and (c) claims for "functional responsibility." Of these, the first factors will not be discussed except to say that they are usually proposed simply to supplement formal organization and the internal formal position and that it is frequently argued that their effective realization requires some latitude of discretion and relaxation of formal controls.[24]

Writers emphasizing internal informal factors would not, of course, rely upon them exclusively. But they often deny that modern governmental organization lends itself easily or naturally to accountability and argue that the conception of formal organization as an orderly hierarchy of governing purposes giving meaning to "efficiency" is misleading. They stress instead that policy-making and change of purposes from within organization are continuous and inevitable, from which follows the impossibility of strict accountability to external agencies through formal organization alone. Often, then, this school is proposing that we reconcile ourselves to deficiencies in accountability and compensate for these by stressing others of our twelve values, though this proposal is seldom stated in just these terms. To the extent that claims are made for "representative" or "functional" accountability the problem is that this can only be a constructive accountability since only a constructive (substantive rather than formal) relationship is involved. This seems to open the internal informal position to serious question on grounds of accountability, though we may find some of our other eleven values well served by one or another variant of the position.

An early statement of the "representative bureaucracy" position was that of J. Donald Kingsley.[25] The position, as he states it, applies chiefly to societies characterized by sharp divisions of social class or status and by a politics more-or-less definitively organized on those divisions. It maintains that in such societies government is not likely to be "responsible" through the normal channels to voters of all classes or parties unless the bureaucracy is recruited on a broadly representative basis. Basically, the theory appears to rest upon two lines of argument. One is the argument noted above and common to all writers in the internal informal camp that in the modern administrative state the value of accountability and the traditional machinery for enforcing it must be discounted, and that we must emphasize more heavily other avenues and other ends of "responsibility." The other line of argument seems fundamentally to be the Marxian theory of "ideology," though in modified form.[26] It is the assumption that formal bureaucratic organization and a related bureaucratic tradition of neutrality and amenability to political direction will not prevail over class-based ideology.[27] The two arguments complement one another. In terms of the framework employed here they lead Kingsley to the conclusion that values such as responsiveness and flexibility, rather than accountability, are the relevant meanings of "responsibility," and that internal informal (representative) administrative arrangements are the critical means of democratic control:

> . . . the essence of responsibility is psychological rather than mechanical. It is to be sought in an identity of aim and point of view, in a common background of social prejudice, which leads the agent to act as if he were the principal. In the first instance, it is a matter of sentiment and understanding, rather than of institutional forms . . .[28]

So far, empirical studies of the problem Kingsley raises remain scarce and perhaps at the most, the theory as it is stated must be limited to classbound societies and political systems.[29]

Contemporary American thinkers have not couched their position in class terms, but have instead stressed (a) the difficulties of definitive representation through purely formal channels in a richly pluralistic society and (b) the inequities and vicissitudes of Congressional and Presidential (especially Congressional) representation.[30] A representative bureaucracy is, in this situation, seen as a useful supplement, or as superior (more equitable, more inclusive) representation to that available through our formal, electoral devices as they are now structured.[31] I think there are two problems not dealt with expressly enough in this literature. These are: (1) who, or what, is represented in the federal bureaucracy, and (2) what values are chiefly gained by this informal, "substantive" representation?

Who or what is represented? As to who is represented, there are two possible views. One, and this seems to be the view of most writers, is that many interests denied effective representation in Congress turn up in the diversity of background to be found among federal government personnel. From this diversity a catholic administrative corps emerges "as a body" to which the original differences of background have contributed.[32] A second view is that the federal bureaucracy constructively represents leading values and traditions of American life because of a generally shared middle class background and liberal university education.[33] The first position implies diversity, the second uniformity (albeit, uniformity of an enlightened sort).

The two positions are not necessarily contradictory, but they may be. Whether they are depends upon three questions. (1) Does American administration typically act "as a body" and apply its diversity of background to particular decisions and programs?[34] (2) Does this presumed diversity have much bearing on general decisions at whatever level taken? (3) What is the pattern of distribution of "constitutional" values in the society, are such values generally engrained in civil servants by education and background even though, as regards "who gets what," their loyalties lie to diverse groups?[35] In fact, it is often unclear whether the representation of groups (interests) or values is intended. This ambiguity can arise because the notion of substantive, rather than formal, representation is a vague one; because of vacillation between the language of "realism" and that of "Platonism"; and because we are not told what values within the rubric of "responsibility" are being pursued through internal informal avenues.

The second major problem, then, is *what* values are maximized through a "representative bureaucracy"? So far as *accountability* is concerned, we still need to know more about what groups are represented within the federal bureaucracy, and *how* this representation is structured within it. That is, we need to know to whom the presumptive accountability lies, and whether it should be viewed as supplementing that achieved (if in limited measure) through our formal electoral and organizational devices, or as distorting and adulterating it. The "representative bureaucracy" position can be better grounded on values other than accountability for, as we have defined it, that value is associated with formality in political institutions, and probably reaches the vanishing point as arrangements become highly informal. In fact, it appears pointless to speak of accountability to *values*.

So far as our other ends are concerned it is, to repeat, important whether we conceive of what is represented in administration as a diversity or a homogeneity or a bit of both. Perhaps the representation of social diversity results in our values of responsiveness, flexibility, competence; perhaps the representation of broadly distributed attitudes results in such values as prudence, due process, stability; and perhaps both types of representation occur together, resulting in some balance of these values. Institutions (especially formal institutions) are difficult to analyze into such elements, but discussions of representative bureaucracy would gain in clarity if the ends in view were made more explicit.

One other aspect of the internal informal position deserves mention, though I shall not deal with it as fully as it deserves. This is the celebrated "fellowship of science" argument of Carl J. Friedrich.[36] It stresses the objectivity of mind and procedure to be found in much professional and disciplinary administrative action, and speaks of responsibility (defined as accountability) to a professional code that sets ethical and intellectual restrictions upon bureaucratic perversion of the public interest. In the terms employed here, "functional responsibility" appeals mainly to competence, probity, and prudence. It is accompanied by reliance upon informal "political responsibility" or, in our terms, responsiveness.[37]

If the position is interpreted as enhancing accountability, then the reservations expressed above about accountability to values seem crucial. Probably it is better understood as discounting the modern likelihood of accountability (as here defined) and as compensatory advocacy of other ends. The extent to which such other ends may be realized in the "fellowship of science" has been much discussed in the literature. Does the term imply a generalized scientific outlook and method or a congeries of special disciplines? Are consistency, prudence and competence here in conflict?[38] Answers depend not only upon what is meant by the fellowship of science, but further upon, the degree to which it is balanced by the responsiveness and flexibility that Friedrich finds in external informal avenues, and by the residue of accountability remaining in our more formal institutions.

This discussion has stressed criticism of internal arrangements, and I should therefore make clear that it is leveled simply against the notion that representation and the "inner check" in administration can achieve much by way of accountability to groups, values, or the "public interest." There may well be gains for others of our twelve values. Which of these are advanced will depend upon the kinds of traditions or moral codes we attempt to instill in bureaucracy, and on patterns of formal organization. One cannot realistically believe that a completely "neutral" or valueless bureaucracy is possible; if we could then we might be concerned for such values as efficacy, prudence and competence. And, if we do not accept the "neutral" bureaucracy, then we should be about determining what are the bureaucratic values we want, or what is the range we shall tolerate. This will include supplemental reliance upon one or another type of "representative bureaucracy."

C. The *Congressional* position. The chief and now classic work supporting a large sphere of Congressional direction and control is that of Charles S. Hyneman.[39] For some, this work is based upon "majority will metaphysics,"[40] for others it is a "search for a golden mean."[41] In my view the study rests upon a theory of political direction and control of administration reflecting a belief in the primary value for policy-making of politics as traditionally conceived and organized in American society, plus implicit emphasis upon accountability as distinguished from others of the values discussed above. The chief theses are: an insistence "that the whole people control the government because [we] dare not let a part of the people do so";[42] that "[if] the political organization of the nation is healthy and the electoral system truly records what the people say they want, then Congress and President . . . will reflect with reasonable accuracy what the people want";[43] that the Presidency may fall into the hands of a poor judge of what the people want, but that "Congress is less likely to offend in these respects, for [it] consists of many men, chosen by segments of the electorate residing in all parts of the nation";[44] that, therefore, in the initial definition of bureaucratic tasks, "Congress should specify in the statute every "guide, every condition, every statement of principle that it knows in advance it wants to have applied in the situations that are expected to arise. This rule derives from a concept of legislative supremacy' ";[45] and that, as regards five other specific subjects of direction and control, Congress is entitled to go far. These subjects, and the proper extent of Congressional activity regarding each, are searchingly analyzed in Part II of Hyneman's book; it is impossible to do justice to that analysis here.

Hyneman's position is basically, then, that popular conceptions of policy and action should govern administrative activity, that our chief reliance to this end should rest with constitutional and formal electoral agencies (though internal and external informal avenues are accepted as supplementary), and that by and large, Congress will be more regularly invested with popularness than will the President. Though Hyneman intends the words "direction and control" to be as one term,[46] there seems to be somewhat more of control than of positive direction in the theory at bottom; for, in reasoning to his ultimate support of Congress within the separation of powers, Hyneman emphasizes Congressional potential as a check upon the Presidency.[47] Here, accountability, in a healthy political system, lies to the whole people (qualification: as represented in Congress); those of our other values most favored would seem to be responsiveness and flexibility; that least favored would seem to be leadership; and as to the others there is no argued difference with proponents of other positions.

Nearly all critics of this approach have stressed a difficulty with its central assumptions about the "representativeness" of Congress.[48] Does Congress represent "segments of the electorate" or the "whole people"? If the latter: at any given time, or over the long run? The debate about the representativeness of Congress is only in part, however, a debate about accountability; primarily, it is a debate about the relative role of other values (e.g., consistency, leadership) in our political system.

On grounds alone of accountability, the case for Congressional direction and control (in some measure) can be more simply stated: it provides an organized external locus of criticism and control of bureaucratic purposes and activities. It provides an external source of direction available against the possibility of bureaucratic inertia. It provides both of these via an organization which promotes the contribution of diverse (if unintegrated) points of view.[49] Congressmen, in turn, are accountable locally through formal elections, and it is at least arguable that these elections yield more accountability than do (national) Presidential elections precisely because the appeal to the constituency is cast in local and hence more specific terms. All this, of course, assumes that some minimum of each of our other values also prevails. Critics can now argue, on grounds other than accountability, that Congressional controls (especially in their informal aspects) result in undue responsiveness to local interests; that Congress as a whole is too slow in responding to movements of national opinion; or that Congressional direction and control are deficient in terms of consistency, efficacy and leadership. Proponents of a substantial Congressional role may dispute the matter of; efficacy, and they will probably argue the need for external prodding and restraint not only for responsiveness and flexibility, but also for the sake of probity, candor, competence, and due process. Those supporting a substantial role for Congress vis a vis administration, e.g., Hyneman, generally stress its value as an external formal control but hold no brief for the frequently informal pattern of Congressional administrative relations.

D. The *Judicial* position. It is in the interest of the last-named values, and the presumed advantage of multiple avenues of accountability, that the protagonists of judicial over administration have taken their stand.[50] There have been those, too, who have sought to serve certain ends of substantive policy and to protect certain social interests through this position, but I am setting this aspect of the question aside. Protagonists of both ample judicial controls and generous Congressional controls have usually stood together in basing their position upon a principle entitled the "rule of Law." For Congressional supporters, this principle has been understood as a corollary of popular sovereignty; for judicial supporters, the principle stands for the contrary aspect of our constitutional system, namely, the conception of "limited government." It seems doubtful whether, if this difference in orientation were explicit, the two companies could march very far together—but the difference has not often been explicit, and protagonists of the courts have frequently maintained that they were also interested in protecting the Congress, as indeed, up to a point, they may be. In the devising and application of standards to govern administrative activity both courts and Congress have sometimes cooperated, as the history (not alone the legislative history, but also the longer pre-history) of the Administrative Procedure Act and its later application attest.[51]

The principle of the "rule of law" has received a host of statements, of which at once the most celebrated and the most criticized was that of A. V. Dicey.[52] Perhaps a representative (if not entirely unambiguous) modern statement by an *amicus curiae* is the following by Bernard Schwartz:

> The concept of the rule of law, conceived of as the safeguard against arbitrary government, rests upon certain constitutional ideas. It presupposes, in the first place, that there are certain legal principles above the State. This is not to go so far as some who assert that the State is limited by a fundamental rule of right and law . . . and that "there is an objective law superior to government." In our sense, we merely assert that there are certain principles which the State, sovereign power though it is, cannot abrogate. These are what we usually comprehend by the expression "individual rights of the person."
>
> What is needed . . . is the assertion of judicial control over administrative excesses . . . for the increased scope of governmental functions will lead to the Power State unless Executive power is controlled by law. Great emphasis should be placed upon the use of the term control. An attempt to make the courts do more than control, an attempt to substitute judicial for Executive justice, will be but a repetition of our errors of the last century. Adequate control of administration is preserved if judicial review can be had to ensure the following: 1) *ultra vires* . . . ; 2) natural justice—that what the Supreme Court has called "the fundamentals of fair play" have been preserved; 3) substantial evidence—that the administrative action is based upon rational evidence of a probative value. In this country there is, of course, the overriding ground of constitutionality. . . .[53]

The basic constitutional theory of judicial control, then, is one of limited government. The "certain legal principles above the State" in the quotation are presumably those comprised in the notion of due process. This, as it has been judicially defined vis à vis administration, seems to accompany heavy emphasis upon values defined above as candor, probity, and competence. But in our own system, with its "overriding ground of constitutionality," due process can be a most comprehensive concern. That it is still not without substantive effect can be seen in the tendency for some liberals who once reprobated judicial intervention in the regulation of business to recommend more intervention today in behalf of civil liberties and economic competition.[54] However the limits of due process are defined, its definition is likely to be cast more in terms of the *lis inter pares* than of values—such as responsiveness, leadership, efficacy, competence—defined with reference to political and administrative experience.[55] Proponents of substantial judicial controls have also stood for further "judicialization" of administration, or at least of the "administrative process." This reform falls within the category of relationships here termed internal formal, but is intended to serve the same ends as judicial (external formal) controls by advancing due process in the administrative process and facilitating accountability to courts. In part it stems from the reluctant conclusion of some that modern courts, unaided by administrative reform, could not be relied upon broadly to define and enforce due process. The reform in question would conflict frequently and directly with Presidential hegemony and with the internal and external informal positions.

The judicial tradition thus tends to minimize several of the values here under discussion, though the Supreme Court has modified the tradition. Advocates of judicial control today could (constitutional rights apart) base their position upon its role in enforcing demonstrable (if marginal) accountability, upon service to the values of candor, competence and due process (conservatively defined), and upon the premise that this supplementary avenue of accountability helps to maintain other avenues by enforcing a certain formality of procedure. This would be a sort of administrative law "preferred position" doctrine in behalf of values deemed essential to public decision and control.

E. The *external informal* position.[56] The manifold patterns of responsibility comprehended in this term all involve an element of public participation in the administrative process. Of the many types of such participation, those most studied are "formalized" and regularized in varying degree, usually through statutory provision or administrative regulation. They are, however, designated "informal" here because they are most often defended for their presumed advantages of popular or group participation and the qualities of identification consensus, status, and stimulation which accompany it.[57] Interpersonal (or intergroup) rather than statutory relationships are emphasized; informal representation is frequently welcomed.

Among the major patterns under review here are: the types of group and citizen participation in regulatory administration studied by, e.g., Leiserson and Redford;[58] the "cooptation" pattern studied by Selznick;[59] the "grass roots democracy" of the farm committee system and the Soil Conservation Service studied by, *inter alia*, Lewis, Frischknecht, Hardin, and Parks;[60] and residually, the other far less "formalized" relations between clientele and agency which are assumed to render or assist in rendering bureaucracy accountable.[61]

Despite their institutional diversity there is a common body of democratic theory upon which external informal arrangements are commended. I believe this theory is rooted in political pluralism, and the relevant aspects of this doctrine include: (1) minimization of the distinction between public and private; (2) "functionalism" in the sense of a belief that most modern problems are best "solved" by functional definition and by the functional cooperation of those publics most directly concerned; (3) distrust of formal, electoral representative arrangements as intellectually (functionally) inept and socially distant; (4) emphasis upon participation, basically of a face-to-face sort, as the basis of community, and upon community as the basis of democracy and, therefore, upon participation as the basis of democracy.[62] But to be clear about it, this is intellectual heritage that stands today in the background and is drawn upon, as a rule, only in part. These propositions can be taken in much more adulterated form and still serve as a collective source of "grass roots democracy" in the shaping of programs, and some measure of "self-regulation" in regulatory administration.

So far as the accountability relationship is concerned, the external informal camp and the internal formal camp lie at opposite ends of contested ground. The principal in the external informal relationship is not a putative national constituency, but a congeries of functional constituencies; the accountability relationship is to be direct, not mediated through formal electoral arrangements and centralized party organization. This, of course, is an extreme statement of the external informal position; one should not ignore the claim that a true national constituency must be pluralistically put together, that it cannot be completely defined in a party system. But the contrary problem, from an accountability standpoint, is the definition of relevant groups or publics as sources of administrative accountability.

Of other desiderata, probably those most unequivocally sought and realized in external informal arrangements are responsiveness and flexibility. Bureaucratic competence may well be enhanced through constant functional contacts, not to mention outright interest group involvement in administration. External informal arrangements are more difficult to assess as regards probity, candor and stability. It is precisely the more informal relationships of this type that have been widely thought to raise serious and subtle problems of administrative ethics.[63] While external informal devices provide disclosure of information and premises of action to particular groups, they may impede disclosure on a broader basis. As regards stability, it is sometimes argued that such devices frustrate executive efforts at policy change based on broad popular demands;[64] or, conversely, that they "conduce to the making of decisions on the basis of immediate situations."[65] On this point the assessment seems especially equivocal. Two values, consistency and leadership, are clearly not to be maximized in external informal institutions. The usual pluralist view of "consistency" is that it is a "formal" value that can be substantively realized only through group participation and involvement. And, as against leadership, the external informal position pits cooperation and consent.

The minimum rationale for external informal arrangements would emphasize their informational value both to bureaucracy and clientele. Playing a limited role they can advance the values of accountability, responsiveness, flexibility, competence, and, perhaps, candor in differing degrees and depending upon how formalized are the arrangements. The position has been set forth here in thoroughgoing terms so as to emphasize the theoretical background, but contemporary advocates of such arrangements are generally not doctrinaire pluralists. External informal institutions are usually proposed as marginal supplements to our representative system. Doubtless many administrators have seen them, in fact, as vehicles of governmental leadership rather than responsiveness, and such, at times, they seem to be. . . .

IV

The framework of administrative responsibility as I have sought to set it forth consists, then, in a number of desiderata (here tentatively defined) that come close to being the specifics of "responsibility," and in an emphasis upon the dimensions of formality-informality, internality-externality that typically relate institutions to the dozen desiderata. Our main traditions of administrative thought can then be analyzed for the emphasis they give to formal-informal, internal-external avenues of direction and control of administration and their probable consequences for the constituent values of "responsibility." Recognizing that, to some extent, three of our five main traditions are constitutionally ordained and the other two practically unavoidable, what will be the probable results for each of our twelve values of incremental changes in emphasis among them? Is this assessment to be made, are changes in emphasis desirable, with respect to governmental activity as a whole, or simply and differently in selected areas of policy? If the latter, for which areas of policy are certain types of arrangements most appropriate; which values should and can be given highest priority in which areas? With what effects upon other areas? What, as an empirical matter, can we expect of various balances of our institutional arrangements; in what ways do revisions in, say, internal informal institutions further and/or frustrate internal formal factors, and so on for the others? These are the questions usually asked in discussions of administrative responsibility. My hope is that the framework for inquiry presented here will help us better to communicate and to direct inquiry toward provisional answers. . . .

Notes

1. Space precludes comprehensive citation of these. Two recent and cogent efforts at clearing and ordering the ground are: Glendon A. Schubert, Jr., " 'The Public Interest' in Administrative Decision-Making," *American Political Science Review* LI (June 1957), 346–368; and Arch Dotson, "Fundamental Approaches to Administrative Responsibility," *Western Political Quarterly* X (September 1957), 701–727. This paper was in draft when these articles appeared, but the author has endeavored to complement rather than overlap them.

2. For a discussion of the term, with ultimate reference to popular control of policy, see Austin Ranney, *The Doctrine of Responsible Party Government* (Urbana, 1954), esp. pp. 12–19; for different and differing points of view, cf., Herbert Spiro, "Responsibility in Citizenship, Government and Administration," in Carl J. Friedrich and J. K. Galbraith, *Public Policy* (Cambridge, 1953), pp. 116–133; Fritz Morstein Marx, *The Administrative State* (Chicago, 1957), pp. 42–45; J. Roland Pennock, "Responsiveness, Responsibility and Majority Rule," *American Political Science Review* XLVI (September 1952), 790–807. The author is grateful to Professor Pennock for helpful suggestions bearing on a number of points in this paper.

3. For a discussion of this value and of the question how "prompt" must acquiescence be to be "responsive," see Pennock, *op. cit.*, p. 791. Some discussion of the notion of "popularness" can be found in William H. Riker, *Democracy in the United States* (New York, 1953), esp. Chs. 1–3.

4. The term "flexibility" is used in the sense of deliberate administrative adjustments in Robert Dahl and Charles E. Lindblom, "Variation in Public Expenditure" in Max F. Millikan (ed.), *Income Stabilization for a Developing Democracy* (New Haven, 1953).

5. Dahl and Lindblom, *op. cit.*, use the term "coordination" with reference to policy. See Morstein Marx, *op. cit.*, pp. 36–37, for use of "rationality" in this sense, among others.

6. For a discussion of this value as an element in "responsibility" see, again, Pennock, *op. cit.*, especially as regards the "authenticity" of public demand. Morstein Marx, *op. cit.*, p. 51, writes of "continuity" in this respect.

7. Discussions of democratic theory seem rarely to include express discussion of this value; it is generally lost sight of in discussions of ultimate popular direction and control of government. See, for example, Ranney, *op. cit.*, pp. 4–5. But discussions of the organization (especially through political parties) of popular direction and control seem usually to assume the "leadership" value; see the same work, pp. 10–19.

8. Cf. Paul Appleby, *Morality and Administration* (Baton Rouge, 1952); N. Grundstein, "Law and the Morality of Administration," *George Washington Law Review* XXI, 265.

9. "Candor" seems to be a value given high priority by many majoritarians, though not always explicitly. See, for instance, Riker, *op. cit.*, Ch. 3 and Henry S. Commager, *Majority Rule and Minority Rights* (New York, 1943). Those who do not accept the majoritarian position sometimes are disposed to pit *consensus*, to some degree, against candor.

10. This is the term used in pretty much the same sense by Morstein Marx, *op. cit.*, pp. 45–51, and by Dahl and Lindblom, *op. cit.*, pp. 355–356. The problem of "objective standards" is discussed in terms of a distinction between "experts" and

"specialists" in Walter Gellhorn, *Individual Freedom and Governmental Restraints* (Baton Rouge, 1956), Ch. 1.

11. This may seem only marginally distinguishable from "competence," but the emphasis here is upon results, rather than on means, in terms of organization, personnel and intellectual outlook. The best known discussion of the problem of "efficiency" is in Herbert A. Simon, *Administrative Behavior* (New York, 1947), Ch. 9. See also Roland S. McKean, "Criteria of Efficiency in Government Expenditures," in U.S. Congress, Joint Economic Committee, *Federal Expenditure Policy for Growth and Stability*, Eighty-fifth Congress, First Session, Washington, D.C., 1957, pp. 252–257. *Cf.*, Edward S. Corwin, *The President: Office and Powers* (3rd Ed., New York, 1948), p. 118, commenting upon the Brownlow Committee: "What the Committee really meant undoubtedly by "responsibility" is capacity for effective action, not accountability to the law . . ."

12. For a discussion of "responsibility" in this sense see Pennock, *op. cit.*, pp. 797ff, and for familiar illustrations of the conception of the "prudent man," see, e.g., Holmes, *The Common Law* (Boston, 1881), *passim*.

13. There have, of course, been shifts in the courts' conception of due process as a requirement upon administration. Some classical statements occur in *ICC v. Louisville and Nashville Ry Co.*, 227 US 88 (1913); *St. Joseph Stockyards Co. v United States*, 298 US 38 (1935); *Railroad Commission v Rowan and Nichols Oil Co.*, 311 US 570 (1941). These discussions, like nearly all in this context, are couched largely in terms of the extent to which due process requires judicial review.

14. Hyneman's terms are to be found in his *Bureaucracy in a Democracy* (New York, 1950), Ch. 3.

15. The citations above to discussions of these values include a good many discussions not directed mainly at the problem of "responsibility." These are cited because they place explicit emphasis on the values under discussion, whereas discussions of "responsibility" are often less explicit.

16. The following are chief meanings provided for "responsibility" in *Webster's Collegiate Dictionary* (Fifth ed., Springfield, Mass., 1947) at 849; "liable to respond; accountable; answerable;" "able to respond or answer for one's conduct . . . ; trustworthy;" "answerable as the primary cause, motive or agent;" and in ethics, "having the character of a free moral agent." Among the synonyms given are: accountable, amenable, liable. Among the meanings given for "responsibility" are: "state or quality of being responsible;" "accountability"; "moral accountability;" and "reliability."

17. Pennock, *op. cit.*

18. It should be emphasized that we are here dealing with five major schools of thought on the institutionalization of administrative responsibility, not with exhaustive description of four categories of institutions. Thus, the descriptive category of internal informal controls properly includes not only Presidential controls, but also such devices as those of the Administrative Procedures Act, and may well include impediments to Presidential control through formal organization of agency independence. For instance, the typical argument for the independent regulatory commission is couched mainly in terms of values listed above as stability, competence, prudence, and due process; and the institutional arguments for the regulatory commission device rest upon a blend of internal formal, external formal, and (frequently) internal informal and external informal relationships.

19. The informal aspects of Congressional control are well discussed in *e.g.*, J. Lieper Freeman, *The Political Process* (New York, 1955), and in V. O. Key, "Legislative Control," in Morstein Marx, *Elements of Public Administration* (New York, 1946.

20. Most of the arrangements here characterized as external informal are in fact formalized in varying degree, and may be so formalized as to border on external formal controls. These arrangements, however, stand outside our more formal constitutional tradition, and the line of advocacy of these arrangements under discussion here commends them chiefly for their informal characteristics.

21. Hyneman, *op. cit.*, pp. 40–43.

22. In this section an attempt is made to state strongly a theory which perhaps not all of the following would accept, *in toto*, since they seldom treat (or treated) all aspects of it systematically. Representative literature includes: Frank Goodnow, *Politics and Administration* (New York, 1900); James M. Burns, *Congress on Trial* (New York, 1949); James M. Burns and Jack W. Pelatson, *Government by the People* (New York, 3rd ed., 1957); Herman M. Somers, "The President as Administrator," *Annals of the American Academy of Political and Social Science* CCLXXXIII (September 1952), 104–114, and "The President, the Congress and the Federal Government Service," in The American Academy, *The Federal Government Service* (New York, 1954); President's Committee on Administrative Management, *Report with Special Studies* (Washington, 1937); Commission on Organization of the Executive Branch of the Government (Hoover Commission), *Concluding Report* (Washington, 1949). The tradition probably begins with the writings and practice of Alexander Hamilton.

23. This assumption appears most strongly in earlier writings. See, e.g., Luther Gulick, "Science, Values and Public Administration," in Gulick and Lydall Urwick (eds.), *Papers on the Science of Administration* (New York, 1937). The problem of the relative impact upon behavior of formal and informal organization is discussed without very definite conclusions, in Simon, Smithburg and Thompson, *op. cit.*, pp. 79–91 and Chs. 24–25.

24. The "representative" and "functional" aspect have recently been thoroughly and provocatively canvassed by Schubert, *op. cit.* His references to the literature of this position are comprehensive.

25. J. Donald Kingsley, *Representative Bureaucracy: An Interpretation of the British Civil Service* (Yellow Springs, Ohio, 1944). The study is aimed chiefly at Britain, not the United States.

26. The same interpretation of Kingsley's argument is drawn by Dwight Waldo in his "Development of a Theory of Democratic Administration," *op. cit.*, p. 91.

27. For a stronger statement of this argument see Harold J. Laski, *Parliamentary Government in England* (London, 1938), Ch. 6.

28. Kingsley, *op. cit.*, p. 282.

29. See Seymour M. Lipset, *Agrarian Socialism* (Berkeley, 1950.) This study does not bear directly upon the Kingsley thesis, since it deals with a bureaucracy without either the form or the tradition of political neutrality. For a sharp criticism of the Kingsley thesis by a proponent of external formal controls, see Herman Finer, *Theory and Practice of Modern Government* (New York, 1949), pp. 616, 784–793. For a discussion of the problem in connection with an interesting typology of bureaucracies, see Morstein Marx, *op. cit.*, Ch. 4, pp. 60–62, 69–71.

30. *Cf.*, Norton Long, "Bureaucracy and Constitutionalism," *American Political Science Review* XLVI (September, 1952), 808–818. Long is critical of Congressional representation, but not of Presidential representation (pp. 811–812).

31. *Ibid.*, pp. 811–814.

32. This is Long's position, *Ibid*. The qualifying phrase, "as a body" is also his, and is used at p. 813.

33. It is difficult to cite anyone in particular as authority for this proposition, though Long at pp. 816–819 seems to take this position regarding attitudes toward "constitutionalism" as a complex of the values discussed above. Some statements in empirical studies might seem ambiguous as to whether the first or second of the two positions above is being adopted, and language sometimes vacillates between the two. See, e.g., Reinhard Bendix, "Who Are the Government Bureaucrats?" in Alvin W. Gouldner (ed.), *Studies in Leadership* (New York, 1950), pp. 330–341, and the language used at p. 335 and pp. 337–338. See also Bendix's *Higher Civil Servants in American Society* (Boulder, Colo., 1949) and Arthur MacMahon and John D. Millett, *Federal Administrators: A Biographical Approach to the Problem of Departmental Management* (New York, 1939) for empirical studies bearing upon this problem.

34. Long recognizes this question at pp. 814–816, and suggests that the answer is a matter of bureaucratic "structure, permanence and processes" (p. 816). His further and most suggestive attempt to deal with it is his "Public Policy and Administration: The Goals of Rationality and Responsibility," *Public Administration Review* XIV (Winter 1954), 22–31.

35. "A truly representative bureaucracy is in its several parts variously representative of special functions and interests, and highly representative altogether of the public at large." Appleby, *op. cit.*, pp. 158–159.

36. Carl J. Friedrich, "Public Policy and the Nature of Administrative Responsibility," in Friedrich and Edward S. Mason (eds.), *Public Policy* I (Cambridge, 1940); and Carl J. Friedrich, *Constitutional Government and Democracy* (Boston, 1941), Ch. 19 and esp. pp. 411–412.

37. It should be emphasized that this discussion focuses upon only *one* aspect of the total approach Friedrich has taken to the subject; that in the article cited above he speaks expressly of a "dual standard" of *functional* and *political* responsibility; that as regards political responsibility he stresses to some extent the "representative bureaucracy" view just discussed above, together with external informal devices; that, finally, this is all a matter of emphasis, and that the role of formal devices is recognized though sharply qualified.

38. Sharp criticism of Friedrich's emphasis upon informal arrangements by an advocate of formal (especially external formal) arrangements may be found in Herman Finer, "Better Government Personnel," *Political Science Quarterly* LI (December 1936), 569–599, and "Administrative Responsibility in Democratic Government," *Public Administration Review* I (1941), 335–350. See also Schubert, *op. cit.*

39. Hyneman, *op. cit.* See also the more majoritarian writings of Herman Finer listed in the note above, which will not be discussed here.

40. Long, "Bureaucracy and Constitutionalism," *op. cit.*, p. 809.

41. Waldo, "Development of a Theory of Democratic Administration," *op. cit.*, p. 97, n. 39.

42. Hyneman, *op. cit.*, p. 12.

43. *Ibid.*, p. 24.

44. *Ibid.*, pp. 24–25.

45. *Ibid.*, p. 81.

46. *Ibid.*, p. 39.

47. *Ibid.*, esp. p. 25.

48. For example, Long in his "Bureaucracy and Constitutionalism," *op. cit.*, and Chester I. Barnard in a review of Charles S. Hyneman's *Bureaucracy in a Democracy*, in *American Political Science Review* XLIV (December 1950), 990–1004.

49. *Cf.*, Roland Young, *The American Congress* (New York, 1957), esp. Chs. 7 and 11; Charles E. Gilbert and Max M. Kampelman, "Legislative Control of the Bureaucracy," *Annals of the American Academy of Political and Social Science* CCXCII (March 1954), 76–87, esp. 77–78.

50. For some statements of this general position, see: The Reports of the Special Committee on Administrative Law of the American Bar Association in the Association's *Annual Reports*, 1934 (pp. 539–564), 1936 (pp. 720–794), 1937 (pp. 789–850), 1938 (pp. 331–368); Report of the Attorney General's Committee on Administrative Procedure, *Administrative Procedure in Government Agencies* (Washington, 1941), the Minority Report at pp. 203ff; Committee on Organization of the Executive Branch of the Government (Second Hoover Commission), Task Force Report on *Legal Services and Procedures* (Washington, 1955).

51. An interesting account of the history, and in itself an example of the "cooperation" referred to, is *Universal Camera Corp. v. National Labor Relations Board*, 340 US 474 (1951).

52. Albert Venn Dicey, *Introduction to the Study of the Law of the Constitution* (3rd Edition, New York, 1939), and the criticism by Sir Ivor Jennings, *The Law and the Constitution* (3rd Edition, London, 1943), Appendix II.

53. Bernard Schwartz, *Law and Executive in Britain* (New York, 1949), pp. 14–23.

54. See, e.g., Gellhorn, *op. cit.*, Ch. 1; and Louis V. Schwartz, "Legal Restriction of Competition in the Regulated Industries: An Abdication of Judicial Responsibility," *Harvard Law Review* LXVII (January 1954), 436–475.

55. Those who literally hold that the rule of law (and of due process of law) "presupposes . . . certain legal principles above the state" will inevitably discount those of our values which are chiefly political or administrative. For holders of this view, the state (*state*, not government) is in the last analysis a creature of the law, not politics; and they are sometimes disposed to reach the last analysis quickly.

56. In general, the strongest protagonists of this theory have not been academicians, but rather persons active in public life, and systematic statements are difficult to come by. See, however, David Lilienthal, *TVA: Democracy on the March* (New York, 1944). Two scholars in whose writings external informal arrangements find high (though not unqualified) favor are: John Guas, "The Responsibility of Public Administration," in Guas, Marshall Dimock and Leonard D. White, *The Frontiers of Public Administration* (Chicago, 1936), and "Public Participation in Federal Programs," in O. B. Conway (ed.), *Democracy in Federal Administration* (Washington, US Department of Agriculture Graduate School, 1956); and John D. Lewis, "Democratic Planning in Agriculture, I and II," *American Political Science*

Review XXXV (April and June 1941), 232–249; 454–469, and "Some New Forms of Democratic Participation in American Government," in Jasper Shannon (ed.), *The Study of Comparative Government* (New York, 1949), pp. 147–176. See also the writings of Friedrich, Note 46 above. Two excellent discussions are Alfred De Grazia, *Public and Republic* (New York, 1951), Ch. 8; and Don K. Price, "Democratic Administration," in Fritz Morstein Marx (ed.), *Elements of Public Administration* (New York, 1946), Ch. 4.

57. For a defense of the more formal ground that such a system of accountability is essential under modern conditions to check, modify, or influence government action which may not easily be remedied after the fact, see Gaus, "The Responsibility of Public Administration," in Gaus, Dimock, and White, *op. cit.*; see also Avery Leiserson, *Administrative Regulation* (Chicago, 1942); and Price, *op. cit.*

58. Leiserson, *op. cit.*; Emmett S. Redford, *The Administration of National Economic Control* (New York, 1952), Ch. 9.

59. David Selznick, *TVA and the Grass Roots* (Berkeley, 1949); Rexford G. Tugwell and Edward C. Banfield, "Grass Roots Democracy—Myth or Reality?" *Public Administration Review* X (Winter 1950), 47–55.

60. J. D. Lewis, "Democratic Planning in Agriculture," *op. cit.*; Charles Hardin, *The Politics of Agriculture* (Glencoe, IL, 1952); Reed L. Frischknecht, "The Democratization of Conservation: The Farm Committee System," *American Political Science Review* XLVII (September 1953), 704–727; Robert E. Parks, *Soil Conservation Districts in Action* (Ames, 1952).

61. For summary discussions, see, e.g., J. D. Lewis, "Some New Forms of Democratic Participation in American Government," *op. cit.*; Don K. Price, *op. cit.*; Walter Gellhorn and Clark Byse, *Administrative Law: Cases and Materials* (Brooklyn, 1954), Ch. 5. The range of such arrangements is great. See Appleby, *op. cit.*, p. 202: "Democratic aspiration . . . has reached variously toward many cooperative arrangements which divide and becloud responsibility. It has propelled us toward means of 'citizen participation' in the operating business of government without much uniformity or clarity of pattern, and without very critical concern for the feasibility or fairness of many of the arrangements . . ."

62. There is, of course, an immense body of literature on this. Two typical American statements are: Mary Parker Follett, *The New State* (New York, 1918); and John Dewey, *The Public and its Problems* (New York, 1927). A study of American pluralism is contained in DeGrazia, *op. cit.*

63. "I suppose that the place where the least ethical performance in . . . subtle terms is to be expected is in places where there is very close and pretty exclusive functional relationship with particular interests." Statement of Paul Appleby, US Senate Special Sub-Committee on the Establishment of a Commission on Ethics in Government, *Hearings*, Eighty-Second Congress, First Session, Washington, DC, 1951, p. 173.

64. *Cf.*, Norton E. Long, "Power and Administration," *Public Administration Review* IX (Autumn 1949), 257–264.

65. Edgar Lane, "Interest Groups and Bureaucracy," *Annals of the American Academy of Political and Social Science* CCXCII (March 1954), 104–110.

CASE E

BENDING RULES

The Happy Valley Hospital healthcare plan covers dependents until age 25 or until a qualifying event occurs. A qualifying event is a divorce, reaching age 19 without student status, end to full-time student status, and, in any case, arrival at age 25. When healthcare coverage is no longer available to dependents under their sponsor's plan, the dependent can be covered under the 1985 Consolidated Omnibus Budget Reconciliation Act (COBRA). By written policy the employee is responsible for notifying the employer when a qualifying event occurs. The employer is then responsible for offering COBRA coverage to the dependent. The rules are quite clear. Failure of the employee dependent to respond within 60 days results in forfeiture of the right to COBRA coverage.

Jane, a senior employee at the hospital, called the personnel office to ask that her daughter Bonnie be placed on COBRA because she was no longer a full-time student. Bonnie had been receiving denials of reimbursement from the health plan insurer. It seems that Bonnie had turned 25 a year previously and thus was no longer eligible for benefits under Jane's plan. Jane claims that she did not know she was required to notify the plan of this event explaining that she misinterpreted the requirements. She thought coverage ended *either* at age 25 *or* when full-time student status ceased.

Procedurally, a student status form is sent to plan recipients specifically at ages 19, 22, and 25. Jane indicates that no student status form was received from the plan insurer or from the hospital. Jane was reminded that ongoing information had been provided regarding responsibilities of the employee concerning notification of a qualifying event.

Since Jane failed to notify the personnel department, or even to contact the insurer about Bonnie's status, benefits automatically were discontinued by the plan insurer. It should be noted that six months previously the hospital had transferred its plan carrier from Blue Cross/Blue Shield to Consolidated Callous. This change of carrier may be connected with some of the administrative difficulties that Jane claims. Nevertheless, according to the regulations, any break in coverage made it impossible to continue coverage under COBRA. However, upon consultation with the personnel director at Happy Valley Hospital, the plan administrator is told that since Jane is a well-respected member of the clinical staff, the hospital will tell Consolidated Callous that the hospital erred. Additionally, the hospital will tell the insurer that it, too, failed to catch this on its end. Thus, Happy Valley Hospital will offer COBRA coverage as if there were no break in coverage. Their mutual failure to monitor more closely may have resulted in no notification being sent to Jane or to Bonnie regarding continuance of coverage. The personnel director states that since the hospital has a self-funded plan, the insurer will follow its directions despite the insurer's contention that coverage is not an option for Bonnie based on COBRA law and the contract.

The Dilemma

I am the plan administrator at the hospital. The dilemma for me is this: Do I follow procedures according to COBRA law and the policies as set forth in the healthcare plan, or do I yield to management and bend the rules as interpreted by the personnel director but which run counter to the insurer's interpretation?

Stakeholders and Values

A stakeholder and values matrix will help me identify the values most at stake (Figure 5.3). A stakeholders' list of powers and controls will help me to clarify where most of the power lies and to what mechanism each is accountable. Identification of these aspects will enable me to brainstorm options. Using another matrix (Figure 5.4), the probable consequences of each option can be identified as they relate to each value. If an option will be positive for the stakeholder, a (+) will be used, and if an option will be negative for the stakeholder a (-) will be used. The option with the most pluses will guide my decision.

These are the values I want to preserve. Each stakeholder has something to lose. COBRA regulations are at stake. Do I adhere to them or bend them at the discretion of administrative authority? Who should bear the economic burden of back premiums? Is it fair to deny Bonnie

Figure 5.3 Values Matrix

| | Values | | | | |
Stakeholders	Law	Cost	Honesty	Fairness	Authority
Jane		X	X	X	
Plan Administrator	X	X		X	X
Employees	X	X		X	
Insurer	X	X			
Personnel Director			X		X

coverage because of her mother's shortcomings? Is it fair to other employees who may have been in a similar situation and lost coverage? Am I accountable to the COBRA law, to the insurer, or to my employer? How will my decision affect the integrity of the law, the hospital, and myself? Whose influence and what controlling mechanisms should I honor? Whose judgment should prevail?

Power and Control

Each stakeholder wields power that affects my resolution of the situation:

- Jane can appeal to higher authority to obtain coverage despite the regulations.
- I can cooperate with my employer, follow the law, or appeal to higher authority.
- The personnel director can override my decision, fire me, or adjust the rules.
- The insurer could refuse to yield and enforce the rules.
- Other employees could complain that they were treated differently.

Formal mechanisms of control affect how stakeholders might use their power. These controls could prevent me from looking at unique

Figure 5.4 Value Choice

| | Consequences | | | | |
	Law	Cost	Honesty	Fairness	Authority
Option A	+	−	+	0	−
Option B	−	−	−	+	+
Option C	0	+	0	+	+

aspects of the situation. If one control is exercised over another it might not be fair to all involved.

Various points of view can be considered as I seek an ethical solution to this situation. Jane contends that her daughter Bonnie should receive coverage since, Jane alleges, she was not aware that she should have reported qualifying events. Although she read her healthcare plan, Jane claims to have misinterpreted the statement regarding age and student status. The insurer counters that COBRA coverage is not warranted since there was a break in coverage time. Administration reasons that Jane's daughter should receive coverage through COBRA retroactively, with the premium being paid by Jane or her daughter. I, however, assert that it was Jane's responsibility to inform her employer about the qualifying event. Continuing coverage is not fair to other employees who have faced this in the past. That their coverage was not continued might appear to have been due solely to their subordinate position. By law, coverage should not be continued and to do so would be in violation of the law. I feel strongly that laws are written to be followed. To break the law based on someone's position in the organization is not ethical. Making an exception would set a precedent and present future problems in efforts to enforce COBRA laws.

Alternatives

The following options occur to me:

Option A. Resist my superior. Do not offer COBRA coverage. Let Bonnie know she will have to find her own coverage due to COBRA regulations and hospital plan rules.

Option B. Defer to my superior. Offer coverage retroactively and ask Bonnie to pay past premiums. COBRA coverage would continue for six months. Tell the insurer that our decision was based on its failure and ours to monitor the plan. Since we have a self-funded plan we can make coverage decisions based on our interpretation.

Option C. Offer coverage retroactively with Bonnie making retroactive payments from the day her mother notified us forward to the current month. The hospital will absorb the remaining retroactive premiums to cover the prior period. Personnel will work more closely with the insurer to monitor accounts and provide proactive informational sessions. Have personnel send mailers and newsletter articles to employees about benefit issues and the responsibilities of the employees. Suggest to the insurer that this decision is not in violation of COBRA law because technically it

> is the employer's responsibility to advise dependents of termination of coverage which in this case may not have occurred in part due to Jane's failure to notify us in a timely manner.

Option A allows enforcement of law and policy. It presents an equitable decision in the eyes of other recipients who face a similar circumstance. However, Bonnie loses coverage. The hospital and the insurer are not accountable for their possible failure to notify Bonnie about coverage termination. The law is upheld.

Option B is somewhat fair to other recipients. They see a precedent being set and believe they will be treated equally if a similar situation arises around their coverage. Bonnie and Jane are not happy because they will face an economic burden. They might question the fairness of the decision. The insurer loses because it, too, faces an economic burden. It will have to pay for denied claims. Loose interpretation of the law prevails.

Option C seems to provide a winning solution for all stakeholders. It is the least detrimental option to all parties involved. Jane and Bonnie see that the hospital is sharing in the responsibility for paying back premiums. Bonnie gets the coverage she needs. The organization and my credibility are maintained due to our reaching a mutually agreeable option. The law, though loosely interpreted, is basically followed and the insurer recognizes that the hospital has discretionary powers. Administrative authority is upheld. All stakeholders share responsibility. Other recipients of coverage might feel the decision is fair in that they can assume that they will receive equal treatment if and when they are in a similar situation. They might feel confident of receiving fair and equitable treatment no matter what their position in the organization. While the decision may cause short-term problems for the organization in that a precedent is being set, the long-term plan to educate staff in an ongoing manner should serve to prevent repeat occurrences.

Organizational structure, legalities, economics, conflicting roles, and societal expectations cause pressure when weighing each option. Organizational structure is key with options B and C. The self-funded plan is one that makes it easier to circumvent the insurer's rules and the COBRA law. It is structured to strong-arm the insurer. This allows for rule-bending.

Legal aspects are key as well. Option A, for example, upholds the law with no negotiating about terms. COBRA law requires the employer to give a dependent notification when coverage will be terminated; yet the only way an employer can be informed about student status or a dependent's turning age 25 is by notification from the employee.

These legalities alone present complications. Economic interests affect judgment in decision-making efforts. A moral decision suggests sharing responsibilities of cost rather than putting the burden on one individual. Thus, the interests of all stakeholders are protected. Money, while a factor, is not the bottom-line motivator.

Another pressure is conflict of authority. Who should be loyal to whom? Where does fiduciary responsibility lie? With option C, responsibilities are not in conflict, but loyalty may be overriding obligation to law. The law is implemented, but creatively. Societal pressures are present in this dilemma. Other employees at the hospital expect the organization to do the right thing. The law was used creatively. Each employee can be assured of future similar and fair treatment. An educational twist included in this option will encourage people to become more aware of their own responsibilities. Education could be a safeguard in preventing similar occurrences. Option C upholds the reputation of the hospital. It promotes trust to do the right thing and sends a message of value.

Adherence to the law is virtuous but the law is unclear at times. In this case the law is broadly interpreted. Laws can be a constraint and can limit a manager's competence. Laws are not always a means by which we can ensure the right decision.

Questions for Discussion

1. Does the plan administrator's reasoning make ethical sense?
2. Is bending the law ethical? Sometimes or always? When? Is *not* bending the law sometimes unethical?
3. How do controls/mechanisms of accountability affect the plan administrator? Do they facilitate or obstruct ethical reasoning and behavior in this case and in your experience?
4. Analyze the case in terms of loyalty and survival; analyze it in terms of the welfare of the individual versus the welfare of the community.
5. Ethically speaking, whose judgment should prevail in this case?

Annotated Bibliography

Arras, J. D., and B. Steinbock. *Ethical Issues in Modern Medicine*, 4th ed. Mountain View, CA: Mayfield, 1995. In discussing macro issues, consistently address various legal, organizational, and other controls that enter the picture.

Cooper, T. *The Responsible Administrator*. San Francisco: Jossey-Bass, 1990. An excellent discussion of external and internal controls (chapter 5 in particular).

Finer, H. "Administrative Responsibility in Democratic Government." In F. Rourke, *Bureaucratic Power in National Politics*. Boston: Little Brown, 1972. Originally published in 1941 as a response to the Friedrich piece cited below, a sophisticated argument for the importance of external controls.

Friedrich, C. "Public Policy and the Nature of Administrative Responsibility." In F. Rourke, *Bureaucratic Power in National Politics*. Boston: Little Brown, 1972. Originally published in 1940, an argument against external controls, favoring instead development of virtue and character in professionals and reliance on them.

Griffith, J. *The Moral Challenges of Health Care Management*. Ann Arbor, MI: Health Administration Press, 1993. An excellent insight to peer control and the value of control by legitimate authority. Reprints the code of ethics of the American College of Healthcare Executives and the ethical conduct guidelines of the American Hospital Association.

Kolenda, K. *Organizations and Ethical Individualism*. Westport, CT: Praeger, 1988. Presents philosophically based arguments for overriding controls by professional judgment.

Trevino, L., and B. Victor. "Peer Reporting of Unethical Behavior." *Academy of Management Journal* 35, no. 1 (March 1992): 38–64. Analyzes the power and variables affecting the exercise of peer controls.

DEVELOPING ETHICAL REFLECTION SKILLS

THUS FAR we have introduced the notion of microethics in health-care and have claimed that its manifestation in reality is based in micro power, guided by conflicting values and influenced by numerous mechanisms of accountability. The next question asks how a healthcare professional can deal skillfully with all this. Clearly, our intellects need to be engaged: chapter 7 discusses approaches to ethical reasoning. And, like it or not, our psyches and emotions are involved, too: chapter 8 brings in this aspect. The present chapter is based on the conviction that our imagination must also be energized if we are to be more ethically mature in dealing with the complicated reality in which we work. Imaginatory reflection, I would argue, is an essential skill undergirding honest intellectual reflection. Using the tool of structured contrast, this chapter attempts to facilitate development of this ethical reflection skill.

Reflection and Moral Imagination

The importance of imaginative reflection to ethical maturity cannot be overstressed. Speaking as a moral philosopher, Daniel Maguire observes that each of us has our own "little method for moral evaluation," but that if we fail to reflect on our method, chances are it will be biased and immature and we will "underestimate our moral freedom." "Moral understanding," he argues, "unfolds in the exquisite power of creative imagination."[1] Writing as a political philosopher, Dennis Thompson contends that skillful reflection is all the more important for public service professionals like us because we are expected, by virtue of the general obligations of professionalism, to foresee, to be aware and to anticipate. "Where the welfare of so many is at stake," he suggests, professionals "must make exceptional efforts to anticipate the consequences of their actions."[2] And, arguing as a nonprofit management specialist, Michael O'Neill maintains that "tapping . . . the reflections of practicing managers may turn out to be a far more effective way of strengthening managerial ethics than trying to impose ethical theories from the outside."[3] So it's important that we healthcare professionals get good at this.

Educator John Dewey used the notion of "deliberation" to explain his understanding of this sort of reflection. He described it as undertaking a "dramatic rehearsal" of the impact of ideas and reasoning.[4] Drawing from Dewey, Terry Cooper uses the term "moral imagination" to describe the skills in reflection we are talking about. Moral imagination develops "the ability to produce a 'movie in our minds' with realistic characters, a believable script and clear imagery." Where ethics is concerned, as he correctly observes, the "movies" we usually produce tend to be black and white on silent screens instead of epic productions of complex sagas in technicolor with Dolby sound: "The more imaginative we can be . . . the more our ethical decision making is enhanced."[5] He is right on.

Structured Contrasts

The next question, then, is how to develop this kind of reflective skill. The simple answer is through experience with practice. A more tangible response is through use of tools such as dialogue, brainstorming, and even sophisticated methods like the Delphi technique. A simple tool that I have found to be most helpful in this regard is what I call structured contrast. It is simply structuring the thought process into a contrasting exploration of seeming opposites.

For example, let's reflect on the contrast of ethics as a matter of **denigrating versus dignifying**. In the daily routine of our healthcare work do we, in fact—not just in theory or in intention—treat our patients, our subordinates, our peers with dignity? Or do we tend to denigrate them by our actions, our words, the tone of our voices. In the hectic hassle of trying to do good do we honor and respect people despite the structure and stress of a situation? Or do we end up subtly or overtly showing disrespect to people in the name of getting the job done?

The centrality of human dignity in normative healthcare ethics is emphasized in numerous treatises. Representative of this is the preamble to the Code of Ethics of the American College of Healthcare Executives: "The fundamental objectives of the healthcare management profession are to enhance the overall quality of life, dignity and well-being of every individual needing healthcare services. . . ."[6] Increasingly, practical healthcare management efforts also emphasize the centrality of dignity. Witness a recent promotion for Continuous Quality Improvement (CQI) in hospitals: Dennis Brodeur argues that a major reason for adopting the CQI paradigm is that it promotes "the dignity of workers above productivity, efficiency, and profits."[7]

The problem is that actually practicing dignity in the day-to-day routine is a major challenge. A descriptive rather than normative ethics study might well suggest that denigration is more the behavioral norm. Do we, for example, in focusing on clinical tasks so that they get done well, treat subordinates and patients as if they were machines? Do we see and appreciate the color of their eyes, or might they just as well be featureless mannequins? Does our paternalism reveal itself in a condescending tone of voice? Do we blithely keep people waiting? And what about the words we use in speaking with and about clients and subordinates? Are they dignifying or denigrating words and tones?

Two recent studies are exceptionally helpful for reflecting on this. One is Robin Lakoff's enlightening exploration of the power of language. While her presentation is relentlessly revealing of how we professionals tend to use language, her most insightful finding may be the one concerning the difficulty we have in realizing how denigrating we can be: "We are reluctant to examine our conversational gambits; first, we get nervous when we have to examine closely behavior that has become habitual and unconscious. . . . Then, too, especially in the area of interpersonal behavior, we like to see ourselves as guileless, our actions as spontaneous."[8] She correctly articulates the difficulty of reflecting on the denigration phenomenon: "To recognize that we are following set patterns, sometimes engaging in strategies to achieve something at the expense of someone else, is to be forced to see ourselves . . . in an ungenerous light."[9]

A second particularly helpful study for contrasting denigrating and dignifying behavior is Yarwood's revealing research on humor in organizations. He found that organizational humor is typically directed against clients and subordinates, that it is often aggressive and hurtful, and that anti-client jokes reinforce anti-client norms.[10] We could well reflect on our humor reality in the day-to-day routine of our own healthcare work. Do we direct denigrating jokes at patients and subordinates? Is this indicative of a behavioral inclination away from the dignity we profess to hold sacred?

The more I reflect using this tool of structured contrast the more I find that, in practice, only a very fine line often separates dignifying behavior from denigrating behavior. My interactions with clients and subordinates often take place in a context of stress, of weariness, of irritation with something or someone. In those contexts I easily slip over the line through abruptness or tone or silence. I make patients wait for my superb clinical care but I don't bother to inform them of the wait. A subordinate asks me a question. I answer "later." I treat them all as inferiors. I know not the color of their eyes even though we have closely interacted. I denigrate them, but in ways so subtle that I am clueless; so I preserve my self-image as a professional who respects and dignifies. Overcoming this blind tendency to denigrate requires imaginative reflection.

Closely related is the structured contrast of **hubris versus humility**. I call myself a care provider, a *servant* of people's needs. I call myself a public *service* professional. But, if the truth were known, am I really a *master* of people? Do I serve the patient's needs or does the patient serve my needs? Do I tend to behave with the hubris of a tyrant or with a humility proper to a servant? And is my ethical responsibility to be a humble servant or a hubristic master making darn sure that healthcare gets delivered?

Hubris is a wonderful Greek word that roughly translates into professional arrogance. Joan Chittister defines it as a self-absorption that values control over equality.[11] Can you relate to that controlling instinct? For myself, especially in the pressures of everyday professional life, I like to be in complete control of the environment, of the agenda, and of the discussion. Is that hubris? And is there something unethical about that? Is it the same thing about which I was so critical of Nurse Ratched in *One Flew Over the Cuckoo's Nest*?

Charles Kelly understands it as "the presumption of superiority, typically by virtue of position, expertise or charisma." It leads, he says, to an "assumed right to persuade, manipulate or coerce others in order to achieve the objectives associated with his or her superior official status."[12] Manfred de Vries warns that the hubris of professionals "is all too familiar" and that "insufficient heed is paid to its dangers."[13] Is he talking about us?

As I reflect more on this I try to take to heart Karen Lebacqz's suggestion that "the trappings of professional life—the books and files, the diplomas on the wall, the clothing worn—can serve to make the one person seem important while the other seems naked and unprotected."[14] Beyond that, everyone calls me "Doctor" or "Professor" or "Sir"; they stand up when I enter the room and listen to what I say and laugh when I laugh. Everything in the environment tends to make me feel important. So, of course, I start to believe it! Subconsciously I sense that I am, indeed, superior. All of the structures and trappings are telling me so. And this sense then leads me into hubristic behavior. I stare down at students. I come in late with neither apology nor explanation. I give my students a marginal grade with hardly a comment. I let them know, usually just by the tone of my voice, that I am without doubt smarter than they. And I actually believe it: I am, indeed, the master! This attitude of hubris tends to come out, as Allinson sees it, in pervasive, subtle, and seemingly little ways such as an unwillingness to ask for, pass on, or receive information. He labels such routine behavior "ethical hubris."[15]

For example, how often have you experienced a scenario similar to that of Dr. Spivey's first encounter with McMurphy in *One Flew Over the Cuckoo's Nest*? Remember how likable Spivey was? Remember how, nonetheless, when McMurphy entered his office, Spivey began to read McMurphy's chart obviously for the first time? He had not even bothered to prepare for the intake interview! That struck me as subtle hubris of the first order and as so subtly denigrating. Then I remembered the many interviews I've had with subordinates, patients, and students without—under the subconscious excuse of time duress—having reviewed their files prior to the meeting. When I was disturbed by Dr. Spivey's behavior, I was actually seeing myself. But it didn't register that way.

The clear suggestion of de Vries is that we well-intentioned healthcare professionals can very easily end up as "victims of hubris." But, he adds hopefully, "such an ending could be avoided if they paid attention to their intrapsychic life, and found help in exploring their blind spots."[16] Hence the importance of developing imaginative reflection skills.

A third helpful structured contrast is **conscience versus consciousness**. Do I follow my conscience? Just what is that? My feelings? My instinct? And how do I form it? By reflex reaction? With grit? With moral principles learned over the years? Or, instead, do I follow my consciousness? And what is that? The things I am aware of? Thoughts that enter my head? How do I form that consciousness? Do I look at what's in front of me? Through cataracts or with corrective lenses? Do I explore what's off to the side? And is it ethical to follow my consciousness? Am I ethically responsible for what my conscience or consciousness intends, or am I responsible for what my conscience or consciousness leads me into whether I am aware of it or not?

Health ethicist Kurt Darr argues that we healthcare managers should be the conscience of the organization and enforce the principle that patient welfare is more important than the financial bottom line of our healthcare facility.[17] Terry Cooper, on the other hand, asserts that the purpose of ethics is to raise experience to a "conscious level."[18] So if Darr's conscience leads us to undermine our organization's solvency, which in turn disfranchises hundreds of patients no longer able to use our facility, is that the ethical thing to do? And are we responsible even though our conscientious intent was patient dignity? And if Cooper's experience-based consciousness leads us—from years of cost-containment pressures—to move patients through the facility expeditiously and occasionally with diminished dignity, is that ethical? Are we free of responsibility for the few who suffer so that more can be served?

Berger and Luckmann maintain that morality is indeed the "content of conscience,"[19] but Milgram found that the shock-givers in his experiments were people of sound conscience and good intentions. Are we, then, responsible for what—in all good conscience and clear consciousness—we intend, or are we healthcare professionals responsible for what we do? A. C. Ewing offers an idea: "The link between virtue and action, being and doing, is not a simple one-to-one correlation in which a right act always indicates a virtuous person and a wrong act always indicates a nonvirtuous person."[20] It is thus possible, according to Ewing's logic, to suggest that a healthcare professional of little conscience might nonetheless be behaving ethically while a peer of great conscience behaves unethically!

Sissela Bok offers another idea on this. She postulates that no one can be blamed for failing to do what he or she did not know needed doing: "Both capacity to act and knowledge that acting is required must be present for there to be moral obligation, and responsibility for its breach."[21] This argument logically flows from the wonderful Judeo-Christian "principle of intentionality," which roughly means that one cannot sin unless one means to sin. I say it's wonderful because it gets me off the hook of responsibility: so long as my intention is good, the bad I do doesn't really count. So I need not worry! But this principle emerged from creative reflections of Augustine, Aquinas, and others on the matter of "culpability" involving *personal* ethics, not *professional* ethics. For a professional healthcare agent are things different? If my good conscience intends only good things, and if my clear consciousness is aware only of good things happening, am I then ethically free and clear? No, says Bok: "At times, even pleas of ignorance do not suffice to acquit one of responsibility. If one has the obligation to remain alert . . . then the fact that one failed to do so gives no excuse." And that is the problem: we healthcare professionals are supposed to be alert, to be aware. That is precisely why they call us professionals and pay us that extra money.

Sabini and Silver piquantly pick up on this: "Assessing a person's responsibility involves considerations of: what he intended to do, what he realized or should have realized, what he could or could not have done, as well as considerations relating to the gravity of the rule transgressed and the priority of competing claims."[22] For us professionals, of course, the key phrase is "what we *should* have realized." Sabini and Silver then put it right to us: "We may *feel* responsibility only for what we intend; we *are* responsible for all that we do. And we know it."

Tom Jones, in the incisive article attached to chapter 7, suggests that the "low moral intensity" of routine, everyday healthcare work results in a low level of deliberation which, in turn, minimizes the level of consciousness of the microethics involved.[23] Is it best, then, to rely on conscience for ethical behavior in the ordinary routine of our professional work? But others argue that, instead, our level of consciousness needs to be elevated. Morgan's extensive research of managers, for example, found a remarkably low level of ethical self-consciousness. Managers, peers, subordinates, and superiors were asked to assess the manager's ethical behavior. His finding: "Self-ratings are significantly more favorable than ratings by superiors, peers, and subordinates."[24]

Jerry Harvey finds that our unconscious thought patterns guide us into justifications for denigrating clients and subordinates. Higher emphasis on consciousness would enable us, he feels, to change these dysfunctional thought patterns.[25] And Bellah's team, in their landmark research, similarly found that our lack of clear consciousness has led our society—healthcare professionals included—into behaviors that emphasize individual success over community and relationships.[26]

As I reflect on my own professional behavior I find myself often led by conscience to admonish unprepared students. My conscientious irritation, however, impedes my consciousness of the tone in my voice or my domineering posture as I stand over the student. There are ways to admonish in good conscience but, without an awakened consciousness, too, those ways easily deteriorate into arrogance and denigration. And my doctor, who regularly has me waiting half an hour beyond my appointment time, is a person of great conscience dedicated to serving all in need. He also is oblivious to the indignity imposed by the unannounced delay. Is he ethical because of his good conscience, or unethical because of his limited consciousness?

A final illustrative structured contrast is that of **rules versus relationship** that can also be described as **contract versus covenant**. In the day-to-day routine of ordinary healthcare what is more ethically important: following established procedures and rules or nurturing relationships with patients, peers, and subordinates? Is it ethically more important to keep the implied contract of a 3:00 p.m. appointment or to honor my covenant of care with previous patients and give more time to them than scheduled? Am I responsible for maintaining the established procedures of my facility and the standards of the Joint Commission, or am I ethically bound to "bend the rules" in response to patient needs and dignity?

Laura Nash urges a "covenantal ethic" emphasis in her discourse to business managers.[27] Covenant involves values and attitudes, she argues, that cannot be accounted for in contracts, rules, and the like. It highlights the welfare of others and views healthcare as "a series of mutually enabling relationships rather than a set of efficiency measures."[28] For Nash, professional ethics entails subordinating rules and procedures to a sense of service and relationships. But, as Michael Bayles contends,[29] isn't it rules and contracts that encourage good relations between clients and professionals? In fact, don't rules, standards, contracts, and procedures actually establish the practice of healthcare and facilitate its goals? Don't rules protect us and our patients from possible errors we would make in exercising our own judgment? Don't they help us cope with the hectic nature of everyday healthcare? Don't they keep us from exhausting ourselves and being unfair? And haven't the rules developed precisely because the healthcare community has found over time that rules and procedures facilitate the best possible results? Aren't our rules sacred?

Think of Nurse Ratched and Randall McMurphy from *One Flew Over the Cuckoo's Nest*. Didn't Mildred have a keen appreciation of rules and procedures? Wasn't her focus on this a key to our negative judgment of her behavior? And wasn't Randall a master at nurturing relationships even to the death of Billy and himself? Had either of them developed a more balanced appreciation of rules *and* relationships, might things have turned out differently?

We need to return to "brass tacks," and thinkers like Gustafson get us there: ethics should not be a choosing of rules over relationships, he points out; rather, professional ethics should be an awareness that rules *and* relationships are involved in every ethical situation.[30] But in our everyday routine of healthcare, are they? Or do we tend to pick and choose: sometimes rules, sometimes relationships?

Is there a way, instead, to blend them? Karen Lebacqz offers a resounding "Yes": the crucial question, she maintains, is not whether the relationships matter or whether the rules matter, but just what the relationship is, how it is defined, and "what rules are appropriately understood to apply to that situation."[31] Relationships and rules are not independent of each other. Perhaps, then, a structured contrast we can call **caring versus coping** is appropriate. Ethics in the ordinary day spent providing healthcare is not just about giving care to patients but rather about creatively coping—intersecting all of those routine rules with all of those rarefied relationships we professionals work amidst.

Pursuing Imaginative Reflection Skills

The development of imaginative reflection skills is part of the growth process to ethical maturity. Gustafson even suggests that in order to act ethically we need to develop an "interpretative capacity that requires imagination."[32] Simple tools, such as the structured contrast just illustrated, can help in the quest. Group dialogue using structured contrast— such as that promoted by Burton Visotzky—can also help enormously. In his intriguing *The Genesis of Ethics*, Visotzky demonstrates how the structured contrast of **sacred versus profane** develops moral imagination. Using group study of the biblical Book of Genesis, he has attracted corporate CEOs, Wall Street financiers, artists, and lawyers apparently because of the reflection skills they have found embryonic in this approach.[33] With such skills in hand we, along with those hot-shots, are much better able to absorb and utilize mentally methodological approaches to ethical reasoning exemplified in the next chapter.

Notes

1. D. Maguire, 1979, *The Moral Choice* (Minneapolis, MN: Winston), p. xv.
2. D. Thompson, 1985, "The Possibility of Administrative Ethics." *Public Administrative Review* 45, no. 5 (September/October 1985): 560.
3. M. O'Neill, 1992, "Ethical Dimensions of Nonprofit Administration." *Nonprofit Management and Leadership* 3, no. 2 (winter): 202.
4. J. Dewey, 1922, *Human Nature and Conduct* (New York: Holt, Rinehart and Winston), p. 190.
5. T. Cooper, 1990, *The Responsible Administrator* (San Francisco: Jossey-Bass), p. 22.
6. American College of Healthcare Executives, 1992, *Code of Ethics* (Chicago: ACHE). It is included as an appendix to this volume.
7. D. Brodeur, 1995, "Work Ethics and CQI," *Hospital and Health Services Administration* 40, no. 1 (spring): 118.
8. R. Lakoff, 1990, *Talking Power* (New York: Basic Books) p. 1.
9. Ibid., p. 2.
10. D. Yarwood, 1995, "Humor and Administration: A Serious Inquiry Into Unofficial Organizational Communication." *Public Administration Review* 55, no. 1 (January/February): 81–89.
11. J. Chittister, 1991, "Humility Could Redeem Us in Sea of Hubris." *National Catholic Reporter* (8 November): 2.
12. C. Kelly, 1988, *The Destructive Achiever* (Reading, MA: Addison-Wesley), p. 26.
13. M. de Vries, 1994, "The Leadership Mystique." *Academy of Management Executive* 8, no. 3 (August): 88.
14. K. Lebasqz, 1985, *Professional Ethics* (Nashville, TN: Abingdon), p. 135.
15. R. Allinson, 1995, "A Call for Ethically Centered Management." *Academy of Management Executive* 9, no. 1 (February): 73.
16. M. de Vries, "The Leadership Mystique."

17. K. Darr, 1991, *Ethics in Health Services Management* (Chicago: Health Professions Press), p. xviii.

18. T. Cooper, 1990, *The Responsible Administrator* (San Francisco: Jossey-Bass), p. 62.

19. P. Berger and T. Luckmann, 1966, *The Social Construction of Reality* (New York: Doubleday), ch. 10.

20. A. Ewing, 1953, *Ethics* (New York: Free Press), ch .8.

21. S. Bok, 1984, *Secrets* (New York: Vintage), p. 66.

22. J. Sabini and M. Silver, 1982, *Moralities of Everyday Life* (New York: Oxford), p. 61.

23. T. Jones, 1991, "Ethical Decision Making by Individuals in Organizations," *Academy of Management Review* 16, no. 2 (April): 366–95.

24. R. Morgan, 1993, "Self and Co-Worker Perceptions of Ethics and Their Relationships to Leadership and Salary," *Academy of Management Journal* 36, no. 1 (February): 209.

25. J. Harvey, 1988, *The Abilene Paradox* (Lexington, MA: Heath).

26. R. Bellah, R. Madsen, W. Sullivan, A. Swidler, and S. Tipton, 1985, *Habits of the Heart* (New York: Harper and Row).

27. L. Nash, *Good Intentions Aside* (Boston: Harvard Business School Press, 1990).

28. Ibid., p. 93.

29. M. Bayles, 1968, *Contemporary Utilitarianism* (New York: Doubleday).

30. J. Gustafson, 1971, "Context Versus Principles." In *Christian Ethics and the Community* (Philadelphia: Pilgrim Press).

31. K. Lebacqz, 1985, *Professional Ethics* (Nashville, TN: Abingdon), p. 23.

32. J. Gustafson, 1974, "Moral Discernment in the Christian Life." In *Theology and Christian Ethics* (Philadelphia: Pilgrim Press), p. 104.

33. B. Visotzky, 1996, *The Genesis of Ethics* (New York: Crown).

READING

The following reading first appeared in one of the finest management journals extant. Although business organization–oriented, it is decidedly generic and, hence, highly relevant to healthcare settings. Moreover, Victor and Cullen have produced one of the more rigorous tools for ethical reflection. While they designed the tool for macro organization analysis, it is nonetheless useful for individual analysis in the micro dimension as well. Their beginning interest is organizational culture and its impact on ethical behavior, an interest that recalls our previous discussion in chapter 5. In this piece they focus on "ethical work climate," a form of moral atmosphere, and its effect on ethical deliberations. As they put it early on, work climates "inform organizational members what one can do and what one 'ought' to do regarding the treatment of others."

By presenting and analyzing a framework for determining ethical climate, the authors provide rich concepts for imaginative reflection on our own professional behavior. The article gets a bit intricate in reporting statistical results of their application of the tool to corporations, but that is not the important part for our purposes. Read this piece to understand a sound structure that can be helpful in developing skill in ethical reflection.

This is a rather sophisticated and comprehensive article. It is also among the best a healthcare professional will find for honing insight to imaginative ethical reasoning in the micro dimension of healthcare, notwithstanding Victor and Cullen's primary concern with the macro dimension of business. Secondarily, the work presented in this article can be professionally useful in evaluating the ethical climate of one's own healthcare organization and group, and one's perceived "fit" with it.

THE ORGANIZATIONAL BASES OF ETHICAL WORK CLIMATES

Bart Victor and John B. Cullen

There is a growing belief that organizations are social actors responsible for the ethical or unethical behaviors of their employees. This trend is reflected in both the bases of legal judgments against corporations (Clinard and Yeager 1980) and in the reactions of society at large to "corporate crime" (Cullen, Maakestad, and Cavender 1987). Consequently, academics (Clinard 1983) and practitioners (Weiss 1986) have shown increasing concern for understanding and managing organizational normative systems that may guide the ethical behaviors of employees. In spite of this growing interest, few methodological and theoretical tools exist with the potential to characterize norms at organizational levels of analysis. One promising mechanism for understanding organizational normative systems is the concept of work climate (Schneider 1983).

A work climate is defined as perceptions that "are psychologically meaningful moral descriptions that people *can agree* characterize a system's practices and procedures" [emphasis added] (Schneider 1975:474). The prevailing perceptions of typical organizational practices and procedures that have ethical content constitute the ethical work climate. For example, when faced with a decision that has consequence for others, how does an organizational member identify the "right" alternative—at least in the organization's view? An important source of this information are those aspects of work climate that determine what constitutes ethical behavior at work.

Employing a broad definition of ethics in developing the concept of an ethical work climate, we encompassed the range of perceptions that answer, for a member of an organization, the Socratic question: "What *should* I do?" Included are the perceived prescriptions, proscriptions, and permissions regarding moral obligations in organizations. For example, in a hiring decision, expectations about whose interests should be considered and/or what codes or laws should be applied would be an aspect of the ethical climate. With such an approach, ethical climates are conceptualized as general and pervasive characteristics of organizations, affecting a broad range of decisions.

Bart Victor and John Cullen, "The Organizational Bases of Ethical Work Climates." *Administrative Sciences Quarterly* 33, no. 1 (March 1988): 101–125. Copyright 1988 by Cornell University. Reprinted by permission. The article is abridged. Bart Victor is professor of management at the University of North Carolina at Chapel Hill. John B. Cullen is professor of management at the University of Rhode Island.

The prevailing epistemology within organizations is explicitly excluded from the concept of ethical climate. How information is discovered (e.g., whether intuition or computation characterizes fact finding in the organization) is not an aspect of ethical climate. Also excluded are conventions, or rules with arbitrary consequences (Lewis 1969; Turiel and Smetana 1984). Organizational decision making that does not have any differential effect on others (e.g., when tradition or current fashion dictates organizational aesthetics) is not part of the ethical climate. Thus, for example, the ethical climate refers to how people in an organization typically decide whether it is right or wrong to pay kickbacks. The ethical climate does not refer to how one determines if the buyer expects a kickback (a question of fact) or whether the kickback should be paid in cash or merchandise (a question of conversation).

We hypothesize that ethical work climates have organization bases separate from individual perceptions and evaluations. We believe that (1) organizations and subgroups within organizations develop different institutionalized normative systems; (2) although not completely homogeneous, these normative systems are known to organizational members sufficiently well to be perceived as a type of work climate; and (3) perceptions of ethical work climate differ from affective evaluations of ethical work climate. Empirically, our assumptions imply two propositions. First, the variation in perceptions of ethical work climate between groups (organizations and subgroups within organizations) is greater than the variation in perceptions of ethical work climate for the individuals within these groups (Drexler 1977). Second, perceptions that describe the ethical work climate are not necessarily correlated with attitudes that evaluate the ethical work climate (Schneider 1975).

Ethical Climates

Work Climates and Organizational Ethics

There is no single type of work climate (Schneider 1975). Researchers have most often studied the existence and extent of autonomy/control, degree of structure, nature of rewards, consideration, warmth, and support (Campbell et al. 1970; Field and Abelson 1982; Schneider 1983; Schneider and Reichers 1983). The majority of these climate types fall into two very broad classifications: aggregated perceptions of organizational conventions regarding forms of structure and procedures for the use of rewards and control; and aggregated perceptions of the existence of organizational norms supporting values such as providing warmth and support to peers and subordinates.

Some of the climate types that represent organizational norms have an ethical basis in that they inform organizational members what one can do and what one "ought" to do regarding the treatment of others. Climate types such as support for conflict resolution (Renwick 1975) and the acceptability of aggression (Lewin, Lippitt, and White 1939) represent perceived norms of an organization or group with an ethical basis. However, at least in the organizational literature, previous researchers did not rely explicitly on any theoretical or philosophical bases to select the types of norms or ethics studied. Different normative themes, including those probably without ethical consequences such as Renwick's (1975) support for creativity, have been studied haphazardly without any clearly stated unifying theoretical scheme. This study differs from earlier work on organizational work climates in that ethical philosophy and theories of ethical behavior guided our selection of ethical issues that possibly form the bases of work climates.

In the literature on individual moral development there is now recognition that individual characteristics alone are insufficient to explain moral and ethical behavior. As such, there is an increasing concern for the impact of social factors on individual moral behavior (e.g., Kurtines 1984, 1986). Even the developmental psychologist Kohlberg and his colleagues (Higgins, Power, and Kohlberg 1984) have introduced the concepts of a "moral atmosphere" and "just community" to consider the social context of moral and ethical behavior. The concept of moral atmosphere is similar to ethical climate in that it represents the prevailing norms of the group and not the individual's level of moral development. However, the focus of Kohlberg's research on moral atmosphere was somewhat narrow, considering only the development of collectiveness norms and valuing of the community, with a prime emphasis on moral education. Kohlberg did not relate his approach, either methodologically or theoretically, to the work climate literature.

Following Schneider's (1983) definition, the existence of an ethical work climate requires that normative systems in the organization be institutionalized. That is, organizational members must perceive the existence of normative patterns in the organization with a measurable degree of consensus. Organizational members are asked to report not on their own behavior and values but, rather, on the practices and procedures that they perceive to exist in their organizations. Thus, we consider respondents to climate questionnaires as a type of observer. However, these observers differ from anthropological informants, members of the culture who provide insider views of culture, often have intensive relationships with the researcher, and provide extreme depth and breadth of information. These observers use a conceptual scheme defined a priori by the researchers and are asked to observe only limited aspects of the practices and procedures of an organization. The strengths of the approach are the large number of observers and the necessity that some consensus exist before aggregated climate perceptions can be said to represent a group or organizational climate.

An institutionalized normative system can be considered an element of culture (Honigmann 1959), although an organizational culture is certainly more comprehensive, including, for example, patterns of behavior, artifacts, ceremonies, and special language (Smircich 1983). Observers of organizational ethical climate report only on those organizational norms concerning practices and procedures with ethical consequences, only a segment of their organizational culture (Ashforth 1985). The climate questionnaire, then, is simply an instrument to tap, through the perceptions of organizational participants, the ethical dimensions of organizational culture. One would also assume that more "developed" (Deal and Kennedy 1982) organizational cultures produce more consensus in perceptions of climate. To the extent that different subgroups within organizations have identifiably different climates, such climates likely indicate the existence of organizational subcultures.

Types of Ethical Climates

This study used a two-dimensional theoretical typology of ethical climates. The first dimension represents the ethical criteria used for organizational decision making (e.g., egoism). The second dimension represents the locus of analysis used as a referent in ethical decisions (e.g., individual interest). Cross-tabulation of the two dimensions results in nine theoretical ethical climate types, as shown in Figure 1. The underlying rationale for these types is presented below.

The ethical criterion dimension. While complex and intricate in its detail, much of moral philosophy can be organized under three major classes of ethical theory: egoism, benevolence, and deontology, or principle (Fritzche and Becker 1984; Williams 1985). These theories differ in terms of the basic criteria used in moral reasoning, i.e., maximizing self-interest, maximizing joint interests, or adherence to principle, respectively. Psychological theories of moral development suggest that individuals use similar criteria in the development of ethical reasoning (see Kohlberg's 1969 review). Perhaps the most influential, the theory proposed by Kohlberg (1967) contains six stages of moral development ranging from egocentric obedience and punishment to universal principle. The six stages of development have three bases of moral judgment, following the three major classes of ethical theory.

Figure 1   Theoretical Ethical Climate Types

LOCUS OF ANALYSIS

	Individual	Local	Cosmopolitan
Egoism	Self-Interest*	Company Profit	Efficiency
Benevolence	Friendship	Team Interest	Social Responsibility
Principle	Personal Morality	Company Rules and Procedures	Laws and Professional Codes

ETHICAL CRITERION

*Typical decision criterion.

Based on this common framework, we assumed that types of organizational ethical climates exist that differ in terms of the three classes of ethical theories. The three types of ethical reasoning compose the Y axis in Figure 1 and are labeled egoism, benevolence, and principle. Because climate is a group or organization concept, types of ethical climates are classifications of groups or organizations only and are not assumed to follow the developmental sequence that is hypothesized for individuals. Moreover, as Kohlberg (1984:87) noted, individuals at various stages of moral development can exist in groups with normative systems that differ from their own level of moral development. However, behavioral compliance with a group or organizational climate incongruent with an individual's level of moral development may lead to adaptive reactions such as stress and whistle blowing.

According to Kohlberg (1984), Gilligan (1982), Haan, Aerts, and Cooper (1985), and others who study individual ethical reasoning, the types of ethical reasoning are relatively incompatible. People who are benevolent tend to be less cognizant of laws or rules and may also be less amenable to arguments employing rules or principles. In contrast, people who are principled tend to be less sensitive to particular effects on others. Given this, organizations might also be expected to develop relatively distinct forms of ethical climates. That is, organizations or subgroups within organizations may be prototypically benevolent, principled, or egoistic. However, although Victor and Cullen (1987) found that there was often a dominant climate type in an organization or a group, organizations did not have single climate types.

The types of ethical climates existing in an organization or group influence what ethical conflicts are considered, the process by which such conflicts are resolved, and the characteristics of their resolution. For example, Kohlberg (1984) believed that the "socio-moral atmosphere" of an organization has a significant impact on the moral decision making of individuals. In discussing the massacre at My Lai, Kohlberg (1984:263) proposed that "the moral choice made by each individual soldier who pulled the trigger was embedded in the larger institutional context of the army and its decision making procedures." In an organization characterized primarily by a benevolent climate, a teleological consideration of the well-being of others may be the dominant reasoning used by employees to identify and solve ethical problems. With a largely principled climate, the application and interpretation of rules or law might be the dominant form of reasoning. In a largely egoistic climate, self-interest might be the dominant consideration.

The locus of analysis dimension. A locus of analysis is a referent group identifying the source of moral reasoning used for applying ethical criteria to organizational decisions and/or the limits on what would be considered in ethical analyses of organizational decisions. Distinct from both moral philosophy and individual moral development, ethical climate is an organizational concept.[1] Therefore, ethical reasoning may vary relative to the use of the concept of organization as a referent (as individual moral reasoning varies relative to the use of the concept of self as a referent). To distinguish possible ethical climate types within each of the ethical criteria noted above, three organizational referents or loci of analysis are conceptualized. The locus of analysis dimension is represented on the X axis of Figure 1 and denoted by three categories: individual, local, and cosmopolitan.

The loci of analysis were derived from sociological theories of roles and reference groups. Merton and others studying roles in social systems identified types of reference groups that help shape the behaviors and attitudes of role incumbents. Merton (1957) distinguished between a local and a cosmopolitan role. For the local role incumbent, the important reference groups or sources of role definitions and expectations are contained within the social system. For the cosmopolitan role incumbent, the sources of role definition are in a social system external to the system in which the actor is embedded. Gouldner (1957) applied this distinction to organizations to show that those holding local or cosmopolitan roles used different reference groups (internal or external to the organization) as sources to define appropriate role expectations.

In the ethical climate typology, the local locus specifies sources of ethical reasoning within the organization, such as the workgroup. The cosmopolitan level specifies organizational sources of ethical reasoning external to the focal organization, such as a professional association or a body of law. Cosmopolitan sources of ethical reasoning can be abstract concepts, generated outside organizations but used inside organizations as part of the institutionalized normative system. The source of profes- sional norms of behavior, for example, is usually external to the work setting, but the norms still become part of the prevailing normative climate of professional work organizations (Kornhauser 1962; Scott 1966). In addition to the cosmopolitan level, another locus external to the focal organization or group was conceptualized. Labeled individual, this locus is external to the focal organization in the sense that the prevailing normative climate supports a referent for ethical reasoning located within the individual. Prevailing norms such as those supporting the use of one's personal ethics or engaging self-interested behavior would be examples of such a climate.

Although the loci of analysis identify the general sources and/or limits of consideration in ethical analyses, the relationships of the loci of analysis with the ethical criteria differ somewhat for each criterion.

In the context of the egoism criterion, the loci of analysis identify the particular "self" (e.g., individual, company) in whose interests one is expected to act. At the individual locus of analysis, the egoism criterion is defined as consideration of the needs and preferences of one's own self (e.g., personal gain, self-defense). At the local locus of analysis, it is defined as considerations of the organization's interest (e.g., corporate profit, strategic advantage). Finally, at the cosmopolitan locus of analysis, it is defined as considerations of the larger social or economic "system's" interest (e.g., efficiency). In each case, the locus of the consideration is a reified, indivisible unit that can be understood to have needs and preferences.

In the context of the benevolence criterion, the loci of analysis both identify for organizational members "who we are" and set the boundaries for "our concerns." This subject-object distinction, and the concomitant obligation for other-regarding, differentiates the benevolent from the egoistic (Gilligan 1982; Haan, Aerts, and Cooper 1985). At the individual locus of analysis, the benevolence criterion is defined as consideration of other people without reference to organizational membership (e.g., friendship, reciprocity). At the local locus of analysis, it becomes consideration of the organizational collective (e.g., esprit de corps, team play). This is in contrast to local egoism, in which a reified organizational construct is the locus of concern. At the cosmopolitan locus of analysis, benevolence is defined as consideration of other constituencies outside the organization (e.g., social responsibility).

In the context of the principle criterion, the loci of analysis define sources of principles expected to be used in the organization. At the individual locus of analysis, the principles are self-chosen. That is, one is expected in this climate to be guided by personal ethics. At the local locus of analysis, the source of principles lies within the organization (e.g., rules and procedures). At the cosmopolitan locus of analysis, the source of principles is extraorganizational (e.g., the legal system, professional organizations). In the local and cosmopolitan climates one is guided by sources of principles apart from the individual and, thus, regardless of one's personal ethical preferences.

To illustrate further the loci of analysis dimension, three climate types might be described along the diagonal of Figure 1. In the upper left corner is individual egoistic reasoning as it might be found among residential real estate brokers or in a telemarketing "boiler room" where each person's sales and commissions are relatively independent and organizational commitment is quite low. In this case, decision making might be characterized as involving mostly considerations of each person's self-interest. For example, recent concern about sales abuses of stockbrokers (and their negative effects on clients and firms) are often attributed to decisions by brokers that are characteristically self-interested (*Wall Street Journal* 1987).

In the center is local benevolent reasoning. This climate might exist in a semiautonomous workgroup or in a research lab in which there is a high need for cooperation and the focus is on jointly produced outcomes. In this case, decision making involves the comparison of each alternative's impact on each member of the team. For example, Peters and Waterman (1982) found a "corporate family" theme in many of the companies they reviewed: the needs of everyone (often including each employee's own family) were considered in company policy decisions.

Finally, in the lower right corner is cosmopolitan principle reasoning as it might exist for a group of lawyers or certified public accountants. In this case, decision making might be dominated by discussion of how law and professional code apply to an issue. For example, in-house corporate counsels often maintain their own organizational structure within a firm. This structure is outside the mainstream of corporate career ladders and incorporates characteristics like the private law firm, such as associate and partner status distinctions. One rationale for this structure is the need for lawyers to adhere to an extraorganizational source of guiding principles (Kalish 1980).

Victor and Cullen (1987) used the 3 x 3 matrix of nine theoretically possible ethical climate themes shown in Figure 1 to develop an ethical climate assessment instrument. The present study used an improved version of their instrument (incorporating changes in language and items suggested by earlier work) and a different sample to examine various organizational bases of work climate.

The Organizational Bases of Ethical Work Climates

Climate researchers focus on two major boundary issues regarding the climate construct. One is the level of aggregation and the second pertains to the belief and affect components of climate.

Organizational or group climate is the aggregated or typical way the organization is perceived by group members (James and Jones 1974; Schneider 1975; Field and Abelson 1982) A variety of factors can form the basis for aggregated perceptions. Howe (1977) identified three types of aggregation, including person variables, situation variables, and joint person-situation variables. Person variables are individual demographics such as age and sex. Situation variables are the organization and its components (e.g., workgroup). Joint person-situation variables are characteristics of the individual with an organizational basis, such as tenure and salary. Since the objective of this research was to establish whether ethical work climates have inter- and/or intraorganizational bases, situation variables and joint person-situation variables were used for aggregation. Thus, the prime interest was whether distinguishable ethical climates arise between different organizations, and/or within organizations, on the bases of organizationally defined groups (e.g., workgroup, job level).

A long-standing debate in the climate literature concerns the redundancy between satisfaction with the work setting and climate perceptions (Guion 1973; LaFollette and Sims 1975). Fortunately, Schneider

(1983; Schneider and Reichers 1983) argued and demonstrated that careful wording of instruments can distinguish between beliefs concerning climates and affective evaluation of climates. However, in spite of appropriate wording, reporting on ethical climates may create enough emotional reaction to confound perceptions with evaluations. To address this possibility directly, the relationships between the dimensions of ethical climate and affective responses to these dimensions were examined for this paper.

Method

Sample

Preliminary discussions with managers concerning a survey of ethical climate revealed a high degree of sensitivity to any study that might examine a company's "ethics." To alleviate fears that the proposed research would identify ethical or unethical companies and to increase the variety of organizational types studied, it was necessary to meet with top company management from many organizations. Toward this end, a seminar on ethics was held (gratis) by our college of business administration and over 40 CEOs (or their representatives) from a midsized midwestern city attended. As part of the seminar, the proposed research project on ethical climate was explained and voluntary organizational participants were requested. Twenty organizations volunteered participation or requested further discussion. From these twenty, the researchers selected four firms that allowed for variance on size and industry and provided favorable terms for conducting the research: a small printing company, a savings and loan, a manufacturing plant, and a local telephone company. In the printing company (33 employees), and in the savings and loan (450 employees), all full-time employees were surveyed. However, due to constraints imposed by the participating organizations, only certain employee groups were surveyed in the other two firms. In the telephone company, all 500 nonunion employees were surveyed. In the manufacturing plant, a random sample of 200 of the managerial employees was surveyed. In all four firms, surveys were distributed with return envelopes addressed to the university. A standardized cover letter from the firms' chief executives described the survey as a study of "corporate work climate" and ensured confidentiality. Return rates were 52 percent from the manufacturing plant *(N = 103)*; 60 percent from the printing company *(N = 20)*; 75 percent from the savings and loan *(N = 338)*; and 84 percent from the telephone company *(N = 411)* for a total of 872 usable surveys returned (74 percent).

Also due to constraints imposed by the participating companies and because of differences in organizational structures different demographic data were gathered for each firm. Respondents from the printing company, the manufacturing plant, and the telephone company identified their functional departments. Respondents from the savings and loan and telephone company identified their level (i.e., officer, manager, supervisor, or nonsupervisor), age (by decade), and tenure in the company. Respondents from the savings and loan and the manufacturing plant identified whether they were located at the home office or one of the branch offices, and respondents from the telephone company listed their salaries. In Howe's (1977) terms, functional department, home/local office, and level are situation variables. Tenure is a person-situation variable, and age is a person variable.

Data from company records allowed us to compare the demographics of the respondents returning surveys with the total population of each company. There were no significant differences in age and tenure.

Climate Measurement

Following Schneider's (1983:111) "climate approach" to research, the Ethical Climate Questionnaire (ECQ) was developed to tap respondents' perceptions of how the members of their respective organizations typically make decisions concerning various "events, practices, and procedures" requiring ethical criteria (Victor and Cullen 1987).[2] The aim of Victor and Cullen's (1987) study was primarily instrument development, and it used a limited sample of MBA students, university faculty, and managers from a trucking firm. The items composing the instrument were written to capture the nine ethical climate types described above. Each of these types represented an a priori class of ethical reasoning in the organization.

The choice of criteria as the basis for operationalizing ethical climate raises the problem of distinguishing between the form and content of ethical reasoning (cf. Kohlberg 1984). As used here, ethical climate refers to the form of ethical reasoning—the structure of decision-making processes—rather than to its content—the range of possible outcome values of the decision.

Form and content are generally conceptualized as independent (Kohlberg 1984), since the same values (content) can arise from different forms of ethical reasoning (ethical criteria). For example, organizational values supporting profitability may be derived from any of the three ethical criteria (i.e., profit is good for me, profit benefits my friends, making profit is what organizations are supposed to do).

To tap the form dimension of ethical reasoning, the ECQ was designed specifically to identify organizational decision-making norms with *direct* links to supporting forms of ethical reasoning. Thus, although an organizational norm might be considered only the content of ethical reasoning, each question in the ECQ contained a direct referent to one of the ethical reasoning criteria. This operationalization was based on the assumption that "what one thinks about the subject matter of ethical thought, what one supposes it to be about, must affect what tests for acceptability or coherence are appropriate to it" (Williams 1985:73). The criteria in use (e.g., the best for each person, the rules, the interest of the organization), then, are observable artifacts of the organizational ethical reasoning process.

Questionnaire items represented each of the nine theoretical ethical climate types shown in Figure 1. Respondents were asked to indicate on a 6-point Likert-type scale how accurately each of the items described their general work climate. The six-point scale had the following verbal anchors: Completely false (0), Mostly false (1), Somewhat false (2), Somewhat true (3), Mostly true (4), Completely true (5). The instructions to the respondents read:

> We would like to ask you some questions about the general climate in your company. Please answer the following in terms of how it really is in your company, not how you would prefer it to be. Please be as candid as possible, remember, all your responses will remain *strictly* anonymous.

Climate questionnaires tap an observer's "description of the forms or styles of behavior in organizations" (Schneider 1975:461). In the present case, the behaviors, procedures, and events were chosen to reflect the use of ethical criteria in organizational decision making. The use of a climate questionnaire assumes that, at least on average, respondents can act as objective organizational observers. However, because perceptions are filtered by individual psychological characteristics and other individual differences, evaluative or affective responses to the organization can confound climate perceptions (Johannesson 1973). To avoid this problem, appropriate instrument design required questions emphasizing description rather than feelings (Schneider 1975, 1983; Schneider and Snyder 1975). Thus, following Schneider's suggestions and as noted by Victor and Cullen for the initial version of the ECQ, the measure of ethical climate did not "focus on whether the respondent believed he or she behaved ethically nor did it emphasize whether the respondent saw the ethical climate as good or bad" (Victor and Cullen 1987:58). . . .

Discussion

The current study investigated the antecedents of ethical work climates in organizations. The specification of such antecedents permits the development of both ethical climate theory and the managerial implications of ethical climate. The major findings of the study, in addition to confirming the multidimensionality of ethical climate (Victor and Cullen 1987) are evidence for at least three distinct sources of ethical climate: sociocultural, bureaucratic-structural, and firm-specific sources.

Ethical Climate as Work Climate

In terms of the more general literature on work climates, the results strengthen two arguments by Schneider (1975, 1983). First, the identification of an ethical climate supports Schneider's argument that there are many types of work climates. Second, the wide range of relationships between the climate types and the evaluations of company ethics supports Schneider's argument that climate differs from affective responses to organizations.

However, differing from the more traditional climate literature in which no systematic theory links the numerous climate types studied, our research examined several possible climate types on the basis of a single theoretical focus. The basis of this theoretical argument was the integration of philosophical ethical theory, psychological theories of moral development, and sociocultural theories of organizations. The results indicate that climates for organizations and groups within organizations are defined primarily in terms of the fundamental ethical criteria described. Only within the principle criterion, however, did the loci of analyses define different climate types. This suggests that, unlike climates emphasizing egoism or benevolence criteria for decision making, ethical climates based on the use of principles or rules have an organization-relative focus generated by the individual, the organization, or by other systems such as the law.

Substantively, these findings and the similarity in satisfaction levels across companies suggest that most workers develop at least a palliative level of satisfaction with their organization's climates. Those who fail to fit in an organization's climate probably turn over while others operate in their "zone of indifference" (Barnard 1938). Future research might consider the impact of fit between the individual's level of moral development and the organization's ethical climates. Lack of fit may produce stress, turnover, or dissatisfaction.

Antecedents of Ethical Climate

From the analysis of variance in climates between and within companies, there is evidence that ethical climates, as normative control systems for organizations, are multidetermined by societal norms, organizational form, and firm-specific factors.

Social norms.   Meyer and Rowan (1977) argued that, to gain legitimacy, organizations develop structures that reflect the myths and rules of society and not just the technical requirements of production. These myths and rules are institutionalized, which "involves the processes by which social processes, obligations, or actualities come to take on rule-like status in social thought and action" (Meyer and Rowan 1977:341). We suspect that climates in organizations, like structures, also reflect, in part, institutionalized societal norms.

The similarity among companies in terms of the caring climate implies that societal norms require organizations to develop at least a minimal caring environment. Although statistically significant, the differences among the companies in terms of instrumentalism were also minimal, suggesting a more general sanctioning of instrumental norms. Not surprisingly, the caring climate was the most preferred by the workers and instrumentalism was both the least dominant and the least preferred climate dimension.

As well as determining similarities between companies, the environment may also specify some between-company differences. With its dominant climate emphasizing the law and codes, the savings and loan company conforms to its highly regulated environmental context. We suspect that another sample of organizational types would show a different mix of dominant climate types. For example, in commissioned sales, a more instrumental climate is socially legitimate and self-interested behavior is the accepted norm. Thus, at least one source of the ethical climate in an organization appears to be the larger social-cultural environment in which it operates and from which it draws its membership.

Organizational form.   A second major determinant of ethical climate may be the organizational form. Both bureaucratic theory (Blau 1970) and economic theory predict a relationship between the normative and technological/structural characteristics of an organization. For example, bureaucratic theory proposes contingent relationships between size and complexity and authority structures (Blau and Meyer 1971). Similarly, transaction-cost economics specifies conditions that give rise to efficient forms of human cooperation and exchange (Williamson 1975). Since ethical climate theory describes the normative structure of the organization, ethical climates may also be determined by organizational form.

The observed variance in ethical climate is consistent with bureaucratic theory. For example, structural differentiation increases the problems of coordination and control (Blau 1970). The climates emphasizing rule and law and code in the geographically separate subunits in the savings and loan and the manufacturing plant may reflect managerial practices designed to deal with spatial differentiation. Blau and Schoenherr (1971) have argued that extensive rules and regulations for local departments substitute for personal control by management and reduce the risk of decentralization of decision making.

The reliance on caring and independence in the printing company may be seen as comparable to the power wielded by the maintenance workers described by Crozier (1964). In the latter case, the uncertainty and complexity of the repair function makes control by rules and direct supervision impossible, forcing control by expertness and group solidarity. In the printing company, the absence of direct supervision and rules results in a similar reliance on caring and independent judgment.

The observed variance between companies in ethical climate is also consistent with recent formulations of transaction-cost economics. For example, Ouchi (1980) identified three ideal-typical transaction forms: markets, bureaucracies, and clans. Markets are governed by price mechanisms, bureaucracies by norms of reciprocity and legitimate authority, and clans by common values and traditions enforced by reciprocal monitoring of group members. The increasing costs of transactions from the simple market to the more involved clan are warranted by an increasing difficulty in assessing exchanges between the individual and the group. Actual organizations have elements of the three basic types of transaction forms.

In an attempt to explain the etiology of organizational culture, Jones (1983:455) argued that transaction forms determine the norms and values associated with an organization's culture: organizational culture emerges "out of the institutional arrangements that are developed to regulate the exchanges or transactions between members of a social group." He reasoned that, when exchanges between the individual and the group are easy to monitor, such as with Ouchi's (1980) markets, the organizational culture emphasizes instrumental behaviors by both employees and employers. When transactions are more difficult to monitor, bureaucratic rules become a dominant cultural focus. Finally, when exchanges are most difficult to monitor, as with highly specialized professional organizations, and similar to Ouchi's clans, shared norms and values become the dominant cultural control mechanism, replacing rules and procedures.

The findings for the ethical climate differences among the companies seem to conform to Jones's expectation for organizational cultures. The savings and loan, telephone company, and manufacturing plant are traditionally bureaucratic organizations, and the individual's economic contribution to the organization is moderately difficult to monitor. Thus, as Jones expected for organizational culture, the climates that govern decisions with consequences for others (i.e., ethical climates) show a focus on rules, laws, and codes and not on the more market-related processes of individual initiative and self-serving behavior.

Interviews with the top-management team in the savings and loan confirmed that it had a long history of successfully controlling ethical behaviors by generating highly specific manuals and regulatory documents. However, many officers of the firm were concerned that laws, codes, and rules might be overemphasized, given the financial industry's new deregulated environment. A new CEO wanted to encourage a greater entrepreneurial and competitive orientation. We hypothesize that such a change would alter the economic governance system and produce more independent and/or instrumental ethical climates.

At the time the survey was conducted, the printing firm had no professional manager, and employees were left to make their own decisions about what was right and what needed to be done to keep the firm viable. Although possibly not the most efficient form of governance for this type of organization, the lack of monitoring for the work processes and outputs might make the transactions between the individuals and the group ambiguous, and a more clan-type governance structure would be predicted (Ouch 1980). Jones (1983) has argued that conditions associated with performance ambiguity result in partnerships and reciprocal monitoring predominating in professional or clan-like settings. He argued further that these conditions usually result for professional workers but may occasionally exist for small teams such as the printing shop. Partnerships bind independent individuals, and reciprocal monitoring controls contribution to the group. This suggests, as was true for the printing firm, that a caring and individual ethical climate should dominate the organizational culture. Earlier research (Victor and Cullen 1987) also showed that an academic organization had strong caring and individual climates but also included a strong orientation toward professional codes.

No organization was studied with a market form of economic governance. We hypothesize that commissioned-sales organizations approach the market conditions and thus would develop more instrumental and individual ethical climates.

However, even in such organizations, caring climates would become a factor to the degree that cooperation among the individuals is required. Regulated-sales industries such as real estate might also include law-and-code-based ethical climates in addition to instrumental and individual climates.

Firm-specific factors.   A third major determinant of ethical climate is the unique characteristics of organizations' histories and individuals' history in the organization. Climates are enhanced by the homogeneity-producing combination of organizational socialization and individual selection, attraction, and attrition (Schneider 1983; Schneider and Reichers 1983). Since different organizational positions are exposed to varied mixtures of these factors, it seems unlikely that organizations have homogeneous climates across subunits, jobs, and tenure levels.

The prime difference between tenure levels occurred for the valued caring climate. Except for very new workers, perceptions of a caring climate increased with tenure. We believe that this result shows an increased feeling of fit with the organizational community for longer tenured workers. Socialization is more extensive and attrition has weeded out those who fit less well with the organization.

Similar to the findings for tenure levels, the differences in caring climate across job levels may be due to a firm-specific factor. In the savings and loan organization, nonsupervisory personnel observed higher levels of caring climates than did officers, managers, and supervisors. Interviews with the top management team of this company revealed that recent officer and management firings inhibited the development of a more caring climate for managerial personnel.

Finally, the lower rule emphasis at the manufacturing plant may have been due to a recent reorganization. For most of its history, the plant had a traditional functional departmentalization. In the year preceding the survey, the plant reorganized into "business teams" with product departmentalization. One of the explicit goals of this reorganization was the reduction of internal rules and standard operating procedures, which was intended to stimulate innovation and flexibility.

Conclusions

Numerous studies have found that various types of work climates affect a range of organizational outcomes from performance and satisfaction (Pritchard and Karasick 1973; Downey, Hellriegel, and Slocum 1975) to research and development innovation (Abbey and Dickson 1983). Since the findings observed here suggest that ethical climates are similar to other types of work climates, ethical climates might affect similar organizational performance factors. Thus, this research adds to the work climate literature by identifying potentially important climate types.

Perhaps more important, however, and because ethical work climates have their basis in ethical reasoning, a consideration of ethical work climates extends organization theory into a new arena of ethical systems and management. If general work climate perceptions identify for organizational participants the key and rewarded behaviors and attitudes (Field and Abelson 1982; Schneider and Reichers 1983), then ethical climate perceptions may influence what ethical issues are considered at work and the types of criteria that are used to resolve these ethical issues. Thus ethical climates identify the normative systems that guide organizational decision making and the systemic responses to ethical dilemmas.

In this study, we employed both organization and economic theory to propose an ethical climate theory. As a result, we believe our work makes two key theoretical contributions. First, ethical climate theory brings ethical content into the mainstream of organization theory. It is our belief that organization theory needs to attend more explicitly to the ethical content in organizational processes. Ethical issues in organizations increasingly preoccupy theoreticians and practitioners. Firms are attempting to control the ethical decision making of individuals, and society is attempting to influence directly the ethical decision making of firms (e.g., through legislation like the foreign corrupt practices act, false claims act, and the racketeering-influenced and corrupt organizations statutes). Organization theory is well positioned to study and inform this process, as we demonstrate in this paper. Second, ethical climate theory provides further data on the relative contribution of environment, transaction efficiency, and firm idiosyncrasies to the nature of organizational normative systems. The procedures developed in this study provide a step toward the systematic understanding of the types and complexities of such normative systems.

Notes

1. The loci of analysis are somewhat similar to Kohlberg's (1984) classification of individual moral reasoning relative to the concept of self. Kohlberg distinguishes levels of moral development within criteria by locating sources of moral reasoning in the self or in a social system (the social perspective dimension in Kohlberg's stage specification). However, given that ethical climate is an organizational rather than an individual construct, the ethical climate typology does not represent Kohlberg's stages of individual moral reasoning nor do we propose a developmental sequence of stages of ethical reasoning as part of the organization or group life cycle. Moreover, outside of the organizational context from which it evolved and is maintained, we are unwilling to judge whether one type of normative system is inherently more moral than another. However, our hesitation to propose either developmental or normative distinctions between climates represents a recognition of the limits of our investigation rather than a theoretical prohibition against such propositions.

2. Copies of the instrument are available from the authors.

References

Abbey, Augustus, and John W Dickson 1983 "R & D work climate and innovation in semiconductors." Academy of Management Journal, 26:362–368.

Ashforth, Blake E. 1985 "Climate formation: Issues and extensions." Academy of Management Review, 10:837–847.

Barnard, Chester A. 1938 The Functions of the Executive. Cambridge, MA: Harvard University Press.

Blau, Peter M. 1970 "A formal theory of differentiation in organizations." American Sociological Review, 35:201–218.

Blau, Peter M., and Marshall W. Meyer 1971 Bureaucracy in Modern Society. New York: Random House.

Blau, Peter M., and Richard A Schoenherr 1971 The Structure of Organizations. New York: Basic Books.

Campbell, John, Marvin D. Dunnette, Edward E. Lawler, and Karl E. Weick 1970 Managerial Behavior, Performance, and Effectiveness. New York: McGraw-Hill.

Clinard, Marshall B. 1983 Corporate Ethics and Crime. Beverly Hills. CA: Sage.

Clinard, Marshall B., and Peter C. Yeager 1980 Corporate Crime. New York: Free Press.

Crozier, Michael 1964 The Bureaucratic Phenomenon. Chicago: University of Chicago Press.

Cullen, Francis T., William J Maakestad, and Gray Cavender 1987 Corporate Crime under Attack. Cincinnati: Anderson.

Deal, Terrence A., and Allen A. Kennedy 1982 Corporate Culture. Reading, MA: Addison-Wesley.

Downey, H. Kirk, Don Hellriegel, and John W. Slocum 1975 "Congruence between individual needs, organizational climate, job satisfaction and performance." Academy of Management Journal, 18:149–155.

Drexler, John A. 1977 "Organizational climate: Its homogeneity within organizations." Journal of Applied Psychology, 62:38–42.

Field, R. H. George, and Michael A. Abelson 1982 "Climate: A reconceptualization and proposed model." Human Relations, 35:181–201.

Fritzche, David J., and H. Becker 1984 "Linking management behavior to ethical philosophy." Academy of Management Journal, 27:166–175.

Gilligan, Carol 1982 In a Different Voice. Cambridge, MA: Harvard University Press.

Gouldner, Alvin W 1957 "Cosmopolitans and locals: Toward an analysis of latent social roles." Administrative Science Quarterly, 2:281–306.

Guion, Robert M 1973 "A note on organizational climate." Organizational Behavior and Human Performance 9:120–125.

Haan, Norma, Elaine Aerts, and Bruce A. Cooper 1985 On Moral Grounds. New York: New York University Press.

Higgins, Ann, Clark Power, and Lawrence Kohlberg 1984 "The relationship of moral atmosphere to judgments of responsibility." In W. Kurtines and J. Gewirtz (eds.), Morality. Moral Behavior and Moral Development: 74–106. New York: Wiley.

Honigmann, John J. 1959 The World of Man. New York: Harper & Row.

Howe, J. G. 1977 "Group climate: An exploratory analysis of construct validity." Organizational Behavior and Human Performance, 19:106–125.

James, Lawrence R., and Allan P. Jones 1974 "Organizational climate: A review of theory and research." Psychological Bulletin, 81:1096–1112.

Johannesson, Russell E. 1973 "Some problems in the measurement of organizational climate." Organizational Behavior and Human Performance, 10:118–144.

Jones, Gareth R. 1983 "Transaction costs, property rights, and organizational culture: An exchange perspective." Administrative Science Quarterly, 28:454–467.

Kalish, Steven E. 1980 "The attorney's role in the private organization." Nebraska Law Review, 59:1–10.

Kohlberg, Lawrence 1967 "Moral and religious education and the public schools: A developmental view." In T. Sizer (ed.), Religion and Public Education: 164–183. Boston: Houghton Mifflin.
1969 "Stage and sequence: The cognitive-development approach to socialization." In David A. Goslin (ed.), Handbook of Socialization Theory and Research: 347–480. Chicago: Rand McNally.
1984 The Philosophy of Moral Development. New York: Harper & Row.

Kornhauser, William 1962 Scientists in Industry: Conflict and Accommodation. Berkeley CA: University of California Press.

Kurtines, William M. 1984 "Moral behavior as rule governed behavior: A psychosocial role-theoretical approach to moral behavior and development." In W. Kurtines and J. Gewirtz (eds.), Morality, Moral Behavior and Moral Development: 303–324. New York: Wiley.
1986 "Moral behavior as rule governed behavior: Person and situation effects on moral decision making." Journal of Personality and Social Psychology, 50:784–791.

LaFollette, William R., and Henry P. Sims, Jr. 1975 "Is satisfaction redundant with organizational climate?" Organizational Behavior and Human Performance, 13:257–278.

Lewin, Karl, Ronald Lippitt, and Ralph K. White 1939 "Patterns of aggressive behavior in experimentally created social climates." Journal of Social Psychology, 10:271–299.

Lewis, David K. 1969 Convention: A Philosophical Study. Cambridge, MA: Harvard University Press.

Merton, Robert K. 1957 Social Theory and Social Structure. New York: Free Press.

Meyer, John W., and Brian Rowan 1977 "Formal structure of organizations as myth and ceremony." American Journal of Sociology, 83:340–363.

Nunnally, Jum C. 1978 Psychometric Theory, 2d ed. New York: McGraw-Hill.

Ouchi, William G. 1980 "Markets bureaucracies. and clans." Administrative Science Quarterly, 25:129–141.

Peters, Thomas J., and Robert H. Waterman, Jr. 1982 In Search of Excellence. New York: Harper & Row.

Pritchard, Robert D., and Bernard W. Karasick 1973 "The effects of organizational climate on managerial job performance and job satisfaction." Organizational Behavior and Human Performance, 9:126–146.

Raelin, Joseph A. 1985 The Clash of Cultures: Managers and Professionals. Boston: Harvard Business School Press.

Renwick, Patricia A. 1975 "Perception and management of superior subordinate conflict." Organizational Behavior and Human Performance, 13:444–456.

Sathe, Vijay 1983 "Implications of corporate culture: A manager's guide to action." Organizational Dynamics, 12:5–23.

Schein, Edgar H. 1984 "Coming to a new awareness of organizational culture." Sloan Management Review 25:3–16.

Schneider, Benjamin 1975 "Organizational climate: An essay." Personnel Psychology, 28:447–479
1983 "Work climates: An interactionist perspective." In N. W. Feimer and E. S. Geller (eds.). Environmental Psychology: Directions and Perspectives: 106–128. New York: Praeger.

Schneider, Benjamin, and Arnon E. Reichers 1983 "On the etiology of climates." Personnel Psychology, 36:19–39.

Schneider, Benjamin, and Robert A. Snyder 1975 "Some relationships between job satisfaction and organizational climate." Journal of Applied Psychology, 60:318–328.

Scott, W. Richard 1966 "Professionals in bureaucracies—Areas of conflict." In Howard M. Vollmer and Donald L. Mills (eds.), Professionalization: 265–275. Englewood Cliffs, NJ: Prentice-Hall.

Smircich, Linda 1983 "Concepts of culture and organizational analysis." Administrative Science Quarterly, 28:339–358.

Turiel, Elliot, and J. G. Smetana 1984 "Social knowledge and action: The coordination of domains." In W. Kurtines and J. Gewirtz (eds.), Morality, Moral Behavior, and Moral Development: 201–281. New York: Wiley.

Victor, Bart, and John B. Cullen 1987 "A theory and measure of ethical climate in organizations." In W. C. Frederick (ed.), Research in Corporate Social Performance and Policy: 51–71. Greenwich, CT: JAI Press.

Wall Street Journal 1987 "Sleepy watchdogs: Regulation of brokers by security industry seems to be faltering." July 27: 1, 17.

Weiss, William L. 1986 "Minerva's owl: Building a corporate value system." Journal of Business Ethics. 5:243–247.

Williams, Bernard 1985 Ethics and the Limits of Philosophy. Cambridge, MA: Harvard University Press.

Williamson, Oliver E. 1975 Markets and Hierarchies: Analysis and Anti-trust Implications. New York: Free Press.

CASE F

SHOULD WE CONTINUE?

Georgia, an occupational therapist, is on contract from a large hospital to a community-based infant development program for the physically handicapped and developmentally disabled. The program serves children from birth through three years, with a variety of disabilities, on an outpatient basis. Family education and counseling is an integral part of the program and at least one parent must accompany the child to therapy.

One patient, a 27-month-old girl named Annie, has been seen in the infant development program for the past 14 months and has been receiving occupational, physical, and speech therapy. Her diagnosis is cerebral palsy with severe to profound mental retardation. Her progress in all areas of development has been minimal and may be attributed to the maturational processes rather than to insufficient therapy.

It has been the program's unwritten policy to refer those children who have not benefited from direct therapeutic intervention—because of severe mental retardation or emotional disturbances—to two other local centers that are better equipped and staffed to meet their needs. The decision to refer a child out of the program is based on the findings of a team that includes occupational, physical, and speech therapists, a social worker, a psychologist, and a pediatrician. In the past two years, since the program's inception, the team has referred at least ten children to the other two facilities. None of these referrals was challenged by the director until the case of Annie.

Annie's referral to a center geared to the needs of retarded children would have been a routine matter if not for her unusual family situation. Last spring, Annie's aunt, who is a local children's television personality, held a benefit concert with the proceeds going to help build a specially designed playground for physically handicapped children at the facility. This event postponed the team's decision to refer Annie out of the program until the summer. Subsequently, Annie's grandfather died and her parents are planning to donate $50 thousand of his estate for the playground. The director has worked very hard to raise money for the playground and has now made it clear that Annie is not to be referred out of the infant program for at least one year (at age three).

Georgia's dilemma is whether or not to continue to provide therapy to this child whom she feels is no longer appropriate for the program, and is not benefiting from the therapeutic intervention.

The organizational and fiscal implications of this case are important considerations. Although not a direct employee of the facility, Georgia is under contract to it. She wants to maintain a good relationship between her hospital and the facility, and to fulfill the terms of her contract. The maintenance of a good relationship between the two facilities is stressed because the contract is renegotiated every year and has, for the past few years, been beneficial for each party. More recently, there has been speculation that the contract might not be renewed. "Rocking the boat" may cause friction on one or both sides, and jeopardize the contract discussions.

Two other organizational issues impinge on the fiscal impact of discontinuing therapy and referring the child out of the center. First, referring Annie out would mean a loss of revenue for the center that is already in financial difficulty. Second, if the child is referred to another center, the parents might change their minds about donating the $50 thousand for the playground. It might take another two years to raise that kind of money. Is it, then, more ethically important that Annie receive the appropriate intervention in the most appropriate setting, or that a playground be built that will benefit many children?

Psychosocial factors are also involved. Annie's parents are currently experiencing marital problems and other emotional stresses that are probably unrelated to their child's problems. Annie's mother has made a link to the center that appears to be a source of stability in her life. Annie is routinely brought to the center by her mother three times a week, where the mother can speak with the therapists and social workers about the family's problems. The parents are aware of the fact that when Annie reaches age three, some decision must be made about her placement; but they are satisfied with her present placement. Referring Annie out of the infant program before the parents are expecting it could place additional stress on the family. In addition, referral to a center that deals with severely retarded children may signify to the parents that all hope for a "normal," or at least functional, child has been abandoned. But is it fair to the parents to be wasting valuable time when their child could be benefiting from a more appropriate program? Do they have the right to know what is professionally considered best for their child? Do they have the right to choose what they think is best for their child regardless of what the "experts" think?

Georgia wonders about the ethics of retaining the child in the program so that the center may benefit from her grandfather's estate. It is true that the playground will be the only one in the county designed especially for the physically handicapped, and that Annie might benefit from it in the future. On the other hand, Annie is at a critical period for learning. Should she be deprived of an appropriate education in order to benefit other handicapped children?

For Georgia it is frustrating, both personally and professionally, to continue treating a child who does not demonstrate progress attributable to the therapy. After exploring all possible avenues of treatment, and consulting with other knowledgeable people in her field, she reaches the conclusion that her specific therapy is not appropriate at this time. Another setting, one that emphasizes education rather than therapy, may be more appropriate for Annie. Professionally, Georgia's job is to provide the most appropriate program for the child, or to see that the child is referred to an appropriate program. Another professional issue is the distribution of resources. If she continues to provide therapy to this child, she will have less time for children who will benefit more. Already, much time has been spent in meetings trying to decide if and when to refer Annie and her family to another center.

Legal factors are also involved. Therapists are required to document a patient's status in the facility every three months. The reports must verify that the child has been making progress in one or more of the therapies; otherwise, state aid for therapy is not renewed. It has been difficult for the therapists involved to write Annie's progress reports because there has been very little progress related to the therapy. In order to keep her on program, they have had to word reports "creatively" to imply that progress was being made.

In order to obtain the various views regarding the situation, Georgia meets individually with the director of the center, the social worker, the consulting pediatrician, and other therapists. The center's director, Mr. Greedle, is of the opinion that Annie's therapy should be continued in the infant development program and that any discussion about referring her to another center should be postponed until she reaches age three. In explaining his rationale, Mr. Greedle discusses the history and original purpose of the center, which was to provide evaluation and therapy to any child with a physical disability, speech impediment, or hearing impairment, regardless of the extent of the child's mental retardation or emotional disturbance. He feels that the center should continue to provide such service to the community. He acknowledges the fact that there now is another facility in the community that serves the needs of the retarded child, and that several other children have been referred from the program to that facility. But he stands firm in his opinion that Annie should remain in her present program and receive therapy. He denies that the family's donation is affecting his decision, and does not wish to discuss the matter further.

The social worker supports this view but offers a somewhat different rationale. She believes that the family situation, specifically the parents' relationship, is too fragile to cope with Annie's transfer to a new facility. The transfer would not only involve their adjustment to a new social worker and new therapists, but to a new group of parents and children as well. These children would be significantly more retarded than the children they are used to seeing. The realization that Annie is at a level comparable to these children may set off another emotional crisis that the family would be unable to handle at this time. She reasons that the parents need more time to adjust to the severity of Annie's situation and that they will accept the situation more easily in an environment with which they are comfortable. In addition, the parents might themselves come to the realization that Annie is not progressing as was initially hoped, and that perhaps an alternative placement should be considered.

The social worker has another reason for supporting the director's point of view. She feels that the good of the community must be considered before a decision is made in the case. A playground for the physically handicapped will not only benefit many children but it will also improve the image of the center and offer more competition to centers in surrounding areas.

An opposing point of view is expressed by the therapists in the infant program. They believe that Annie's therapy should be discontinued in order to facilitate referral to another, more appropriate agency. The consulting pediatrician expresses her support of this decision. Their first concern is Annie's overall development. They feel that they are serving neither the child's nor the parents' best interests by maintaining her in a program that is not designed to meet her special needs. Since the parents have not been informed of these recommendations, the therapists feel that they are deceiving them by providing false hopes of progress. They believe that the parents have a right to know about Annie's status and the alternatives available to them. Both the therapists and the parents are discouraged about Annie's lack of progress. It is the therapists' and pediatrician's professional judgment that an alternative placement would greatly benefit both the child and her family, and facilitate their acceptance of the severity of Annie's disabilities.

Their second point of contention with the opposing view is the ethics of maintaining the child in the program based on financial gain to the center. While recognizing the importance of building the playground, they feel strongly that the benefits to the child should outweigh the benefits to the organization. They see themselves in service professions and in programs designed to meet the needs of every child on an individual basis. They conclude that they cannot meet this child's needs adequately, and are therefore professionally obligated to refer her to a program where her needs can be better met. In addition, they have referred several children out of the program in the past. By keeping Annie in the program they would be treating this case unequally compared to the other cases. In the other cases, they had prioritized the child's needs to be first; in this case they would be placing the higher priority on financial gain. These inconsistencies would hinder the regularization of formal referral policies and would run counter to established practice.

Questions for Discussion

1. What should Georgia ethically do? Why?
2. Should rules or relationships prevail in this case? How is the issue of denigration versus dignity involved?
3. Which is more ethically important: the good of each individual or the good of the whole?
4. Whose judgment should prevail ethically?
5. What options does Georgia have, and what are their probable consequences?

Annotated Bibliography

Bellah, R., R. Madsen, W. Sullivan, A. Swidler, and S. Tipton. *Habits of the Heart.* New York: Harper and Row, 1985. A landmark macro analysis of societal values and habits that can be well adapted to reflection on microethics.

Block, P. *Stewardship: Choosing Service Over Self-Interest.* San Francisco: Berrett-Koehler, 1993. Although extremely macro in perspective, this book provides reflective fodder for contrasting control and consistency with partnership and choice.

Harvey, J. *The Abilene Paradox.* Lexington, MA: Heath, 1988. Offers a creative structured reflection on the absurdities of organizational life.

Kellman, H., and V. Hamilton. *Crimes of Obedience.* New Haven, CT: Yale University Press, 1989. An insightful macro analysis that can be highly useful for ethical reflection at the micro level.

Lakoff, R. *Talking Power.* New York: Basic Books, 1990. A sensational reflection on the subtleties of language; it offers wonderful insight for ethical reflection.

Morgan, R. "Self and Co-Worker Perceptions of Ethics and Their Relationships to Leadership and Salary," *Academy of Management Journal* 36, no. 1 (February 1993): 200–14. The empirical evidence presented prods reflection on our self-image versus our actual behavior.

Visotzky, B. *The Genesis of Ethics*. New York: Crown, 1996. An insightful illustration of imaginative reflective skill applied to analysis of biblical ethical dilemmas.

APPROACHES TO ETHICAL ANALYSIS: TOOLS AND METHODS

IN ADDITION to moral imagination skill, ethical maturity requires keen reasoning. As Sidney Callahan maintains, ethical maturity consists of an integration of our creative, affective, and reasoning capacities.[1] This chapter probes the reasoning aspect.

Ethical reasoning, Harron, Burnside, and Beauchamp remind us, contrasts with intuition and casuistry. Intuitionism assumes that professionals of good character and educated minds instinctively know what ethically to do; we don't need to reason things out. Casuistry assumes that there is a rule for every situation, hence, no need to think things through. Ethical reasoning, on the other hand, "assumes that rules, principles and concepts must be pursued in an orderly way to be useful in finding answers to new questions."[2] The key word is *orderly*. Ethical reasoning attempts to bring rigor, discipline, and structure to complexity that might otherwise be confusing, even chaotic. In Maguire's words: "Early impressions, in ethics and elsewhere, come to us in largely undifferentiated globs. Reason and analysis break them up and sort them out so that we can know what it really is that we are talking about."[3] Moreover, Bok is correct: without discipline and rigor in our thinking, "bias, self-deception, even sleight of hand" easily take over.[4] We need to be *systematic* in our reasoning, and we need to be doing this in the micro dimension of healthcare, not just in macroethics.

Process versus Decision

The structure, rigor, and discipline I am stressing here have nothing to do with ethical decisions *per se*; rather they have to do with the *process* of discerning decisions. The former is the focus of what is often called the "moral education" model for ethical development, while the latter is typically referred to as the "ethical reasoning" model.[5] Ethical reasoning stresses step-by-step, participative approaches to ethical discernment. Clarity and balance are its hallmarks; broadened awareness is its quest. As London has argued, the "key to mastery" is that set of higher brain processes that produces an "ethic of awareness."[6] But the process of getting there requires going beyond conscience into a state of consciousness appropriate to anyone paid to be a healthcare professional; it goes beyond one's "internal thought experiment" to dynamics such as asking friends, elders, and colleagues for advice, looking up precedents, and conversing with stakeholders.[7]

A mature ethical reasoning process, I am convinced, is characterized by (1) community collaboration and (2) systematic methodology. Glaser eloquently portrays what he calls the "community of concern" in healthcare ethics. Any process of ethical decision making is flawed, he argues, if the proper community is not part of the process: "To weigh complex values, we need complex, first-hand experience, as well as adequate analysis of that experience."[8] Marilyn Ray concurs. In her extensive research of nursing ethics she finds that "communal moral interaction" is key to the development of ethical maturity.[9]

This communitarian aspect of any ethically mature reasoning process is surprisingly stressed by Stephen Carter in his recent treatise on *Integrity*. Dialogue, he contends, is essential to sound ethical reflection, which is essential to true integrity.[10] Visotzky, in putting this community dialogue emphasis into practice, has found remarkable development of ethical reasoning skill with participants in his workshops.[11] Both authors seem to embrace Harmon's recent argument that "responsible decisions, which are by definition social products, cannot be made alone."[12]

The message of all of these ethicists is that a single-minded ethical reasoning process inevitably degenerates and debilitates judgment.[13] Remember our friend, Diane the medical director, back in chapter 4, who discovered some apparently unsafe conditions? The point is that had Diane single-mindedly jumped to expose the firm, chances are the company would have moved south, causing economic harm to the very employees she was presumably protecting. Had she similarly caved in and simply deferred to her superiors, chances are the unhealthy conditions would have lingered longer. By opening up dialogue in her reasoning process, she helped to reconcile what had seemed an inalterable conflict.

Methodologies

The second key to sound ethical reasoning is systematic methodology. Methodologies are simply road maps, guideposts, or organizers to help the thought process generate and order ideas. They can be viewed as crutches that help us bear the weight of complexity and time constraints in the ordinary routine of healthcare, and as catalytic tools to help open airways for ideas that otherwise might be clogged or overlooked. A good methodology—customized to each healthcare professional's thinking traits—opens the mind, frees reasoning capacity, and broadens awareness; a poor methodology closes the mind, constrains reasoning, and limits awareness. In the hectic hubbub of everyday healthcare, we all need help with discernment; we all need an ethical reasoning system. The trick is to find the method that helps *me*, the individual, to test it, to customize it, and to refine it until it becomes habitual. As John Mitchell crisply puts it: "Good ethics is not a matter of luck; ethical behavior is not in the hands of fate. Ethics is work. . . . [Healthcare professionals] enjoy the prospect of acting ethically when they are willing to subject themselves to the discipline of an adequate methodology."[14] The following illustrative methodologies are intended to help professionals design a method suited to their individual talents and situations.

Check Lists offer a simple and flexible methodological approach. It was in navy pilot training that I first learned the brilliance of the check list methodology. There was a check list for everything, and the first thing our flight instructors taught us was to use them always, rigorously, without exception! Developed over years of experience, they not only kept us out of trouble, they saved our lives. The simple check lists made sure we did not forget something important. They made the complexity of flying a jet a whole lot simpler. Some of us would add items, but all of us would religiously check off each standard item.

Check lists are reminder notes. In ethics they help us to remember to factor into our reasoning items we may tend to forget. A simple example is as follows:

_____ Get the facts.

_____ Specify the stakeholders.

_____ Describe your feelings.

_____ Clarify the values involved.

_____ Imagine the options beyond either-or.

_____ Describe the control mechanisms operating.

_____ Articulate probable consequences of options.

_____ Discuss with someone.

_____ Choose your response.

Check lists like this can be easily customized and modified. With practice they can become second nature. The use of them in naval aviation has prevented many a crash. The use of them in healthcare ethics might well prevent many an unethical behavior.

Similar to the check list approach is the *questions* methodology. Daniel Maguire maintains that failure to ask the right questions is the most common cause of ethical error. The art of ethics, he insists, resides in the ability to ask the "reality revealing" questions.[15] His question methodology has four elements:

1. *What?* This seeks the facts and factors at hand.
2. *Who, when, where, why,* and *how?* This question illuminates the actors, places, and timing involved, as well as the means, style, purposes, and motives.
3. *What might happen if?* This question pursues foreseeable effects of current actions and decisions.
4. *What are the viable alternatives?* Here we seek options.

Laura Nash has espoused a 12-question ethical reasoning methodology which she views as "a way to articulate an idea of the responsibilities involved and to lay them open for examination."[16] While her target is macroethics, her questions can be adapted to microethics concerns as well. Her items are as follows:

1. Have you defined the problem *accurately?*
2. How would you define the problem if you stood on the *other* side of the fence?
3. *How* did this situation occur in the first place?
4. To whom and to what do you give your *loyalty* as a person and as a member of the corporation?
5. What is your *intention* in making this decision?
6. How does this intention compare with the probable *results?*
7. Whom could your decision or action *injure?*
8. Can you *discuss* the problem with the affected parties before you make your decision?
9. Are you confident that your position will be as *valid* over a long period of time as it seems now?
10. Could you *disclose* without qualm your decision or action to your boss, your CEO, the board of directors, your family, society as a whole?
11. What is the *symbolic potential* of your action if understood? If misunderstood?

12. Under what conditions would you allow *exceptions* to your stand?

A third example of the question methodology is a values-based list in which questions are specifically linked to the values at stake. The following is one variation:

Competence
_____ Do I have the skills my position assumes?
_____ Do I generate options and ideas?

Fairness
_____ Do I follow due process?
_____ Do I listen to other views?
_____ Do I follow procedures?

Legality
_____ Do I know the laws and policies involved?
_____ Do I bend the rules?

Responsiveness
_____ How do I identify with the clients?
_____ What provision do I make for input from them?
_____ Is my response affected by client power, race, size, etc.?

The beauty of the question methodology is that it can be so readily adapted to each professional's needs, blind spots, and triggers. For some it could effectively be as simple as the question, "Whose judgment should prevail?" which we broached in chapter 5; for others it might involve a sophisticated barrage.

A third possible moral reasoning methodology is the *principles* approach that draws from the normative philosophical tradition of ethics. A fairly straightforward illustration of this method is Marcia Bacon's distinction between the duty of *justice* and the duty of *benevolence*.[17] The former is a duty we owe to everyone; the latter is a duty we are not able to afford everyone. When these are in conflict the duty of justice overrides the duty of benevolence.

A more involved example of this approach is Hosmer's "first principles" method.[18] He identifies four basic principles as particularly useful in ethical reasoning. One is the *utilitarian* principle: always act to generate the greatest good with the least harm. Second is the *universalism* principle: do unto others as you would have them do unto you. The third is the principle of *distributive justice*: always act such that the least empowered are benefited in some way. And the fourth he calls the *personal liberty* principle: act such that the ability of others to lead dignified lives is enhanced. This methodology recognizes that, because each principle expresses only a portion of truth, any ethical situation needs to be examined from all four dimensions: "Though this increases the complexity of moral reasoning, it leads to valuable insight and understanding."[19]

Hosmer recently developed a much more involved illustration of the principles methodology.[20] In attempting to capture the bulk of our normative tradition, he has derived ten ethical principles to use in ethical reasoning deliberations:

1. *Self-Interests*: Never take any action that is not in the long-term self-interests of yourself and the healthcare organization to which you belong.
2. *Personal Virtues*: Never take any action that is not honest, open, and truthful, and which you would not be proud to see reported widely in national newspapers and on television.
3. *Religious Injunctions*: Never take any action that is not kind, and that does not build a sense of community.
4. *Government Requirements*: Never take any action that violates the law.
5. *Utilitarian Benefits*: Never take any action that does not result in greater good than harm in your healthcare facility.
6. *Universal Rules*: Never take any action that you would be unwilling to see another healthcare professional take in similar situations.
7. *Individual Rights*: Never take any action that abridges the agreed-upon rights of others.
8. *Economic Efficiency*: Always act to maximize profits subject to legal and market constraints and with full recognition of external costs.
9. *Distributive Justice*: Never take any action in which the least among us are harmed in some way.
10. *Contributing Liberty*: Never take any action that will interfere with the rights of others for self-fulfillment.

Hosmer and others argue that the reflection which this principles-based methodology engenders leads to greater moral reasoning.

A fourth approach, for those whose minds are better opened with a nudge from numbers, is the *decision science* methodology. It employs matrices, multi-attribute utility models, performance tables and the like to help organize information and thoughts in ethical reasoning. For example, this methodology would organize information gleaned from the power/values/controls reality prism (see chapters 3 through 5) as shown in Figure 7.1.

Using this matrix general assessments are made of the strength or weakness of each alternative at each criterion. This requires filling in the

Figure 7.1 Matrix of Alternatives

CRITERIA (Values)

ALTERNATIVES	A	B	C	D	E
1					
2					
3					
4					
5					

performance table with assessments of how each alternative ranks with respect to each criterion. Employing a modified Likert scale, rankings could range from very low to low, neutral, high, and very high. These involve a subjective judgment, of course, but they can help a professional consider more clearly how each value is affected by each option identified. The process helps to organize or structure thinking.

These general assessments can then be converted into quantitative measures reflecting utility. Each cell of the performance table is given a point value that forces the thinking process to refine further the assessment of relationship between alternatives and values. "Weighted utilities" can then be calculated, which will suggest which alternative action holds "maximum utility" in terms of the values criteria. Decision science buffs understand the mechanics of this approach. The net result is a systematic ethical reasoning process for evaluating alternative possible responses to complex situations.

Finally, there are simple methodologies such as those focused on *consequences*. Sometimes identified with utilitarianism, it has been a favored approach to the macroethics of healthcare. A consequentialism methodology emphasizes specific identification of outcomes from various alternatives and a comparative analysis of those anticipated results. John Casey is one proponent of this approach: "Responsible decisions require that people and groups that may be affected have been correctly identified, and the consequences of the contemplated actions anticipated." It is particularly important, he stresses, "that ethical decision-makers see the negative consequences—the harm, the dislocations—of their decisions."[21]

But identifying consequences can be easier said than done. So tools are often employed with this method. Illustrative is the simple matrix shown in Figure 7.2.

Figure 7.2   The Likelihood of Consequences

	Consequences	
Likelihood	Positive	Negative
Possible		
Probable		
Certain		

Tools like this matrix can help organize the thinking process. They can, of course, be refined, and can help provide clarity. For example, a matrix like this one can help us analyze possible positive consequences versus certain negative consequences, and so forth.

Conclusion

Good ethical reasoning requires the creative energy of community dialogue and the discipline and structure of a methodological system. Most of us need these road maps to keep us from getting lost and to guide us safely to our destinations. Dialogue and method can help healthcare professionals to identify and utilize the resources needed to advance ethical maturity. Although following a communitarian process and a rigorous methodology does not ensure that good ethical choices will always result—the limitations of process and methodology are numerous—the lack of dialogue and method undoubtedly makes for a more difficult and less mature ethical roadway.

Notes

1. S. Callahan, 1990, *Good Conscience: Reason and Emotion in Moral Decision Making* (San Francisco: Harper).

2. F. Harron, J. Burnside, and T. Beauchamp, 1983, *Health and Human Values* (New Haven, CT: Yale), p. 4.

3. D. Maguire, 1978, *The Moral Choice* (Minneapolis, MN: Winston), p. 262.

4. S. Bok, 1979, *Lying* (New York: Vintage), p. 57.

5. D. S. Lee, 1993, "Ethical Decisionmaking: Lessons To Be Learned from Temptation." *Public Voices* 1, no. 1 (fall): 45–53.

6. P. London, 1971, *Behavior Control* (New York: Harper and Row), ch. 1.

7. S. Bok, *Lying*, p. 101.

8. J. Glaser, 1994, *Three Realms of Ethics* (Kansas City, MO: Sheed and Ward), p. 26.

9. M. Ray, 1994, "Communal Moral Experience as the Starting Point for Research in Health Care Ethics." *Nursing Outlook* 42, no. 3 (May/June): 104–109.

10. S. Carter, 1996, *Integrity* (New York: Basic Books), pp. 22ff, 59.

11. B. Visotzky, 1996, *The Genesis of Ethics* (New York: Crown).

12. M. M. Harmon, 1995, *Responsibility as Paradox* (Newbury Park, CA: Sage).

13. See S. Bok, 1984, *Secrets* (New York: Vintage), p. 25, for views as far back as Lord Acton on this matter.

14. J. Mitchell, 1980, "Ethics in Business Today." *Journal of Business Education* 4 (November): 62.

15. D. Maguire, 1979, *The Moral Choice* (Minneapolis, MN: Winston), pp. 128ff.

16. L. Nash, 1981, "Ethics Without the Sermon." *Harvard Business Review* 59, no. 6 (November/December): 79–90.

17. M. Bacon, 1984, *The Moral Status of Loyalty* (Dubuque, IA: Kendall/Hunt).

18. L. Hosmer, 1987, "Making Ethical Decisions." *Health Management Quarterly* 9, no. 3 (third quarter): 7–8.

19. Ibid., p. 8.

20. L. Hosmer, 1994, *Moral Leadership in Business* (Homewood, IL: Irwin). See also his article "Trust: The Connecting Link Between Organizational Theory and Philosophical Ethics." *Academy of Management Review* 20, no. 2 (April 1995): 379–403.

21. J. Casey, 1989, "Ideals Aside, Ethics Are Practical." *The New York Times* (25 June), p. 8-1.

READING

As Thomas Jones correctly observes, examinations of ethical decision-making methods are in relatively short supply. The following article from the generic management literature significantly raises the level of discourse. Using the rich concept of "moral intensity," the author offers a practical approach to improving our skills at ethical reasoning. Once again, although Jones' focus seems to be the macro dimension, his insights are salient and germane to our microethics interest. Note his definition of a moral issue as an action that harms or benefits others even when the actor is unaware that a moral issue is at stake.

After critically presenting a useful overview of recently proposed models for ethical decision making, Jones introduces his notion of moral intensity as a means of raising our consciousness of ethical "timing" and of ways in which we deal with the ethical dimension of our work. If we take the six components of moral intensity that the article discusses and apply them to the routine situations of our daily workplace, we might develop an enlightened perspective on the micro dimension of our everyday healthcare settings. In particular, his four propositions about high moral intensity feed our argument that the micro dimension—that area of such low, subtle moral intensity—is painfully underappreciated and underanalyzed in healthcare ethics dialogue. Finally, what about Jones' closing sentence? Would you agree that this is a problem in that the question of what is substantively important in ethics has not been raised regarding microethics?

ETHICAL DECISION MAKING BY INDIVIDUALS IN ORGANIZATIONS: AN ISSUE-CONTINGENT MODEL

Thomas M. Jones

Reasons for increased societal focus on ethics in organizations are many. Insider trading on Wall Street; defense contractor scandals, involving both private and public sectors; rental car repair overcharges; and the resignation of over 100 Reagan administration officials have helped keep ethical issues in the public eye. Institutions have responded to these challenges in a variety of ways. Corporations have established or updated codes of ethics, and some business schools have responded with increased offerings in business ethics. Academe has also produced a greatly expanded literature on the subject of ethics, including textbooks and two scholarly journals—the *Journal of Business Ethics* and the *Business and Professional Ethics Journal.* An entire volume of *Research in Corporate Social Performance and Policy* has been devoted to business ethics and values (Frederick 1987).

Despite this increased attention to ethics in organizations, theoretical and empirical examinations of ethical decision making in organizations are in relatively short supply. Trevino (1986) offered a general theoretical model whereas Ferrell and Gresham (1985), Hunt and Vitell (1986), and Dubinsky and Loken (1989) offered models that focus on marketing ethics. Rest (1986) presented a theory of individual ethical decision making that can easily be generalized to organizational settings. Among the empirical contributions to date are the works of Hegarty and Sims (1978, 1979) Fritzsche and Becker (1983), Frederick (1987), Laczniak and Inderrieden (1987), Fritzsche (1988), Dubinsky and Loken (1989), and Weber (1990). One reason for this relative paucity of theoretical and empirical work in ethics may be that few scholars are interested in both ethics and organizational behavior and decision making. The models that have emerged are the products of scholars in psychology or psychology-based disciplines, including organizational behavior and marketing. In addition, organizational scholars may be reluctant to study value-based issues because of ideological reasons or because methodological problems are considered difficult to surmount. Although this article is grounded in social psychology, it also contains elements of moral philosophy and applied ethics.

Thomas M. Jones, "Ethical Decision Making by Individuals in Organizations: An Issue-Contingent Model." *Academy of Management Review* 16, no. 2 (April 1991). 366–95. Copyright 1991, the Academy of Management. Reprinted by permission. Thomas M. Jones is professor of organization and environment at the University of Washington.

The purpose of this article is to introduce concepts not present in prior models and to offer a model that supplements, but does not replace, other models. The article argues that moral issues vary in terms of their moral intensity and that an issue-contingent model of ethical decision making and behavior can add significantly to the understanding of moral processes This is an initial attempt to identify, not empirically validate, the issue-related components of ethical behavior on which future research may be based. It attempts to build a nomological net of constructs and theory, which can be formally validated and tested in future studies. The validity of the proposed constructs is here limited to content validity based on logic, observation, and, in some cases, empirical analogy. The article also advances and discusses four general research propositions.

Definitions

Three definitions are central to the article. First, a moral issue is present where a person's actions, when freely performed, may harm or benefit others (Velasquez and Rostankowski 1985). In other words, the action or decision must have consequences for others and must involve choice, or volition, on the part of the actor or decision maker. The definition is broad, decisions frequently have some consequences for others and volition almost always present, although the costs of certain choices may be high. In sum, many decisions are moral decisions simply because they have a moral component. Second, a moral agent is a person who makes a moral decision, even though he or she may not recognize that moral issues are stake. This feature of the definition is important because a central element of the moral decision-making model presented here is recognizing moral issues. (In this article, the terms moral and ethical are considered equivalent and will be used interchangeably, depending on context.)

Third, an ethical decision is defined as a decision that is both legal are morally acceptable to the larger community. Conversely, an unethical decision is either illegal or morally unacceptable to the larger community. The definition follows from Kelman and Hamilton's (1989) definition of crimes obedience and is consistent with the definitions used, either explicitly or implicitly, by some other authors in the field of ethics. Although the definition is admittedly imprecise and relativistic, it is adequate for the purposes of this article. Some authors, including Ferrell and Gresham (1985), Trevino(1986), Hunt and Vitell (1986), and Dubinsky and Loken (1989) did not provide substantive definitions of the terms ethical and unethical. Discussions regarding the difficulty of establishing substantive definitions for ethical behavior can be found in Cavanagh, Moberg, and Velasquez (1981), Beauchamp and Bowie (1979), and Jones (1980).

Existing Models

Rest (1986) proposed a four-component model for individual ethical decision making and behavior, whereby a moral agent must (a) recognize the moral issue, (b) make a moral judgment, (c) resolve to place moral concerns ahead of other concerns (establish moral intent), and (d) act on the moral concerns. He argued that each component in the process is conceptually distinct and that success in one stage does not imply success in any other stage. For example, a person with a well-developed sense of moral reasoning (Component 2) will not necessarily have great resolve to act morally (Component 3). Much of the empirical research conducted in the context of this model has involved either Component 2, called moral development by Kohlberg (1976) and Rest (1979, 1986), or the relationship between Components 2 and 4, moral development and action. Rest (1979) developed an instrument for measuring moral development that can be administered in groups and scored relatively easily, which probably accounts for the dozens of empirical studies involving this stage of the process.

Although Trevino (1986) did not directly address Rest's model, she offered a competing model, which implicitly builds on it. Her person-situation interactionist model begins with the existence of an ethical dilemma and proceeds to a cognitions stage, wherein Kohlberg's cognitive moral development model becomes operative. Moral judgments made in the cognitions stage are then moderated by individual and situational factors. Individual factors include ego strength, field dependence, and locus of control. Situational factors include elements of immediate job context, organizational culture, and characteristics of the work. Moral judgments, thus moderated, affect ethical or unethical behavior.

Ferrell and Gresham (1985) proposed a contingency framework for ethical decision making in marketing. In this model, an ethical issue or dilemma emerges from the social or cultural environment. The contingent factors that affect the decision maker are both individual (knowledge, values, attitudes, and intentions) and organizational (significant others and opportunity). The effect of significant others is supported in this model by differential association theory (Sutherland and Cressey 1970) and role-set theory (Merton 1957). Opportunity (to behave unethically) as a variable stems from the work of Cloward and Ohlin (1960) and, in Ferrell and Gresham's model, is related to the existence (or nonexistence) of professional codes, corporate policy, and rewards and punishment. The decision that emerges from this process leads first to behavior and next to evaluation of behavior, which, in turn, is the starting point for a feedback loop to individual and organizational factors.

Hunt and Vitell (1986) proposed a general theory of marketing ethics that consists of several stages. A substantially simplified summary of this model is offered here. Environmental factors (cultural, industrial, and organizational) and personal experiences affect perceptions of the existence of an ethical problem, alternatives, and consequences. In turn, these perceptions, along with deontological norms and an evaluation of consequences, lead to both deontological and teleological evaluations, which, in turn, lead to ethical judgments. Judgment affects intentions, which, along with situational constraints, affect behavior. A feedback loop leads from behavior to actual consequences and back to personal experiences.

Dubinsky and Loken (1989) presented an ethical decision-making model based on the theory of reasoned action (Fishbein and Ajzen 1975). Their model begins with behavioral beliefs, outcome evaluations, normative beliefs, and motivation to comply. The first two of these variables affect attitude toward ethical or unethical behavior; the latter two variables affect subjective norms toward ethical or unethical behavior. Finally, attitude and subjective norms lead to intentions to engage in ethical or unethical behavior which, in turn, affect actual behavior, ethical or unethical. No feedback loop is present.

Although they did not add to present theory, Ferrell, Gresham, and Fraedrich (1989) developed a five-stage synthesis of other models. Awareness (of ethical issues), cognitions (moral development), moral evaluations (deontological and teleological judgments), determination (intentions), and actions (ethical or unethical behavior) constitute the sequential order of their model. They also featured a feedback loop with behavioral evaluation of consequences leading to awareness, cognitions, moral evaluations, and determination.

Brommer, Gratto, Gravender, and Tuttle (1987) also claimed a model of ethical decision making, but it actually distills to a catalog (albeit a thorough one) of factors that influence ethical decision makers. Environmental factors (work, personal, professional, governmental, legal, and social) join individual attributes to affect the ethical decision process. In all, over 20 variables are expected to be relevant to ethical decision making in this formulation.

Each of these models has something to contribute to the understanding of ethical decision making. None, however, does more than hint that characteristics of the moral issue itself will affect the moral decision-making process. Ferrell and Gresham (1985) noted that the consensus regarding proper ethical conduct will be likely to change as the issue changes. They suggested that fewer people would endorse embezzling company funds than would endorse padding an expense account. Their model, however, includes no acknowledgement that issue differences affect ethical decision making. Hunt and Vitell (1986) added a teleological evaluation stage, wherein the consequences of the moral decision are evaluated, but they did not suggest a systematic relationship between consequences and subsequent elements of the model—intentions and behavior. Dubinsky and Loken (1989) implied that attitudes may vary according to the behavior being evaluated, but they made no attempt to explain how this variation would occur. In sum, existing models do not adequately account for differences in ethical issues.

A rough synthesis of existing models is useful for assessing their collective strengths and weaknesses. This synthesized model, shown in Figure 1, is necessarily simplified (e.g., feedback loops are omitted), and it uses Rest's (1986) four-stage model as a foundation.

The process begins with the environment, which typically includes

Figure 1 Synthesis of Ethical Decision-Making Models

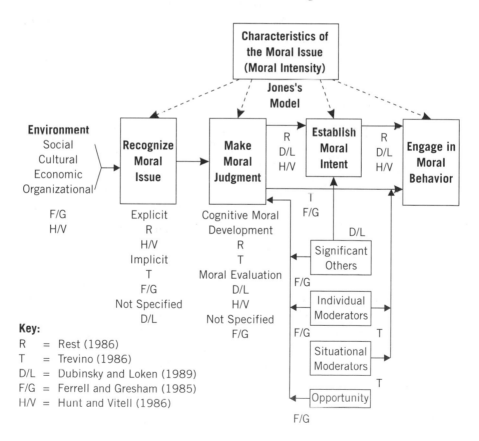

economic, social, cultural, and organizational factors (Ferrell and Gresham 1985; Hunt and Vitell 1986). From the environment emerge ethical issues (Ferrell and Gresham 1985; Hunt and Vitell 1986). Hunt and Vitell (1986) acknowledged that not all moral issues may be recognized by their use of the term perceived ethical problem, whereas Rest (1986) made recognition of moral issues an explicit element of his model. Trevino (1986) and Ferrell and Gresham (1985) left this step implicit, but Dubinsky and Loken (1989) did not include it.

Four of the five models contain some form of moral judgment stage. In Rest's (1986) and Trevino's (1986) models, cognitive moral development is the critical element in the judgment phase. For Hunt and Vitell (1986) and Dubinsky and Loken (1989), moral evaluation (teleological and deontological) takes place. Ferrell and Gresham (1985) did not specify a process for this step.

Rest (1986), Dubinsky and Loken (1989), and Hunt and Vitell (1986) explicitly included a step whereby the ethical decision maker establishes moral intent before engaging in moral behavior. Trevino (1986) and Ferrell and Gresham (1985) postulated a direct transition from the moral judgment phase to moral behavior. Moderating variables include significant others (Dubinsky and Loken 1989; Ferrell and Gresham 1985), individual moderators (Ferrell and Gresham 1985; Trevino 1986), situational moderators (Trevino 1986), and opportunity (Ferrell and Gresham 1985).

Despite the fact that collectively these models are reasonably comprehensive, this synthesized model clearly shows that none of the previous models of ethical decision making explicitly includes characteristics of the moral issue itself as either an independent variable or a moderating variable. If the models making up this synthesized model are taken at face value, the moral decision-making and behavior process of individuals in organizations is identical for all moral issues. For example, people will decide and behave in the same manner whether the issue is the theft of a few supplies from the organization or the release of a dangerous product to the market. As the relationships represented by dotted lines (see Figure 1) indicate, the model presented here and explained in detail in the following sections explicitly rejects that view and formally includes characteristics of the moral issue itself as an independent variable affecting all four stages of moral decision making and behavior.

Specifically, ethical decision making is issue contingent; that is, characteristics of the moral issue itself, collectively called moral intensity, are important determinants of ethical decision making and behavior. The issue-contingent model presented here owes its genesis to intuitive, observational, and empirical factors. Intuitively, people tend to become much more concerned about moral issues that affect those who are close to them rather than those with whom they have little or no contact. Individuals also seem to react more strongly to injustices that have immediate effects as opposed to those that have effects in the distant future.

In terms of observational evidence, the quotation of a militiaman for one of Beirut's factional forces explains his reasoning that as long as the victims are strangers, the killing doesn't bother him: "Those I do not know, I don't care about," and "for bloody and tough battles, I take other fighters, not the ones I have here. These are my friends. I don't want a guilty conscience if something happens" (*Newsweek* 1989, 58). Similarly, the Soviet invasion of Afghanistan, though recognized by Americans as horrible, registered "only at the fringes of our consciousness," according to Kaplan (1989, 29). This occurred, he argued, because "the war in Afghanistan—in addition to being difficult to report—happened too far away, to an alien people with few ethnic compatriots in America" (Kaplan 1989, 29). These observations suggest that distance (physical, psychological, cultural, or social) affects the manner in which human beings view moral issues. In an organizational context, it can be noted that some employees, who would not consider stealing from individual strangers, pilfer supplies from their firms or make personal long-distance calls on company phones. Dispersion of effect seems to play a role in these moral decisions.

Empirically, Fritzsche and Becker (1983, 297), who conducted a survey of managerial attitudes toward the appropriate responses to various ethical vignettes, rejected the hypothesis that "the behavior of marketing managers is invariant across categories of ethical problems." Further, respondents "would act more ethically in the dilemmas posing serious consequences than they would in less risky situations" (1983, 297). Similarly, Fritzsche (1988) found that marketing managers responded differentially to ethical vignettes where the magnitude of the consequences was varied. In some of the vignettes, the variation was related to the magnitude of the consequences. Additionally, Weber (1990) offered evidence that corporate managers use different modes of moral reasoning for different types of moral issues.

The previous evidence suggests that human beings may respond differentially to moral issues in a way that is systematically related to characteristics of the issue itself. This article, drawing on theory from social psychology, argues that six characteristics of the moral issue (magnitude of consequences, social consensus, probability of effect, temporal immediacy, proximity, and concentration of effect) will be positively related to moral decision making and behavior. These characteristics of moral issues, collectively called moral intensity, are integral parts of an issue-contingent model of moral decision making and behavior. This model is discussed in detail, following an elaboration of the moral intensity construct.

Moral Intensity

Central to the issue-contingent model presented here is the notion of moral intensity. Moral intensity is a construct that captures the extent of issue-related moral imperative in a situation. It is multidimensional, and its component parts are characteristics of the moral issue such as magnitude of consequences, social consensus, probability of effect, temporal immediacy, proximity, and concentration of effect. Moral intensity does not include traits of moral decision makers, such as moral development (Kohlberg 1976); ego strength, field dependence, or locus of control (Trevino 1986); or knowledge or values (Ferrell and Gresham 1985). It also does not include organizational factors, such as organizational culture (Trevino 1986) or corporate policies (Ferrell and Gresham 1985). In sum, moral intensity focuses on the moral issue, not on the moral agent or the organizational context.

Moral intensity is likely to vary substantially from issue to issue, with a few issues achieving high levels and many issues achieving low levels. The probable reliability and stability of moral intensity are unknown, but these parameters could be established empirically.

The construct of moral intensity is not found in the literature of descriptive models of moral decision making. It is derived, in part, from the normative arguments of moral philosophers who differentiate levels of moral responsibility based on proportionality. Proportionality is related to:

1. The type of goodness or evil involved.
2. The urgency of the situation.
3. The certainty or probability of effects.
4. The extent of the moral agent's influence on events.
5. The availability of alternate means. (Garrett 1966, 9–10)

Wirtenberger (1962) offered a similar expansion of proportionality in terms of cooperation in evil acts.

Legal concepts also serve as precedents for the concept of moral intensity. One of the functions of penalties in criminal law is retribution (Packer 1968), and the extent of retribution is often proportional to the evil perpetrated. Thus, the range of sentences for murder is more severe than the range of sentences for petty larceny. This legal principle is analogous to moral intensity in ethical decision making.

The argument for validity of the moral intensity construct is based on logic, analogy, and, in the case of some of its components, observations from prior research. According to Schwab, construct validation is often a sequential process. The scientist typically begins with a construct, probably ill defined. She/he suspects (hypothesizes) that this construct is related to other constructs in some sort of theoretical model which is probably also ill defined. At this point, a measure of the construct is typically developed (1980, 9).

Because both the moral intensity construct and the issue-contingent model are in preliminary stages of development, the validation process suggested by Schwab will be approximated.

Only content validity can currently be claimed for the moral intensity construct. The argument for content validity is based on the observations that (a) moral intensity varies from issue to issue, (b) individuals can make judgments of moral intensity, and (c) these judgments, although often subject to error and systematic bias (Kahneman, Slovic, and Tversky 1982), are sufficiently accurate for a person to make critical distinctions.

Moral philosophers are not the only ones to make judgments of proportionality on moral issues; ordinary citizens do so as well. The legal system of the United States provides evidence that human beings can and do make such distinctions. Trained individuals (judges) and untrained individuals (jury members) are repeatedly called upon to render legal judgments regarding guilt, liability, sentencing, and damages in the court system. Although legal issues and moral issues do not completely overlap, legal principles are often based on moral principles. Judgments of moral intensity are certainly analogous to judgments that are routinely made in courts of law. If human beings were unable to make such judgments reasonably well, the legal system would have collapsed long ago.

Another approach to construct validation is elaboration of the theoretical framework that includes the construct. According to Schwab (1980), this elaboration serves two purposes. The theorized interconstruct linkages provide clarification of the construct of interest and serve as input for subsequent establishment of validation procedures. Finally, empirical testing of the hypothesized relationships among constructs can strengthen the case for construct validity of the focal construct (Schwab 1980). Discussion of the issue-contingent model in later sections of this article will also serve to help validate the moral intensity construct.

Components of Moral Intensity

This article postulates that every ethical issue can be represented in terms of its moral intensity, a construct that includes six components:

magnitude of consequences, social consensus, probability of effect, temporal immediacy, proximity, and concentration of effect. Definitions and examples of these components and a rationale for their inclusion in the construct follow.

Magnitude of Consequences

The magnitude of consequences of the moral issue is defined as the sum of the harms (or benefits) done to victims (or beneficiaries) of the moral act in question. For example:

1. An act that causes 1,000 people to suffer a particular injury is of greater magnitude of consequence than an act that causes 10 people to suffer the same injury.
2. An act that causes the death of a human being is of greater magnitude of consequence than an act that causes a person to suffer a minor injury.

The inclusion of magnitude of consequences in the moral intensity construct is based on common-sense understanding and observation of human behavior and empirically derived evidence. First, the definition of moral issue is broad; decisions involving consequences for others and volition on the part of the moral agent have a moral component. However, many moral issues are quite trivial in terms of consequences. For example, most people are unlikely to become morally outraged when a co-worker is denied a desired vacation at a time when others also want to take their vacations; the consequences don't warrant it. Further, because moral issues are present in most organizational decisions, people concerned with minor issues would be morally agitated most of the time. Because people are not constantly agitated over moral issues, it is assumed that many moral issues fail to reach a threshold of magnitude of consequences.

Empirically derived clues (described above) include Fritzsche and Becker's (1983) judgment that when moral dilemmas are faced, serious consequences are more likely to prompt ethical behavior than are modest consequences. Further, Fritzsche (1988) found some support for a positive link between serious consequences and the ethical responses of marketing managers to vignettes containing moral dilemmas. Also, Weber (1990) discovered a link between decision consequences and moral reasoning patterns. Finally, York (1989) determined that subjects were more likely to make judgments of sexual harassment where job consequences for the victim were more severe.

Social Consensus

The social consensus of the moral issue is defined as the degree of social agreement that a proposed act is evil (or good). For example:

1. The evil involved in discriminating against minority job candidates has greater social consensus than the evil involved in refusing to act affirmatively on behalf of minority job candidates.
2. The evil involved in bribing a customs official in Texas has greater social consensus than the evil involved in bribing a customs official in Mexico. (Nehemkis 1975)

Social consensus is included in the moral intensity construct for logical and empirical reasons. Logically, it is difficult to act ethically if a person does not know what good ethics prescribes in a situation; a high degree of social consensus reduces the likelihood that ambiguity will exist. Empirically, Laczniak and Inderrieden (1987) determined that subjects in an ethical judgment experiment rejected illegal decisions with far greater frequency than they rejected unethical (but not illegal) decisions. Although this result may suggest that legal penalties play a role in moral decision making, it may also be that the social consensus that is implied by legal prohibition of a practice reduces moral ambiguity for the moral agent. Indeed, these authors seemed to agree: "In order for individuals to respond appropriately to a given situation, agreement must exist as to whether or not the behavior is appropriate" (Laczniak and Inderrieden 1987, 304).

Probability of Effect

The probability of effect of the moral act in question is a joint function of the probability that the act in question will actually take place and the act in question will actually cause the harm (benefit) predicted. For example:

1. Producing a vehicle that would be dangerous to occupants during routine driving maneuvers has greater probability of harm than producing a vehicle that endangers occupants only during rear-end collisions.
2. Selling a gun to a known armed robber has greater probability of harm than selling a gun to a law-abiding citizen.

Probability of effect is included in the moral intensity construct for reasons of logic. The expected value of, for example, a financial gain is the product of the magnitude of the gain and its probability of occurrence. Similarly, the expected consequences of a moral act would be the product of the magnitude of consequences, the probability that the act will take place, and the probability that the act will cause the harm (benefit) predicted. Moral acts of given magnitude of consequences will thus be "discounted" if either of the probabilities mentioned is substantially less than 1.00. To be sure, individuals are not good at estimating probabilities (Kahneman, Slovic, and Tversky 1982), but imperfect estimates may be adequate to make rough assessments of expected consequences of moral acts.

Temporal Immediacy

The temporal immediacy of the moral issue is the length of time between the present and the onset of consequences of the moral act in question (shorter length of time implies greater immediacy). For example:

1. Releasing a drug that will cause 1 percent of the people who take it to have acute nervous reactions soon after they take it has greater temporal immediacy than releasing a drug that will cause 1 percent of those who take it to develop nervous disorders after 20 years.
2. Reducing the retirement benefits of current retirees has greater temporal immediacy than reducing retirement benefits of employees who are currently between 40 and 50 years of age.

Temporal immediacy is a component of the moral intensity construct for two related reasons. First, as economists know well, people tend to discount the impact of events that occur in the future. The value of a dollar today is greater than the value of a dollar promised in two years. The greater the time period, the greater the discount. Hence, the magnitude of consequences will be discounted in accordance with the temporal distance of the predicted effects. Second, as the time period between the act in question and its expected consequences expands, the probability that the act will actually cause the predicted harm declines. Assuming that all else remains constant, additional time creates additional possibilities for moral interventions, by either the moral agent or by another person and, hence, reduces the moral urgency of the immediate problem.

Proximity

The proximity of the moral issue is the feeling of nearness (social, cultural, psychological, or physical) that the moral agent has for victims (beneficiaries) of the evil (beneficial) act in question. For example:

1. Layoffs in a person's work unit have greater moral proximity (physical and psychological) than do layoffs in a remote plant.
2. For U.S. citizens, the sale of dangerous pesticides in U.S. markets has greater moral proximity (social, cultural, and physical) than does the sale of such pesticides in Latin America.

The moral intensity construct includes proximity for intuitive and empirical reasons. Intuitively, people care more about other people who are close to them (socially, culturally, psychologically, or physically) than they do for people who are distant. The words of the Beirut militiaman quoted previously are evidence of this claim. The proximity element of the construct is highlighted in the historical novel, *Schindler's List*, by Thomas Keneally (1982). In his book the author recounts the courageous efforts of the German industrialist Oskar Schindler to move the Jews who had worked at his factory near Crakow to his new factory in Moravia, where he could continue to protect them. The women prisoners had been routed to the death camp at Auschwitz, where camp authorities offered him 300 "fresh" inmates for his factory. Schindler, however, insisted on employing his original workers, despite the fact that most, after weeks in Auschwitz, had lost all value as industrial workers.

Empirically, a series of obedience experiments by Milgram (1974) supports the inclusion of proximity in the moral intensity construct. Milgram's subjects ("teachers") were ordered by the experimenter to administer (what the teacher thought were) increasingly powerful shocks to a "learner" (an actor working with the researcher) when the learner failed to answer certain questions correctly. The experiment was designed "to find out when and how people would defy authority in the face of a clear moral imperative" (1974, 4). Milgram found that increased physical proximity of the teacher and the learner significantly reduced the incidence of complete obedience. In an experimental variation that required actual physical contact with the victim, complete subject obedience dropped from 62.5 percent in the baseline condition to 30 percent.

Proximity also plays a role in relationships in legal contexts. The legal scholar Charles Fried (1976) argued that not only do attorneys often tend to develop close (proximate) relationships with their clients, but also that these relationships are morally appropriate. He paraphrased Mill (1961) and Sidgwick (1907) in the following sentence: "Our propensity to prefer the interests of those who are close to us is in fact perfectly reasonable because we are more likely to be able to benefit those people" (Fried 1976, 1067). This utilitarian argument is part of Fried's "lawyer as friend" analogy in justification of zealous pursuit of client interests by attorneys. Proximity seems to be linked to morality in legal relationships as well. Thus, the case for including proximity in the moral intensity construct becomes even more compelling.

It must be conceded that proximity is really four variables; that is, social, cultural, psychological, and physical proximity could be separately analyzed. These variables are combined here because of their conceptual similarities and in order to simplify the discussion of components in this exploratory paper.

Concentration of Effect

The concentration of effect of the moral act is an inverse function of the number of people affected by an act of given magnitude. For example:

1. A change in a warranty policy denying coverage to 10 people with claims of $10,000 has a more concentrated effect than a change denying coverage to 10,000 people with claims of $10.00.
2. Cheating an individual or small group of individuals out of a given sum has a more concentrated effect than cheating an institutional entity, such as a corporation or government agency, out of the same sum.

Concentration of effect has been included in the moral intensity construct mainly for intuitive reasons. People who have a sense of the paramount importance of justice for the individual (Rawls 1971) will abhor immoral acts that result in highly concentrated effects. This sentiment is well captured in Ursula LeGuin's "The Ones Who Walked Away from Omelas" (1975), where some inhabitants of a mythical paradise reject a social order that depends on the abject suffering of a single individual. Concentration of consequences is also included in the moral intensity construct for the sake completeness.

Moral Intensity and Its Component Parts

Because the intent of this article is to identify some possible components of ethical decision making and behavior for future research, it is impossible to precisely specify (a) the relationships between the moral intensity construct and its components, including their relative importance, and (b) the relationships among the components. Such determinations must be made empirically at a future date. A few comments are in order, however. First, there are two reasons for aggregating these components into a single construct: (a) the components are all characteristics of the moral issue itself and (b) the components are expected to have interactive effects, at least at some levels, as suggested by the expected relationships that will be described is the following sections. Second, moral intensity is generally expected to increase (monotonically) if there is an increase in any one (or more) of its components, and it is expected to decrease if there is a decrease in any one (or more) or its components, assuming the remaining components remain constant. Interactive effects among components are quite likely, however. For example, some threshold of proximity may have to be reached before differences in magnitude significantly affect moral intensity; the precise death toll of violence in Azerbaijan is probably of little consequence to most Americans because the proximity of the event is so low. Indeed, it is expected that threshold levels of all components must be reached before moral intensity begins to vary significantly.

Measurement of moral intensity and its components is probably possible only in terms of relatively large distinctions. For example, acts resulting in death will have greater magnitude than acts resulting in injuries, all else being equal. Magnitude of economic harm is an exception, however, where the continuous "money metric" (harm measured in dollars) can be employed.

An Issue-Contingent Model

Because the primary purpose of this article is to introduce a new construct into the discourse on ethical decision making, the underlying framework presented here includes only the major components of ethical decision making present in earlier models. Other scholars have adequately made the case for the relevance of other components, and their arguments will be repeated or expanded upon only as they become germane to the formulation presented here.

Rest's (1986) four-component model (recognizing moral issues, making moral judgments, establishing moral intent, and implementing moral actions) is a worthy starting point. It is parsimonious, yet it contains all the key elements of moral decision making and behavior. Important contributions by other theorists will be noted and discussed, as the explanation of the issue-contingent model requires. The model is graphically depicted in Figure 2; its component parts and the research propositions derived from it are discussed in the following sections.

Much of the theoretical foundation of the issue-contingent model presented here is the complex set of theories and relationships grouped under the general heading of social cognition (Fiske and Taylor 1984). The elements and processes of social cognition are not fully understood. Models of various processes and relationships overlap, and semantic differences among them make integration difficult; no single model is universally accepted. This article assumes a simplified model of cognitive processes that retains elements critical to the understanding of single-event moral decision making and eliminates elements that may shape moral decision making over time. The discussion of the model also includes some individual difference variables, which, though important to moral decision making in general, are not vital to the issue-related factors of concern here.

In the simplified model assumed here, stimuli from the environment vie for attention through an encoding process. Attention influences attributions, inferences, memory, affect, judgments, intentions, and be-

Figure 2   An Issue-Contingent Model of Ethical Decision Making in Organizations

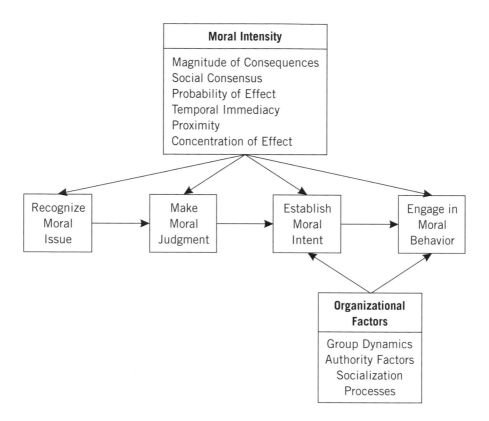

havior. Attributions underlie inferences, judgments, intentions, and behavior. Elements of social cognition that are assumed to remain constant over the course of single-event moral decision making include schemata and attitudes. The following analysis points out the effects of moral intensity on various elements of social cognition and, in turn, on moral decision making and behavior.

The Moral Issue

Human decision-making processes are often activated by the presence of a problem that requires a solution or response and often some form of action (Bazerman 1986). Moral decision making is no exception; the process begins with a problem, which includes a moral component. The moral component of the problem, or moral issue, can be characterized in terms of its moral intensity.

Recognizing Moral Issues

For the moral decision-making process to begin, a person must be able to recognize the moral issue. Although many decisions are moral decisions, decision makers do not always recognize the moral element of their decisions. Recall that, according to Velasquez and Rostankowski (1985), moral issues are present if a person's actions, when freely performed, may harm or help others. Therefore, recognizing moral issues involves two elements. A person must recognize that his or her decision or action will affect others (decisions or actions have consequences for human beings) and some choice must be involved (the person has volition). In sum, the person must recognize that he or she is a moral agent. As discussed more fully at the end of this section, a person who fails to recognize a moral issue will fail to employ moral decision-making schemata and will make the decision according to other schemata, economic rationality, for example.

Moral intensity will affect the recognition of moral issues through its impact on the individual's recognition of the consequences of decisions. Moral intensity will affect the selective aspects (as opposed to the effort aspects) of attention, that is, salience and vividness. Stimuli are salient to the extent that they stand out from their backgrounds. Moral issues of high intensity will be more salient than those of low intensity because (a) their effects are more extreme (greater magnitude of consequences), (b) their effects stand out (higher concentration of effect), or (c) their effects involve significant others (greater social, cultural, psychological, or physical proximity) (Fiske and Taylor 1984, 187).

Stimuli are vivid to the extent that they are emotionally interesting, concrete and imagery provoking, and proximate in a sensory, temporal, or spatial way (Nisbet and Ross 1980). Fiske and Taylor (1984) argued that, although the empirical case for vividness effects is not strong, vivid stimuli may well dominate pallid stimuli under certain real-world conditions where differential attention is important. Moral issues of high intensity will be more vivid than those of low intensity because (a) their effects are emotionally interesting (greater magnitude of consequences or greater concentration of effect), (b) they are more concrete (more extensive social consensus or higher probability of effect), or (c) they are more proximate, that is, socially, culturally, psychologically, physically (proximity), or temporally (temporal immediacy). In sum, because high-intensity moral issues are salient and vivid, they will be more likely to catch the attention of the moral decision maker and will be recognized as having consequences for others, a vital component of recognizing moral issues.

Vivid information also elicits more information from memory than does pallid information. Because the information added from memory is likely to be similar to the vivid stimulus, according to the laws of association (Nisbett and Ross 1980), inferences of consequences for others are likely to be magnified. Therefore, recognition of moral issues is rendered more probable.

A study by Rothbart, Fulero, Jensen, Howard, and Birrell (1978) suggests that magnitude of consequences and salience are linked. These researchers found that subjects judged the proportion of criminals in a sample to be greater if the severity of the individual offenses was greater. Apparently severe offenses were more salient than mild offenses. Recognition of moral issues should be similarly affected by magnitude of consequences.

Another factor that may exaggerate the impact of moral intensity on moral judgment and behavior is the tendency of people to utilize simplifying heuristic principles to evaluate the likelihood of uncertain events. In particular, the availability heuristic, in which people use the ease with which instances can be brought to mind to assess the probability of an event, causes people to overestimate the risks present in various situations if these risks are vividly portrayed (Tversky and Kahneman 1982). Because issues of high moral intensity tend to be more vivid, people will tend to exaggerate the probability of their effect, further heightening the moral intensity and subsequent impact on moral decision making and behavior. The salience of high-intensity moral issues may have a similar effect (Nisbett and Ross 1980; Taylor 1982).

Volition is another element in the recognition of moral issues; a person must acknowledge that he or she has choice. Heider's (1958) work on perceptions of responsibility for outcomes is relevant here. Heider postulated four levels of responsibility for an individual's actions. The first three (intentional, foreseeable, and causal) are of no concern here, but the most removed level of responsibility, associational, is relevant. Associational responsibility occurs when a person is held accountable for an action, even though he or she is not causally involved. For example, if, in a fit of anger, a worker verbally abuses his boss and is fired, he may hold a co-worker responsible for failing to restrain him, even though the co-worker saw that he was angry. The co-worker's attribution of personal responsibility will be associational in this case. Moral intensity will influence attributions of associational responsibility, and, hence, perceived volition, in three ways. A person will assume little responsibility (a) if the consequences affect someone psychologically or physically removed from him or her (low psychological and physical proximity), (b) if the consequences are expected to occur in the distant future (low temporal immediacy), and (c) if the consequences are unlikely to occur (low probability of effect).

Volition and moral intensity may also be linked by what has been called the defensive attribution hypothesis: greater personal responsibility is attributed to perpetrators of accidents that hold severe, rather than mild, consequences (Fiske and Taylor 1984). Moral issues of greater magnitude of consequences or concentration of effects would therefore elicit attributions of greater responsibility. Research by Walster (1966) and Shaver (1970a,b) supports the defensive attribution hypothesis.

Volition will also be related to self-attributions of freedom. Attributions of freedom are related to "perceptions that an action was chosen from a set of available options and not forced on one by circumstances" (Fiske and Taylor 1984, 103). Hence, attributions of freedom depend on context. Contextual factors that enhance attributions of freedom include the availability of positive outcome options and certainty on the part of the decision maker regarding a desirable outcome (Wortman 1975). Two components of moral intensity (magnitude of consequences and social consensus) are relevant here. Moral issues of great magnitude will make clear the availability of positive options (enhanced benefit or decreased harm). High levels of social consensus will enhance the certainty of the decision maker (moral agent) regarding the desirability of the chosen outcome. Thus, moral intensity will influence self-attributions of freedom and, hence, perceived volition.

Individual difference variables will also play a role in the recognition of moral issues. Rotter's (1966, 1971) concept of locus of control posits that some people, called internals, credit themselves with substantial control over events, whereas others, called externals, see events as largely under the control of luck, chance, or other individuals. Internals are masters of their fate; externals are pawns of other forces. Locus of control may be related to perceived volition and, hence, to recognition of moral issues.

Individuals also differ in terms of their responses to unpleasant events, which moral choices often are. Repressors avoid psychological threats and often ignore the initial signs of unpleasant situations. Sensitizers tend to investigate such threats, mull them over, and explain them intellectually (Fiske and Taylor 1984). The repression-sensitization dimension also may affect a person's ability to recognize moral issues.

Overarching all of these attributional factors that may be theoretically linked to volition is the actor-observer effect, whereby people rely heavily on situational factors, as opposed to dispositional factors, in explaining their own behavior (Fiske and Taylor 1984). They tend, in effect, to underestimate their own volition. Presumably, this bias will be constant over moral issues of all levels of intensity; moral intensity will still affect volition differentially, as described above. These theoretical and empirical observations lead to Proposition 1.

Proposition 1. Issues of high moral intensity will be recognized as moral issues more frequently than will issues of low moral intensity.

The recognition of moral issues is related to moral decision making and behavior in an important way. Moral decision making and behavior can be thought of in terms of schemata. Schemata are cognitive structures "that represent organized knowledge about a given concept or type of stimulus. A schema contains both the attributes of the concept and the relationships among the attributes" (Fiske and Taylor 1984, 140). Event schemata, or scripts, are "structures that describe appropriate sequences of events in well-known situations" (Fiske and Taylor 1984, 167). Role schemata are norms and behaviors appropriate to certain social roles. The moral decision-making process is an event schema; the moral decision maker is a role schema. The recognition of moral issues triggers schemata that are relevant to moral issues, that is, the moral decision-making process (event) and the moral decision maker (role). Issues of great moral intensity will positively affect the recognition of moral issues and, therefore, will increase the likelihood that moral decision-making schemata will be employed.

Moral Development and Moral Judgments

Once a person recognizes that a moral issue exists, he or she must make a moral judgment. Component 2 of Rest's (1986) model relates to the question, "How do people make moral judgments?" At this point, Kohlberg's (1976) model of moral development becomes relevant. Kohlberg postulated that human beings make moral judgments in some combination of six analytically distinct ways. Children and morally immature adults have predominantly preconventional orientations. In Stage 1, Obedience and Punishment, the individual obeys rules to avoid punishment; in Stage 2, Instrumental Purpose and Exchange, the individual obeys rules only to further his or her own interests. Most adults operate at conventional levels of moral development. In Stage 3, Interpersonal Accord, Conformity, and Mutual Expectations, the individual adapts to the moral standards of his or her peers; in Stage 4, Social Accord and System Maintenance, the individual adopts the moral standards of society, particularly its laws. Some adults reach a postconventional level of moral development. In Stage 5, Social Contract and Individual Rights, the individual is aware of the relativity of values and upholds rules because they conform to the social contract; in Stage 6, Universal Ethical Principles, the individual chooses his or her own ethical principles and follows them, even if they run counter to laws. Rest (1979) subdivided the basic categories somewhat, but mainly followed Kohlberg's model. These authors agreed that individuals vary considerably in terms of their approaches to moral issues and that some form of cognitive-development perspective is appropriate.

Although many researchers have regarded moral development as a relatively stable individual difference variable, some, including Rest (1979), argued that many individuals operate within a range of moral development stages. Higgins, Power, and Kohlberg (1984, 103) offered empirical evidence of the effect of context ("moral atmosphere") on individual moral reasoning: "These students did not use their highest or best moral reasoning when thinking about real-life dilemmas in the context of their own schools." Weber (1990) also found evidence that organizational context affects moral reasoning. Levine (1979) argued that individuals may perform at moral development levels lower than their potential and discussed conditions under which this phenomenon may occur. Finally, Trevino (1986) postulated that managers will use lower levels of cognitive moral development in actual work environments compared to hypothetical situations, such as those found on tests designed to measure moral development. These authors have suggested that moral development, or at least the levels at which people actually reason, may be context dependent.

This article argues that moral reasoning is issue dependent. The argument is intuitive, theoretical, and empirical. From an intuitive perspective, because moral reasoning takes time and energy (e.g., gathering facts, applying moral principles, and making moral judgments [Velasquez 1982]), it is likely that moral agents will economize on efforts devoted to moral reasoning when moral stakes are low. Fiske and Taylor (1984, 146) captured this view well in terms of social cognition in general: "People dedicate more effort to social understanding when the stakes are higher. They think more, if not more accurately."

Theoretically, social cognition provides a number of supporting perspectives for the postulated link between moral intensity and stage of moral reasoning. Some of these theoretical perspectives are based on the "cognitive miser" principle, whereby people adopt cognitive strategies that simplify complex problems. "The capacity-limited thinker searches for rapid adequate solutions, rather than slow, accurate solutions" (Fiske and Taylor 1984, 12). Efficiency is stressed at the expense of accuracy. The argument presented here focuses on conditions under which efficiency will be sacrificed for more thorough understanding.

A study by Taylor (1975) suggests that the magnitude of consequences of decisions influences the amount of time and information that a person will bring to bear on cognitive processes. People may make use of external cues when stakes are low, but they will rely on self-perception processes more fully when the stakes are higher. Moral cognitive processes should be similarly affected by this component of moral intensity.

Weber (1990) presented empirical evidence that suggests a link between moral intensity and stage of moral reasoning. He noted that subjects responded differentially to three moral dilemmas that vary in what this article calls moral intensity. Mean stage level for a dilemma that pits human life against obedience to the law (Kohlberg's "Heinz" dilemma) was 3.84; two other dilemmas (of his own design), involving personal career goals versus personal integrity, and professional duty versus obedience to a superior, elicited mean stage scores of 3.22 and 3.35, respectively (1990, 695). Although Weber conceded that organizational context factors might account for part of these differences, he added that "the nature of the moral issue confronting the individual may influence the respondent in determining if postconventional or conventional moral reasoning is appropriate" (1990, 698). This empirical evidence strongly suggests that moral reasoning patterns not only vary from issue to issue, but also may vary in rough proportion to moral intensity as postulated in this article. Issues of high moral intensity may elicit more sophisticated moral reasoning. This empirical evidence and the theoretical considerations discussed above lead to Proposition 2.

Proposition 2. Issues of high moral intensity will elicit more sophisticated moral reasoning (higher levels of cognitive moral development) than will issues of low moral intensity.

Cognitive moral development has been linked to ethical behavior in several studies. Blasi (1980, 11) reviewed 15 studies of moral reasoning and delinquency and found "a degree of congruency" between moral reasoning and delinquent behavior. Also, with respect to 17 studies on cheating, he determined that "it is not unreasonable to conclude that the hypothesis of a significant positive relation between level of moral thinking and resistance to temptation is supported" (Blasi 1980, 25). Similarly, he found a positive link between moral stage and resistance to conformity, based on an examination of five studies. Blasi also found that moral development was not conclusively linked to altruistic behavior or "real-life behavior." Overall, he concluded that considerable support exists for a positive link between moral reasoning and moral action. In a review of several studies of moral development and behavior that utilized the Defining Issues Test (Rest 1979), Thoma and Rest (1986, 135) concluded that "generally there is a link between moral judgment and behavior," although "the strength of the relationship is only moderate."

Trevino (1986, 602) strengthened her case for a person-situation interactionist model of ethical decision making in organizations by arguing that cognitive moral development "strongly influences" ethical judgments. Further, she marshaled empirical evidence that linked moral development and cheating (negative relationship) (no reference given), obedience to harmful authority (negative relationship) (Kohlberg 1969), and helping behavior (positive relationship) (Kohlberg and Candee 1984) to support her contention that moral development and ethical behavior are linked. This evidence helped to validate her interactionist model. Similarly, it should help to validate the issue-contingent model presented here.

Moral Intent

Once a person has made a moral judgment, a process that is dependent on his or her cognitive moral development (Kohlberg 1976; Rest 1986), he or she must decide what to do. A decision about what is morally "correct," a moral judgment, is not the same as a decision to act on that judgment, that is, to establish moral intent. The term intent is functionally equivalent to the word intentions, which is found in some of the social psychology literature (e.g., Fishbein and Ajzen 1975). At this stage, the moral agent balances moral factors against other factors, notably including self-interest (Rest 1986). For example, a supervisor may determine that refusing to fire a senior employee is the "right" thing to do (a moral judgment), but may decide to fire him or her anyway (failure to establish moral intent) for reasons of career advancement or organizational pressures. In his autobiographical account of the "Aircraft Brake Scandal," Kermit Vandivier (1972) never considered "blowing the whistle" on his own company, even though the firm was about to deliver a dangerously unsafe product. He knew what was "right," but intended to do nothing meaningful about it.

Moral intensity may also play a role in establishing moral intent. Attributions of responsibility are related to perceived control over an event; the greater the perceived control, the greater the attributed responsibility (Fiske and Taylor 1984). Proximity, an element of moral intensity, is likely to affect perceived control and, in turn, attributions of responsibility. For example, a person usually cannot be held responsible for events that are physically distant. Because people seek to avoid negative attributions of responsibility, they will establish positive moral intent more frequently when the moral issue is proximate.

Further, this desire to avoid aversive consequences will influence moral intent in situations where social consensus is high. Because low social desirability of behavior often reveals underlying dispositions (Jones and McGillis 1976), people will attempt to behave appropriately when the social consensus is high regarding the desirability of certain moral behavior.

Moral intensity may also influence moral intent profoundly through its influence on affect (emotions, feelings, and mood). Stimuli that are vivid and salient often heighten emotions and feelings, which, in turn, intensify both cognitive and behavioral responses (Fiske and Taylor 1984). In particular, people may commit themselves to (moral) actions (establish moral intent) while emotionally excited, and they may retain the commitment even after the intense feelings have died down (Bryant and Zillman 1979). The moral commitment established in an emotionally aroused state may carry through to actual moral behavior, the next step in the process. Indeed, affect may be a critical element in overcoming the organizational impediments to moral action (discussed in a later section). These theoretical observations lead to Proposition 3.

Proposition 3. Moral intent will be established more frequently where issues of high moral intensity are involved than where issues of low moral intensity are involved.

The establishment of moral intent is important to the moral decisionmaking and behavior model presented here because intentions are important determinants of behavior. Fishbein and Ajzen argued that "the best predictor of a person's behavior is his intention to perform the behavior" (1975, 381), especially when the intention and behavior are measured at the same level of specificity. Moral intent and moral behavior should be similarly related. Indeed, Dubinsky and Loken (1989) and Hunt and Vitell (1986) explicitly included a link between moral intent and moral behavior in their models.

Moral Behavior

The fourth component of Rest's model involves acting on a person's moral intentions, that is, engaging in moral behavior. In Rest's words, "Executing and implementing a [plan] of action . . . involves . . . working around impediments and unexpected difficulties, overcoming fatigue and frustration, resisting distractions and allurements, and keeping sight of the original goal" (1986, 15). Establishing moral intent is not enough; colloquially, "The road to Hell is paved with good intentions."

Social cognition is also useful in establishing theoretical links between moral intensity and moral behavior. Attributions of controllability influence how people respond to others, particularly those in need of help (Weiner 1979, 1980). A person is more inclined to help someone whose predicament is uncontrollable than one whose predicament is controllable through, for example, increased effort. Help is less likely to be forthcoming to those who are responsible for their predicaments. Similar research by Ickes and Kidd (1976) on the effect of intentionality on helping behavior and Berkowitz (1969) on the effect of internal (personal) versus external (environmental) factors on helping behavior supports this conclusion.

These findings, when coupled with research results examined by Burger (1981), also link moral intensity with behavior. Burger concluded that subjects attribute less responsibility to perpetrators of accidents as the severity of consequences increased when subjects and perpetrators were situationally and personally similar. When subjects and perpetrators were dissimilar, more responsibility was attributed to perpetrators as accident severity increased. These findings suggest that proximity (personal and situational similarity), a component of moral intensity, is negatively linked to attributions of responsibility. If attributions of responsibility are negatively linked to helping behavior, as discussed in this section, it is likely that proximity will positively influence helping behavior.

Even attributional biases may favorably affect the link between moral intensity and behavior. The fundamental attribution error is the tendency to attribute the behavior of others to dispositional qualities, as opposed to situational factors. People tend not to see that situational forces influence the behavior of others; instead, they see the behavior of others as freely chosen. "Victims of situational forces may be held more accountable for their situations than they should be" (Fiske and Taylor 1984, 74).

In sharp contrast, people explain their own behavior more in situational terms and attribute it much less to dispositional factors. In sum, they hold themselves less accountable for their behavior than they would hold others in the same situation. This self-serving attributional bias is thought to be related to two factors: differential salience (a person cannot observe him- or herself behaving) and differential information (Fiske and Taylor 1984). The latter of these factors is relevant here. People know their own attitudes, feelings, and intentions toward an event and, hence, can attribute their behavior to situational factors about which outside observers have no knowledge. The observer therefore tends to attribute behavior more to dispositional factors than does the actor. This phenomenon is called the actor-observer effect (Fiske and Taylor 1984).

Moral intensity may play a role in the distribution of attributions between dispositional and situational factors in the following way. Information about a person and a situation will be influenced significantly by proximity. People tend to know more about other people and situations that are proximate (socially, culturally, psychologically, and physically) compared to people and situations that are distant. Greater knowledge would tend to reduce the gap between actor attributions (the actor him- or herself being the ultimate in proximity) and observer attributions. Hence, the tendency to make dispositional attributions would decline as proximity increased; greater knowledge would increase the incidence of situational attributions.

Further, as discussed in this section, people are more inclined to help those whose predicaments are uncontrollable (attributed to situational factors) compared to those whose predicaments are controllable (attributed to dispositional factors). It follows that proximity, a component of moral intensity, will positively influence helping behavior.

Kelman and Hamilton, in their examination of destructively obedient behavior, *Crimes of Obedience* (1989), argued that an individual's tendency to challenge authority is based on the interplay of two opposing forces: binding forces, which tend to reinforce the authority structure, and opposing forces, which heighten resistance to authority. When opposing forces are stronger than binding forces, the person will tend to challenge authority. Important among these opposing forces are physical and psychological distance; as these distances increase, opposing forces decrease. In moral intensity terms, proximity is inversely related to distance. Therefore, as proximity (physical and psychological) increases, opposing forces increase, challenges to authority become more probable, and the incidence of immoral behavior in authority situations should decrease. Milgram's (1974) obedience studies also demonstrated the importance of physical distance to obedience. His subjects resisted authority more fully when the physical distance between learner and teacher was reduced (ultimately, to actual contact).

Kilham and Mann (1974), using a variant of the Milgram experiment, divided the teacher's role into two parts: a person who was a "transmitter" and a person who was an "executant." The transmitter informed the executant when to push the switch. Obedience among transmitters was significantly higher than that among executants. This result lends further credence to the importance of proximity in moral behavior; the hierarchically more proximate executants showed greater moral restraint.

These empirical findings, coupled with the theoretical arguments discussed above, lead to Proposition 4.

Proposition 4. Ethical behavior will be observed more frequently where issues of high moral intensity are involved than where issues of low moral intensity are involved.

Biases in Assessing Moral Intensity

The preceding discussion has highlighted the differential effects of various cognitive processes on moral issues of varying intensity. Some cognitive processes will affect moral decision making and behavior in general, without regard to the moral intensity of the issue itself.

Some of these cognitive processes create biases against the recognition of moral issues and, hence, against the engagement of moral decisionmaking processes. Included in this first group is the inability of people to conceptualize events that have not occurred (Ross and Anderson 1982). In the case of moral issues, where events are often prospective, bias in risk perception (Slovic, Fischoff, and Lichtenstein 1982) may be particularly important; people may fail to recognize risky future situations because they are less imaginable. According to Nisbett and Ross, "Such 'null' information tends to be overlooked and underappreciated" (1980, 48).

Individuals are also poor at detecting covariation. True covariation plays a limited role in the perception of covariation in the social domain; preexisting theories play a much larger role (Jennings, Amabile, and Ross 1982; Nisbett and Ross 1980). The failure to detect covariation may affect a person's ability to recognize early symptoms of various problems (Jennings, Amabile, and Ross 1982), a particularly important element in moral decision making. Even when covariation is detected, its causes may be difficult to analyze correctly; "prior theories of causality may override the implications of the covariation pattern" (Nisbett and Ross 1980, 10). Prior theories may not include moral elements, thus biasing the causal inference process against moral considerations.

Individuals may tend not to perceive themselves as independent agents in moral situations. Kelman and Hamilton (1989), in their analysis of the Milgram (1974) obedience studies, argued that some subjects felt that they did stop administering shocks, even though their hands were still manipulating the switches. These subjects regarded the decisions and the responsibility for those decisions as being entirely in the hands of the experimenter. This ceding of responsibility was total in some cases; one subject could not imagine conditions under which he would have stopped administering shocks (Kelman and Hamilton 1989). Apparent ceding of responsibility was also present in the responses of subjects in a study conducted by Derry (1987). Many (33%) of her subjects reported that they never faced a moral conflict at work, despite evidence to the contrary. Some of this group of subjects accepted the organization's authority structure in moral matters, whereas others saw their roles as employees as limited to matters of efficiency and effectiveness. Clearly, not all people see themselves as independent moral agents in work situations.

Bias favorable to the recognition of moral issues may also be present in cognitive processes. Langer (1982) discussed the illusion of control, wherein people overestimate their personal control in situations involving substantial chance. Where moral issues are involved, this tendency would bias individuals toward attributions of personal responsibility and away from situational attributions. In essence, this tendency would bias moral agents toward judgments of personal volition, an important element of moral decision making and behavior.

On balance, the net effect of these biases in cognitive processes on moral decision making is unknown. However, they are expected to affect all moral situations equally and not apply differentially to moral issues of differing intensity.

Organizational Factors

Organizational settings present special challenges to moral agents. Moral decision making and behavior at the individual level, though often difficult, at least are not complicated by major organizational factors. Trevino discussed several such factors under the heading of "situational variables" (1986, 603). Ferrell and Gresham (1985), Ferrell, Gresham, and Fraedrich (1989), and Hunt and Vitell (1986) included organizational factors in their models under significant others and opportunity, organizational culture, and organizational environment, respectively. Higgins, Power, and Kohlberg (1984) provided empirical evidence that moral atmosphere affects moral reasoning and moral judgment.

Smith and Carroll (1984) presented a detailed argument that organizational factors often create impediments to individual ethical behavior. In their view, socialization processes, environmental influences, and hierarchical relationships collectively constitute a "stacked deck," which impedes moral behavior. Research conducted on small group conformity behavior (Asch 1951, 1955, 1956), obedience to authority (Milgram 1963, 1974), and groupthink (Janis 1972) also suggests that organizational factors may distort the ethical intentions of individuals.

Kelman and Hamilton (1989) described the dynamics of challenging organizational authority in considerable detail. In order to overcome macrolevel obstacles to challenging authority (those anchored in institutional and social structures), an individual must redefine the authority relationship and the demand as illegitimate. Conflicts between individual morality and macro-level authority are often acted out on the micro level, however. At this level, the interplay of binding forces (immediate presence of authority, consequences of disobedience, fear of embarrassment, and the actions of comparable others) and opposing physical and psychological forces (proximity of the victim and perceptions of personal causation) help determine the individual's behavior (Kelman and Hamilton 1989).

Organizational factors are likely to play a role in moral decision making and behavior at two points: establishing moral intent and engaging in moral behavior. Implicit organizational pressures may be sufficient to determine the person's moral intent (e.g., the previous Vandivier [1972] example). Explicit organizational factors may cause unethical (or ethical) behavior to result despite good (or bad) intention.

Conclusions and Implications

Existing theoretical models have ignored the effect of characteristics of the moral issue itself on ethical decision making and behavior in organizations. Taken at face value, these models suggest that individuals will decide and behave in the same manner regardless of the nature of the moral issue involved. An employee of a drug manufacturer would view the release of a dangerous drug by his or her firm with the same alarm (or lack of alarm) that he or she viewed the theft of a few diskettes from the company supply cabinet by a fellow employee. The issue-contingent model proposed here explicitly rejects this view and suggests that the moral intensity of the issue itself has a significant effect on moral decision making and behavior at all stages of the process. If this model is found to have empirical support, the testing of other models would be significantly affected. Controlling for issue traits would become an integral part of a meaningful test of Trevino's (1986) person-situation interactionist model, for example; the relative importance of personal factors and situational factors might vary considerably, from issue to issue. Similarly, issue characteristics could alter the balance of teleological and deontological considerations in the moral evaluation stage of Hunt and Vitell's (1986) general theory model of marketing ethics.

Perhaps the most important potential impact of an empirical finding that ethical decision making and behavior are issue contingent involves the applicability of the models themselves. Moral intensity is expected to play a major role in the recognition of moral issues and, hence, in the actual engagement of moral decision-making processes instead of, or in addition to, other decision-making schemata. Simply stated, the details of moral decision-making and behavior processes become irrelevant if the person does not recognize that he or she is dealing with a moral issue. Future models of ethical decision making should include some consideration of the effect of the moral agent's failure to recognize the moral issue.

Moral intensity is also relevant to the general applicability of Kohlberg's (1976) theory of cognitive moral development. If moral development is issue contingent, as this article and some emerging empirical evidence suggest, then Kohlberg's theory would have to be substantially revised, and much of the research based on it would have to be reappraised. Future research based on his developmental theory would have to control for traits of the moral issues involved.

From a practical point of view, issue contingency is important to normative judgments of moral decisions and of the people who make them. Many of the elements of moral intensity (magnitude of consequences, probability of effect, temporal immediacy, and concentration of effect) are directly related to judgments of the importance of moral issues. If these elements of moral intensity are found to be positively linked to moral behavior, it can be concluded that people generally behave better when the moral issue is important than they do when it is unimportant. Regardless of a person's views regarding the overall moral tenor of society or its alleged decline in recent years, he or she could easily be encouraged by the finding that people's best moral behavior is inspired by issues of substantial importance.

References

Asch, S. E. 1951. Effects of group pressure upon the modification and distortion of judgments. In H. S. Guetzkow (ed.). *Groups, leadership and men*: 177–190. Pittsburgh: Carnegie Press.

Asch, S. E. 1955. Opinions and social pressure. *Scientific American*, 193: 31–35.

Asch, S. E. 1956. Studies of independence and conformity: I. A minority of one against a unanimous majority. *Psychological Monograph* 70(9), no. 416: 1–70.

Bazerman, M. H. 1986. *Judgment in managerial decision making* New York: Wiley.

Beauchamp, T. L., & Bowie, N. E. (eds.). 1979. *Ethical theory and business*. Englewood Cliffs, NJ: Prentice-Hall.

Berkowitz, L. 1969. *Roots of aggression: A reexamination of the frustration-aggression hypothesis*. New York: Atherton.

Blasi, A. 1980. Bridging moral cognition and moral action: A critical review of the literature. *Psychological Bulletin* 88: 1–45.

Brommer, M., Gratto, C., Gravender, J., & Tuttle, M. 1987. A behavioral model of ethical and unethical decision making. *Journal of Business Ethics*, 6: 265–280.

Bryant, J., & Zillmam, D. 1979. Effect of intensification of annoyance through unrelated residual excitation on substantially delayed hostile behavior. *Journal of Experimental Social Psychology*, 15: 470–480.

Burger, J. M. 1981. Motivational biases in the attribution of responsibility for an accident: A metaanalysis of the defensive-attribution hypothesis. *Psychological Bulletin*, 90, 496–512.

Cavanagh, G. F., Moberg, D. J., & Velasaquez, M. 1981. The ethics of organizational politics. *Academy of Management Review*, 6: 363–374.

Cloward, R. A., & Ohlin, L. E. 1960. *Delinquency and opportunity*. Glencoe, IL: Free Press.

Derry, R. 1987. Moral reasoning in work-related conflicts. In W. C. Frederick & L. E. Preston (eds.), *Research in corporate social performance policy*, vol. 9 25–49. Greenwich, CT: JAI Press.

Dubinsky, A. J., & Loken, B. 1989. Analyzing ethical decision making in marketing. *Journal of Business Research*, 19(2): 83–107.

Ferrell, O. C., & Gresham, L. G. 1985. A contingency framework for understanding ethical decision making in marketing. *Journal of Marketing* 49(3): 87–96.

Ferrell, O. C., Gresham, L. G., & Fraedrich, J. 1989. A synthesis of ethical decision models for marketing. *Journal of Macromarketing*, 9(2): 55–64.

Fishbein, M., & Ajzen, I. 1975. *Belief, attitude, intention and behavior: An introduction to theory and research*. Reading, MA: Addison-Wesley.

Fiske, S. T., & Taylor, S. E. 1984. *Social cognition*. New York: Random House.

Frederick, W. C. (ed.). 1987. *Research in corporate social performance and policy* (vol. 9). Greenwich, CT: JAI Press.

Fried, C. 1976. The lawyer as friend: The moral foundations of the lawyer-client relation. *Yale Law Journal*. 85: 1060–1091.

Fritzache, D. J. 1988. An examination of marketing ethics: Role of the decision maker, consequences of the decision, management position, and sex of the respondent. *Journal of Macromarketing*, 8(2): 29–39.

Fritzache, D. J., & Becker, H. 1983. Ethical behavior of marketing managers. *Journal of Business Ethics*. 2: 291–299.

Garrett, T. M. 1966. *Business ethics*. Englewood Cliffs, NJ: Prentice-Hall.

Hegarty, W. H., & Sims, H. P., Jr. 1978. Some determinants of unethical decision behavior: An experiment. *Journal of Applied Psychology*. 63: 451–457.

Hegarty, W. H., & Sims, H. P., Jr. 1979. Organizational philosophy, policies and objectives related to unethical decision behavior: A laboratory experiment. *Journal of Applied Psychology*, 64: 331–338.

Heider, F. 1958. *The psychology of interpersonal relations*. New York: Wiley.

Higgins, A., Power, C., & Kohlberg, L. 1984. The relationship of moral atmosphere to judgments of responsibility. In W. M. Kurtines & J. L. Gewirtz (eds.), *Morality, moral behavior and moral development*: 74–106. New York: Wiley.

Hunt, S. D., & Vitell, S. 1986. A general theory of marketing ethics. *Journal of Macromarketing*, 6(1): 5–16.

Ickes, W. J., & Kidd, R. F. 1976. Attributional analysis of helping behavior. In J. H. Harvey, W. J. Ickes, & R. F. Kidd (eds.), *New directions in attribution research*. vol. 1: 311–334. Hillsdale, NJ: Erlbaum.

Janis, I. L. 1972. *Victims of groupthink*. Boston: Houghton Mifflin.

Jennings, D. L., Amabile, T. M., & Ross, L. 1982. Informal covariation assessment: Data-based versus theory-based judgments. In D. Kahneman, P. Slovic, & A. Tversky (eds.), *Judgment under certainty: Heuristics and biases*: 211–230. Cambridge: Cambridge University Press.

Jones, E. E., & McGillis, D. 1976. Correspondent inferences and the attribution cube: A comparative appraisal. In J. H. Harvey, W. J. Ickes, & R. F. Kidd (eds.), *New directions in attribution research*, vol. 1: 389–420. Hillsdale, NJ: Erlbaum.

Jones, T. M. 1980. Corporate social responsibility revisited, redefined. *California Management Review*. 22(3): 9–67.

Kahnemam, D., Slovic, P., & Tversky, A. (eds.). 1982. *Judgment under certainty: Heuristics and biases*. Cambridge: Cambridge University Press.

Kaplan, R. D. 1989. Afghanistan postmortem. *The Atlantic.* April: 26, 28, 29.

Kelman, H. C., & Hamilton, V. L. 1989. *Crimes of obedience.* New Haven, CT: Yale University Press.

Keneally, T. 1982. *Schindler's list.* New York: Penguin Books.

Kilham, W., & Marm, L. 1974. Level of destructive obedience as a function of transmitter and executant roles in the Milgram obedience paradigm. *Journal of Personality and Social Psychology.* 29: 696–702.

Kohlberg, L. 1969. Stage and sequence: The cognitive developmental approach to socialization. In D. A. Goslin (ed.), *Handbook of socialization theory and research.* 347–490. Chicago: Rand McNally.

Kohlberg, L. 1976. Moral stages and moralization: The cognitive-development approach. In T. Lickona (ed.), *Moral development and behavior: research and social issues.* 31–53. New York: Holt, Rinehart & Winston.

Kohlberg, L., & Candee, D. 1984. The relationship of moral judgment to moral action. In W. M. Kurtines & J. L. Gewirtz (eds.), Morality, moral behavior and moral development. 52–73. New York: Wiley.

Laczniak, G. R., & Inderrieden, E. I. 1987. The influence of stated organizational concern upon ethical decision making. *Journal of Business Ethics.* 6: 297–307.

Langer, E. I. 1982. The illusion of control. In D. Kahneman, P. Slovic, & A. Tversky (eds.), *Judgment under uncertainty: Heuristics and biases.* 231–238. Cambridge: Cambridge University Press.

LeGuin, U. K. 1975. The ones who walked away from Omelas. *The winds twelve quarters* New York: Harper & Row.

Levine, C. G. 1979. Stage acquisition and stage use: An appraisal of stage displacement explanations of variation in moral reasoning. *Human Development.* 22: 145–164.

Merton, R. K. 1957. The role set. *British Journal of Sociology.* 8 (June): 106–120.

Milgram, S. 1963. Behavioral study of obedience. *Journal of Abnormal and Social Psychology.* 67: 371–378.

Milgram, S. 1974. *Obedience to authority.* New York: Harper & Row.

Mill, J. S. 1961. Utilitarianism. In M. Cohen (ed.), *The philosophy of John Stuart Mill.* New York: Modern Library.

Nehemkis, P. 1975. Business payoffs abroad: Rhetoric and reality. *California Management Review.* 18(2): 5–20.

Newsweek. 1989. Beirut days: Life and death. November 13: 58–59.

Nisbett, R., & Ross, L. 1980. *Human inference: Strategies and shortcomings of social judgment.* Englewood Cliffs, NJ: Prentice-Hall.

Packer, H. L. 1968. *The limits of the criminal sanction.* Stanford, CA: Stanford University Press.

Rawls, J. 1971. *A theory of justice.* Cambridge, MA: Harvard University Press.

Rest, J. R. 1979. *Development in judging moral issues.* Minneapolis: University of Minnesota Press.

Rest, J. R. 1986. *Moral development: Advances in research and theory.* New York: Praeger.

Ross, L., & Anderson, C. A. 1982. Shortcomings in the attribution process: On the origins and maintenance of erroneous social assessments. In D. Kahnemam, P. Slovic,

& A. Tversky (eds.), *Judgment under uncertainty: Heuristics and biases.* 129–152. Cambridge: Cambridge University Press.

Rothbart, M., Fulero, S., Jensen, C., Howard, J., & Birrell, B. 1978. From individual to group impressions: Availability heuristics in stereotype formation. *Journal of Experimental Social Psychology.* 14: 237–255.

Rotter, J. B. 1966. Generalized expectancies for internal versus external control of reinforcement. *Psychological Monographs: General and Applied.* 80(1), Whole No. 609: 1–28.

Rotter, J. B. 1971. External control and internal control. *Psychology Today.* June: 37–42, 58–59.

Schwab, D. P. 1980. Construct validity in organizational behavior. In B. M. Staw & L. L. Cummings (eds.), *Research in organizational behavior.* vol. 2. 3–43. Greenwich, CT: JAI Press.

Shaver, K. G. 1970a. Defensive attribution: Effects of severity and relevance on the responsibility assigned for an accident. *Journal of Personality and Social Psychology.* 14: 101–113.

Shaver, K. G. 1970b. Redress amd conscientiousness in the attribution of responsibility for accidents. *Journal of Experimental Social Psychology.* 6: 100–110.

Sidgwick, H. 1907. *The methods of ethics* (7th ed.). Indianapolis: Hackett.

Slovic, P., Fischoff, B., & Lichtenstein, S. 1982. Facts versus fears: Understanding perceived risk. In D. Kahneman, P. Slovic, & A. Tversky (eds.), *Judgment under uncertainty: Heuristics and biases.* 463–489. Cambridge: Cambridge University Press.

Smith, H. R., & Carroll, A. B. 1984. Organizational ethics: A stacked deck. *Journal of Business Ethics.* 3: 95–100.

Sutherland, E., & Cressey, D. R. 1970. *Principles of Criminology* (8th ed.). Chicago: Lippincott.

Taylor, S. E. 1975. On inferring one's own attitudes from one's behavior: Some delimiting conditions. *Journal of Personality and Social Psychology.* 31: 126–131.

Taylor, S. E. 1982. The availability bias in social perception and interaction. In D. Kahneman, P. Slovic, & A. Tversky (eds.), *Judgment under uncertainty: Heuristics and biases*: 190–200. Cambridge: Cambridge University Press.

Thoma, S. J., & Rest, J. R. 1986. Moral judgment, behavior, decision making, and attitudes. In J. R. Rest (ed.), *Moral development: Advances in research and theory*: 133–175. New York Praeger.

Trevino, L. K. 1986. Ethical decision making in organizations: A person-situation interactionist model. *Academy of Management Review.* 11: 601–617.

Tversky, A., & Kahneman, D. 1982. Judgment under uncertainty: Heuristics and biases. In D. Kahneman, P. Slovic, & A. Tversky (eds.), *Judgment under uncertainty: Heuristics and biases.* 3–20. Cambridge: Cambridge University Press.

Vandivier, K. 1972. The aircraft brake scandal. *Harper's Magazine.* April: 45–52.

Velasquez, M. G. 1982. *Business ethics: Concepts and cases.* Englewood Cliffs, NJ: Prentice-Hall.

Velasquez, M. G., & Rostankowski, C. 1985. *Ethics: Theory and practice.* Englewood Cliffs, NJ: Prentice-Hall.

Walster, E. 1966. Assignment of responsibility for an accident. *Journal of Personality and Social Psychology*. 3: 73–79.

Weber, J. 1990. Managers' moral reasoning: Assessing their responses to three moral dilemmas. *Human Relations*, 43: 687–702.

Weiner, B. 1979. A theory of motivation for some classroom experiences. *Journal of Educational Psychology*. 71: 3–25.

Weiner, B. 1980. *Human motivation*. New York: Holt, Rinehart & Winston.

Wirtenberger, H. I. 1962. *Morality and business*. Chicago: Loyola University Press.

Wortman, C. B. 1975. Some determinants of perceived control. *Journal of Personality and Social Psychology*. 31: 282–294.

York, K. M. 1989. Defining sexual harassment in workplaces: A policy-capturing approach. *Academy of Management Journal*. 32: 830–850.

CASE G

WHISTLE WHILE YOU WORK

A fellow hospital pharmacist comes to work while apparently under the influence of alcohol. Should his peer get involved or ignore the situation?

Paul Pleasance has been a pharmacist at Compassionata Hospital for nine years. Within the past six months he has regularly detected the scent of alcohol on another pharmacist's breath during working hours. Neal Tippler—the other pharmacist—often arrives at work with bloodshot eyes, and flushed face; he's loud, overly friendly, and talkative, and has a distinct smell of alcohol. During Secretaries' Week the pharmacy staff took the secretarial staff out to lunch. The director of pharmacy joined the pharmacists and secretarial staff for the event. The secretaries ordered cocktails for themselves as did Neal. Paul and the director ordered soda. Neal ordered two additional alcoholic drinks before the end of the luncheon and then returned to work. Nothing was said about the drinking.

On another occasion Neal arrived red-faced, loud, and smelling of alcohol. He began to joke with the director in an unprofessional manner. The director said nothing.

Paul has always tried to act and perform in a professional manner. He has known Neal from their college days when they were students and fraternity brothers. Neal was known to be a heavy drinker and user of drugs in college. Their relationship at the hospital pharmacy has been strictly professional. They have communicated freely and have worked well together.

Neal has worked at Compassionata Hospital for the past seven years. Previous to this he had difficulty holding a job. A strong personality, he has seldom been reprimanded by his supervisors. His wife and both sons have a genetic disease that usually results in early death. Last year, as a result of this stress, his wife apparently came close to an emotional breakdown.

The pharmacy staff includes six pharmacists all of whom are aware of the pressure in Neal's life. Three of these pharmacists are junior to Neal. Frank Rabbitt has been the chief pharmacist for eight years. He suffers from a stomach ulcer and tries to avoid conflict. Bob Bumbleson is director of the pharmacy. He and Neal socialize and play golf together.

Compassionata Hospital's pharmacy policies and procedures state that any employee reporting to work under the influence of alcohol or narcotic drugs is subject to suspension and/or termination. Richard Ebenezer, director of personnel, has stated that it is the policy of the hospital to suspend such employees for three days or, depending on circumstances, to have the employee terminated after due process procedures. The hospital also offers an option that allows employees confidential counseling through the employee assistance program.

Statutory provisions of Title VIII of the state Education Law, subarticle 3 §§ 6509 states that practicing the profession of pharmacy while the ability to practice is impaired by alcohol, drugs, physical disability, or mental disability will be considered professional misconduct. The penalties under §§ 6511 for misconduct include: (1) censure or reprimand; (2) suspension of license; (3) revocation of license; (4) annulment of license or registration; (5) limitation on registration or issuance of any further license; and (6) a fine not to exceed $500 or probation.

In addition to disciplinary action by the Education Department, an impaired pharmacist is liable for civil and criminal charges. Further, supervising pharmacists and the hospital itself are held accountable for the actions of their employees. This, too, can involve disciplinary action by the Education and Health Departments as well as civil and criminal suits.

In this context, Frank Rabbitt simply tells others that Neal will eventually hang himself. Bob Bumbleson apparently refuses to acknowledge that any real problem exists. The staff pharmacists have refused to confront the issue or initiate action, perhaps fearing reprisal from Neal or their supervisors.

Recently, Paul used the informal network of the pharmacy to communicate his concern to Frank. Paul spoke to one of the pharmacy secretaries who is a personal friend of Rabbitt. The secretary responded a few days later that Frank was aware of the situation and that no corrective action would be instituted. The secretary reported that Frank feels that if he ignores the problem it may go away by itself or, if it worsens, Tippler will eventually commit a flagrant incident resulting in corrective action. Frank also indicated to the secretary that Pleasance should ignore the problem as well and leave any responsibility for intervention to Bumbleson.

Paul is concerned that Neal's problem may result in severe damage or even death to a patient. But, if he pursues the issue, he knows that he may experience harassment, social ostracism from peers, scheming from supervisors, and even possible dismissal. His professional career—which has been advancing successfully to this point—and thus his family's welfare could be put into jeopardy. He is angry at the situation and at his supervisors' laissez-faire attitude. He is fearful for patients and for himself. He is frustrated by the whole thing!

Questions for Discussion

1. Should Paul report Neal? Should he blow the whistle? Why? What is your ethical reasoning?
2. Is it ethical for Paul Pleasance to disregard his supervisor's request to back off?
3. What is Paul's ethical obligation? To report to his superiors and leave it to them? Or to ensure that Neal is removed? Whose judgment should prevail?
4. What values are at stake in this case? What powers does Paul have for addressing the situation? What about mechanisms of accountability?
5. Evaluate this case in terms of its "moral intensity."

CASE H

NO HARM, NO ALARM

Sam Lazarus, a 66-year-old retired businessman, has been admitted to the hospital for metastatic cancer. Five years prior to this hospitalization, he was diagnosed as having prostate cancer, was treated surgically, and was discharged following an uneventful recovery. One month before this current admission he developed progressive weakness in both legs. Now on admission he is paralyzed from the waist down, his mind is clear, memory and orientation intact. (The doctor, after extensive testing, has diagnosed Sam as having bony metastasis involving the vertebrae.) After two weeks of conservative treatment—medications and physical therapy—the physician begins sending the patient for daily cobalt (radiation) therapy. After three weeks of treatment, the patient now has sensation in the lower half of his body, yet no noticeable movement of the extremities. Now Sam requires frequent pain medication and has developed an open, deep sore on his back from five weeks of bedrest.

After two more weeks, Sam's doctor—among the most respected in the community—arrives on the floor and orders 200 units of regular insulin to be injected into Sam's present intravenous bottle and, when that runs out, to start another bottle with 200 more units.

The head nurse, upon questioning the physician regarding these orders, is told to "forget them, just draw up 200 units of regular insulin in a syringe, and I'll be back to see the patient." The doctor returns and speaks to the nurse in private, saying: "You know what I'm doing. The man is suffering. He asks me daily how much longer. His wife is pressuring me. She can no longer bear to see her husband in such pain. Do you think it's fair he has to suffer like this? What else can I do? Only the two of us have to know about this." The head nurse tells the physician he has no right to play God, and that she would report this, and any like incident involving a patient, to the nursing supervisor. The doctor says "forget the whole thing" and leaves the unit.

At 11 o'clock that night the physician returns and injects the insulin directly into Sam's vein. The patient survives the night, with the nursing staff giving him food continuously throughout to counteract the physician's attempt to "end the patient's misery."

The patient does survive. Should the head nurse report the physician to the Medical Board (even though she actually agrees with the expected outcome of his actions)? Or should she forget the incident and risk the chance that the physician may return again and take the same action? The doctor is, in fact, being pressured by the patient and his wife to speed up his death. Their request has created a difficult and controversial situation for the physician. By accelerating death the physician feels that he is being more merciful than by waiting for painful and expensive complications such as infection, renal failure, or starvation to occur.

At one time a nurse who second-guessed a physician on diagnosis or treatment may have been legally overstepping her or his authority. But judicial decisions have turned that traditional concept around, making it easier for nurses to report actions of physicians. Now there is more of an expectation that a nurse will report any obvious inadequacy or irregularity of treatment, regardless of the nature of the patient's illness. A severe error may be more likely to result in litigation than a minor matter, but the nurse's duty is the same. However, "socially acceptable" means of providing dying patients with a comfortable death have also emerged. Among these is the practice—often called "snowing"—of medicating the patient with painkillers around the clock, depressing their vital systems, and eventually depressing the respiratory system to the point of stopping it.

The head nurse consults with colleagues who were working on the unit at the time Sam was a patient. All agree that the physician is wrong in the way he handled the situation. Most prefer the "snowing" method of providing a comfortable death. They all feel that direct injection of an abnormal dose of a medication is outright killing of the patient. Even though the final outcome is the same, these colleagues reason that snowing is the humane way of helping the patient to a comfortable, pain-free death. All agree that the doctor should be reported.

The head nurse does report the physician. He is called before the medical board and his privileges are suspended at the hospital. Sam Lazarus' care—to his distress—is assumed by another physician who orders pain medication around the clock. Sam dies ten days later.

Questions for Discussion

1. Did the head nurse behave ethically? What ethical reasoning process leads you to your judgment?
2. Was it ethical to have the patient's wishes obstructed, thus prolonging his suffering?
3. Does the subtlety of snowing—versus the flagrancy of lethal injection with insulin—make it a more ethically acceptable behavior? Or does its subtlety just make it less "morally intense" and easier to rationalize?
4. Compare the outcome of Sam's death, so soon after the incident, with the outcome that his original physician—who was so respected—was suspended from treating patients for the long term. Does this calculation enter into your judgment of the head nurse's ethical responsibility?
5. Given recent experiences involving Dr. Kevorkian, and the U.S. Supreme Court's consideration of the legality of assisted suicide, evaluate the head nurse's action in terms of law and ethics. Are they the same or different? If the laws on assisted suicide change, should that also change the head nurse's ethical reasoning? Would it affect her ethical responsibility?

Annotated Bibliography

Allen, D., and M. Fowler. "Cognitive Moral Development Theory and Moral Decisions in Health Care." *Law, Medicine and Health Care* (February 1982): 20–23. Provides useful insight on the process of ethical reasoning using Kohlberg's schema.

Harron, F., J. Burnside, J. and T. Beauchamp. *Health and Human Values*. New Haven, CT: Yale University Press, 1983. Presents a first-rate example of the application of a principles-based methodology to ethical reasoning.

Hosmer, L. "Trust: The Connecting Link Between Organizational Theory and Philosophical Ethics." *Academy of Management Review* 20, no. 2 (April 1995): 379–403. A wonderful compendium of first principles applied to ethical reasoning processes.

Lebacqz, K. *Professional Ethics*. Nashville, TN: Abingdon, 1985. Illustrates how a very simple methodology can be employed with sophistication in ethical reasoning.

Maguire, D. *The Moral Choice*. Minneapolis, MN: Winston, 1979. Certainly the best written discourse on ethical reasoning that is out of print.

Nash, L. "Ethics Without the Sermon." *Harvard Business Review* 59, no. 6 (November/December 1981): 78–90. A well-written illustration of the question methodology.

Ray, M. "Communal Moral Experience As the Starting Point for Research in Health Care Ethics." *Nursing Outlook* 42, no. 3 (May/June 1994): 104–109. An up-to-date presentation of research on community process approaches to ethical reasoning.

CONCLUSION: MICROETHICS AS MARATHON

A S WE conclude, let's come back to the question with which we began. What is ethics in the micro dimension of healthcare and how does a healthcare professional do it? We have suggested that it concerns the power we wield over people in the ordinary routine of our daily healthcare work; that acting ethically—doing it—requires responsible attention to the sacred values of the healthcare community; that doing it is both assisted and complicated by numerous mechanisms of accountability in our work; and that imaginative reflection and ethical reasoning skills are keys to doing it well.

This final chapter attempts to focus the "reality prism" more sharply by recognizing that, in fact, even with a well-developed ethical maturity, doing healthcare microethics is tough. For us runners, it can seem very much like a marathon race. We train, we try. But it still hurts, and along the way the route often seems endless. Sometimes we don't make it to the finish line.

The reality is that the more ethically mature we try to become, the more wearying and frustrating the task sometimes seems. Just the basic premise of this book—the suggestion that the micro dimension of healthcare, every hour of every day, is filled with ethical content—can be alarming. We have enough to do just getting through each day without the added burden of ethical deliberation! The emphasis on being aware of the power we wield constantly is daunting. The challenge to reconcile conflicting expectations in our daily routine is easily intimidating. We might well mutter, "Give me a break!" And the notion that we should be alert and careful with all the controls in our environment seems a bit preposterous. Furthermore, the effort to grow our reflective imagination and to hone our ethical reasoning skills is draining. On top of all this, the more steps we take the more gaps we see in our ethical maturity. We find ourselves asking questions like: Who needs this? Why bother? And, will I ever get it right? In effect, there are emotional and psychological realities in this quest for ethical maturity, just as there are in a marathon run. Why run the microethics marathon in the first place, then?

Good Ethics and Good Business

For perspective in dealing with this experiential phenomenon that we all encounter, it is important to conclude with some tempering observations. First, let's come down from the rarefied air of lofty moral heights and breathe some sea-level oxygen. Working toward ethical maturity is much more a practical matter that is part and parcel of professionalism than it is a weighty panacean obligation. More and more researchers and practitioners are uttering the words "Good ethics is simply good business." It is not an extra burden, it is not a "value-added" nicety. It is part of the job of being a healthcare professional. It may help to consider that we need ethical maturity to be more *productive* healthcare providers.

At least this is what ethicists like Hosmer[1] and management scholars like Kotter and Heskett[2] are saying. The former argues the connection theoretically, the latter empirically. Susan Harrington found corporate CEOs concurring.[3] Drawing from Frank's extensive research,[4] Jones maintains that the connection is relational: "[G]ood ethics, made manifest in the context of economic relationships with others, is also good business."[5] Laura Nash supports his contention: "[S]ubordinating the pursuit of efficiency to a sense of service and relationships, managers will increase the possibilities of being able to sustain their personal ethical norms and build business strength."[6] These contentions have been resoundingly sustained in a recent American Medical Association report that concludes the more productive doctors are those who develop relational, not just clinical, skills.[7]

I would maintain that the connection is specifically the sense of dignity that ethical maturity conveys to clients and subordinates. Charles Garfield vehemently and convincingly contends this.[8] Kelly's interviews sustain it.[9] Conger and Kanungo's exhaustive studies of empowerment support it.[10] The message is strong and clear. Quinn and Jones put it succinctly: "Enlightened self-interest leads managers to 'ethical' behavior."[11] So remember: the reason we run the ethics marathon is that impressive medal they put over our head at the finish line just for completing the course!

Tolerating Human Limitations

Second, dealing with the microethics of modern healthcare is little different from dealing with most other aspects of healthcare. We study and train. We do our best. We try to stay current. Sometimes we get it right. Sometimes we get it partially right. And sometimes we have a real bad day. Doing microethics well and maturely requires that we develop tolerance of our own limitations. Simply put, in the micro dimension of our healthcare work we do not and will not always get it ethically right. We need to acknowledge that and accept it while, at the same time, proceeding to develop *greater* ethical maturity each day in our profession.

Donaldson and Dunfee can help us appreciate this. They realistically articulate the *limitations* of our human capacity for ethical reasoning. "Moral rationality is bounded," they assert; "[O]therwise rational moral agents, when applying moral theory to actual situations, confront confining limits."[12] Specifically, they note, we confront our own finite capacity "to comprehend and absorb all details relevant to ethical contexts." Thus, in the daily routine of healthcare, we are doomed to confront ethical risk that we will not always be able to resolve. To paraphrase Donaldson and Dunfee, healthcare professional life is more confusing than we would hope.

But ethical reasoning capacity is not our only limitation. Our moral imagination is also bounded, making it inevitable that we will sometimes just not be able to figure out an ethically mature response to a certain situation. Maguire correctly observes that we often circumscribe the ethical dimension of our daily work by the limited options we are able to perceive. Accordingly, he concludes, many of our responses are based on that segment of reality that our limited imaginations allow us to envision. Consequently, realistic ethical possibilities are often likely to be missed.[13]

Gustafson specifically comments that in healthcare "good is sought under conditions of finitude."[14] In another context Fritz Morstein Marx has formulated the logical consequence of such finitude: "One cannot commandeer responsibility. One can only cultivate it, safeguard its roots, stimulate its growth, and provide it with favorable climatic conditions."[15] Remembering this might give us more tolerance of our own microethics limitations while at the same time prompting us to cultivate and stimulate our ethical maturity.

Some years ago while I was giving an ethics seminar at Mother Teresa's headquarters in Calcutta, this issue of limitations emerged starkly. Mother Teresa's order has a sacred rule that at prescribed times of the day the sisters stop their work to pray. The purpose is not only spiritual but psychological and physical as well in view of the difficult work they do in caring for the poorest of the poor. But a consequence of this rule is, for example, that hundreds of suffering people waiting for help sometimes have the door literally closed on them while the sisters go off in prayer. Is this ethical, we reflected? "What would you have us do, Professor?" wondered one of the superiors. After brainstorming ideas like rotating prayer time, coordinating with other care providers in the area, and so forth, one of the sisters commented that while the sisters are unable to meet all the physical needs of all the suffering at the door, they can spiritually help "carry the cross they bear." She explained that it is one thing to close the door for prayer oblivious to the pain that remains outside; it is another thing to be sensitive to that continuing pain and to bring it to prayer.

While the sister's response reflected a deep spiritual theology, it was also a brilliant observation on ethical maturity within the reality of human limitations. In the daily routine of my healthcare work, where I am sometimes unable to reconcile competing claims, I can be aware of and sensitive to the pain I cause, or I can be oblivious to it. The former can be difficult and, taken too far, can lead to stress and burn-out; the latter is certainly much easier and bearable. But which is more ethically mature, which is more professional? There may, indeed, be something enriching in that sister's comment. Ethical maturity may well involve the development of *tolerance* both of the pain I cause, given my limited capacities, and of the pain I am able and willing to feel in communion with those subjected to it.

This reality of human limitations is well captured by Griffith, and his articulation of it sets a sobering and sensible standard: "The challenge presents itself to managers as a continuous series of individual tests that are often difficult enough to frighten beginners and perplex the most accomplished. Any manager can expect to fail some of these tests but also to succeed."[16]

From Either–Or To Win–Win

A key to dealing effectively with human limitations and growing in ethical maturity is surrender of the "either–or" ethics syndrome and embracing of the "win–win" paradigm. We professionals, especially in the hectic routine of daily healthcare delivery, too easily let ourselves be captured by the either–or syndrome: either efficiency or responsiveness, either this patient or that one, either honesty or survival, either make patient Paul wait or rush client Clara. The either–or mindset is extremely powerful. With ethical maturity, however, a win–win paradigm can be cultivated and used to expand our ethical capacities. Is there a way to be both responsive and efficient, to give both Paul and Clara dignified treatment? The paradigm does not always produce ethically desirable results, but the either–or syndrome *never* does. In running a marathon some athletes end up either breaking the four-hour milestone or not finishing at all. Others make that four-hour goal but severely damage their knees in the process. Experienced, mature marathoners know their limitations and just seek to finish the course with their personal best effort; and they know the win–win feeling at the finish line as that medal— heavy with meaning—is draped over the shoulders of every runner who completes the 26 miles.

The marathon analogy is helpful in synthesizing the nature of ethical maturity in the micro dimension of healthcare. We healthcare professionals train and prepare for our work, just like the marathoner trains for the run. We, too, equip ourselves. Over time we improve and learn how to manage the course better. There is risk, and along the way we can and sometimes do get hurt. We fear what might happen. During the race it usually helps to run in groups for better pacing and support, and to accept the water offered at stations, and to absorb the cheering and encouragement of people along the neighborhood sidelines. So, too, dialogue and community are helpful in ethics. Along the way we struggle, we think strategy, we feel discouraged, we experience elation. And we perspire a lot. So, too, I think, in the ethics marathon.

In the end, two recollections stand out. One, it is so much fun. Both along the route and in finishing the course a marathon—even in the midst of the ordeal—is wonderful. Two, we amaze ourselves when we realize that we have actually done it, actually completed the 26 miles and lived to tell about it! The microethics marathon is similarly—even in the midst of the ordeal—fun and amazing. Go for it!

Notes

1. L. Hosmer, 1995, "Trust: The Connecting Link Between Organizational Theory and Philosophical Ethics." *Academy of Management Review* 22, no. 2 (April): 400.

2. J. Kotter and J. Heskett, 1992, *Corporate Culture and Performance* (New York; Free Press).

3. S. Harrington, 1991, "What Corporate America Is Teaching About Ethics." *Academy of Management Executive* 5, no. 1 (February): 21–30.

4. R. Frank, 1988, *Passions Within Reason: The Strategic Role of Emotions* (New York: Norton).

5. T. Jones, 1995, "Instrumental Stakeholder Theory: A Synthesis of Ethics and Economics." *Academy of Management Review* 20, no. 2 (April 1995), p. 417.

6. L. Nash, 1990, *Good Intentions Aside: A Manager's Guide To Resolving Ethical Problems* (Boston: Harvard Business School Press), p. 243.

7. W. Levinson, D. Roter, J. Mullooly, V. Dull, and R. Frankel, 1997, Physician-Patient Communication: The Relationship with Malpractice Claims Among Primary Care Physicians and Surgeons." *Journal of the American Medical Association* 277, no. 7 (19 February): 553–559.

8. C. Garfield, 1992, *Second To None: How Our Smartest Companies Put People First* (Homewood, IL: Irwin).

9. C. Kelly, 1988, *The Destructive Achiever* (Reading, MA: Addison-Wesley), p. 164.

10. J. Conger and R. Kanungo, 1988, "The Empowerment Process: Integrating Theory and Practice." *Academy of Management Review* 13, no. 3 (December): 471–482.

11. D. Quinn and T. Jones, 1995, "An Agent Morality View of Business Policy." *Academy of Management Review* 20:1 (January): 27.

12. T. Donaldson and T. Dunfee, 1994, "Toward a Unified Conception of Business Ethics." *Academy of Management Review* 19, no. 2 (April): 256.

13. D. Maguire, 1979, *The Moral Choice* (Minneapolis, MN: Winston), p. 170.

14. J. Gustafson, 1990, "Moral Discourse About Medicine." *Journal of Medicine and Philosophy* 15, no. 2 (April): 141.

15. F. Marx, 1940, *Public Management in the New Democracy* (New York: Harper), p. 121.

16. J. Griffith, 1993, *The Moral Challenges of Health Care Management* (Chicago: Health Administration Press), p. 3.

READING

In two disparate ways, Richard Nielsen lends a sobering tone to this concluding chapter. On the one hand, he deals superbly with the behavioral problem common to those who have raised their own level of ethical consciousness. The problem is that, in seeing more clearly instances of ethical immaturity around us and in our organizations, we may often be inclined to leap self-righteously onto a white horse like a shining knight out to conquer dragons. Nielsen's article, drawing from actual cases, offers a mature perspective for dealing with this existential condition. On the other hand, in focusing on the ethics of others in our organizations and profession, Nielsen contributes to the problem that this book struggles to overcome: namely, the strong proclivity to be alert to the ethics of others but blind to the ethics of ourselves. Indeed, fascination with the behavior of others becomes a pull away from reflection on our own ethical maturity and behavior. Moreover, Nielsen is rigorously interested in the extraordinary, macro-level case. But his promotion of the win–win paradigm is excellent. As we conclude, we can apply his useful notions to the micro dimension we have been probing.

CHANGING UNETHICAL ORGANIZATIONAL BEHAVIOR

Richard P. Nielsen

To be, or not to be: that is the question:
Whether 'tis nobler in the mind to suffer
The slings and arrows of outrageous fortune,
Or to take arms against a sea of troubles,
And by opposing end them?

—William Shakespeare, *Hamlet*

What are the implications of Hamlet's question in the context of organizational ethics? What does it mean to be ethical in an organizational context? Should one suffer the slings and arrows of unethical organizational behavior? Should one try to take arms against unethical behaviors and by opposing, end them?

The consequences of addressing organizational ethics issues can be unpleasant. One can be punished or fired; one's career can suffer, or one can be disliked, considered an outsider. It may take courage to oppose unethical and lead ethical organizational behavior.

How can one address organizational ethics issues? Paul Tillich, in his book *The Courage to Be*, recognized, as Hamlet did, that dire consequences can result from standing up to and opposing unethical behavior. Tillich identified two approaches: *being* as an individual and *being* as a part of a group.[1]

In an organizational context, these two approaches can be interpreted as follows: (1) Being as an individual can mean intervening to end unethical organizational behaviors by working against others and the organizations performing the unethical behaviors; and (2) being as a part can mean leading an ethical organizational change by working with others and the organization. These approaches are not mutually exclusive; rather, depending on the individual, the organization, the relationships, and the situation, one or both of these approaches may be appropriate for addressing ethical issues.

Richard P. Nielsen, "Changing Unethical Organizational Behavior." *The Academy of Management Executive* 3, no. 2 (May 1989): 123–130. Copyright 1989, the Academy of Management. Reprinted by permission. Richard P. Nielsen is a management professor at Boston College.

Being as an Individual

According to Tillich, the courage to be as an individual is the courage to follow one's conscience and defy unethical and unreasonable authority. It can even mean staging a revolutionary attack on that authority. Such an act can entail great risk and require great courage. As Tillich explains, "The anxiety conquered in the courage to be . . . in the productive process is considerable, because the threat of being excluded from such a participation by unemployment or the loss of an economic basis is what, above all, fate means today. . . ."[2]

According to David Ewing, retired executive editor of the *Harvard Business Review*, this type of anxiety is not without foundation.

> There is very little protection in industry for employees who object to carrying out immoral, unethical or illegal orders from their superiors. If the employee doesn't like what he or she is asked to do, the remedy is to pack up and leave. This remedy seems to presuppose an ideal economy, where there is another company down the street with openings for jobs just like the one the employee left.[3]

How can one be as an individual, intervening against unethical organizational behavior? Intervention strategies an individual can use to change unethical behavior include: (1) secretly blowing the whistle within the organization; (2) quietly blowing the whistle, informing a responsible higher-level manager; (3) secretly threatening the offender with blowing the whistle; (4) secretly threatening a responsible manager with blowing the whistle outside the organization; (5) publicly threatening a responsible manager with blowing the whistle; (6) sabotaging the implementation of the unethical behavior; (7) quietly refraining from implementing an unethical order or policy; (8) publicly blowing the whistle within the organization; (9) conscientiously objecting to an unethical policy or refusing to implement the policy; (10) indicating uncertainty about or refusing to support a cover-up in the event that the individual and/or organization gets caught; (11) secretly blowing the whistle outside the organization; or (12) publicly blowing the whistle outside the organization. Cases of each strategy are considered below.

Cases

1. Secretly blowing the whistle within the organization. A purchasing manager for General Electric secretly wrote a letter to an upper-level manager about his boss, who was soliciting and accepting bribes from subcontractors. The boss was investigated and eventually fired. He was also sentenced to six months' imprisonment for taking $100,000 in bribes, in exchange for which he granted favorable treatment on defense contracts.[4]

2. Quietly blowing the whistle to a responsible higher-level manager.

When Evelyn Grant was first hired by the company with which she is now a personnel manager, her job included administering a battery of tests that, in part, determined which employees were promoted to supervisory positions. Grant explained:

> There have been cases where people will do something wrong because they think they have no choice. Their boss tells them to do it, and so they do it, knowing it's wrong. They don't realize there are ways around the boss. . . . When I went over his [the chief psychologist's] data and analysis, I found errors in assumptions as well as actual errors of computation. . . . I had two choices: I could do nothing or I could report my findings to my supervisor. If I did nothing, the only persons probably hurt were the ones who "failed" the test. To report my findings, on the other hand, could hurt several people, possibly myself.

She quietly spoke to her boss, who quietly arranged for a meeting to discuss the discrepancies with the chief psychologist. The chief psychologist did not show up for the meeting; however, the test battery was dropped.[5]

3. Secretly threatening the offender with blowing the whistle.

A salesman for a Boston-area insurance company attended a weekly sales meeting during which the sales manager instructed the salespeople, both verbally and in writing, to use a sales technique that the salesman considered unethical. The salesman anonymously wrote the sales manager a letter threatening to send a copy of the unethical sales instructions to the Massachusetts insurance commissioner and the *Boston Globe* newspaper unless the sales manager retracted his instructions at the next sales meeting. The sales manager did retract the instructions. The salesman still works for the insurance company.[6]

4. Secretly threatening a responsible manager with blowing the whistle outside the organization.

A recently hired manager with a San Francisco Real Estate Development Company found that the construction company his firm had contracted with was systematically not giving minorities opportunities to learn construction management. This new manager wrote an anonymous letter to a higher-level real estate manager threatening to blow the whistle to the press and local government about the contractor unless the company corrected the situation. The real estate manager intervened, and the contractor began to hire minorities for foremen-training positions.[7]

5. Publicly threatening a responsible manager with blowing the whistle.

A woman in the business office of a large Boston-area university observed that one middle-level male manager was sexually harassing several women in the office. She tried to reason with the office manager to do something about the offensive behavior, but the manager would not do anything. She then told the manager and several other people in the office that if the manager did not do something about the behavior, she would blow the whistle to the personnel office. The manager then told the offender that if he did not stop the harassment, the personnel office would be brought in. He did stop the behavior, but he and several other employees refused to talk to the woman who initiated the actions. She eventually left the university.[8]

6. Sabotaging the implementation of the unethical behavior. A program manager for a Boston-area local social welfare organization was told by her superior to replace a significant percentage of her clients who received disability benefits with refugee Soviet Jews. She wanted to help both the refugees and her current clients; however, she thought it was unethical to drop current clients, in part because she believed such an action could result in unnecessary deaths. Previously, a person who had lost benefits because of what the program manager considered unethical "bumping" had committed suicide: He had not wanted to force his family to sell their home in order to pay for the medical care he needed and qualify for poverty programs. After her attempts to reason with her boss failed, she instituted a paperwork chain with a partially funded federal agency that prevented her own agency from dropping clients for nine months, after which time they would be eligible for a different funding program. Her old clients received benefits and the new refugees also received benefits. In discussions with her boss she blamed the federal agency for making it impossible to drop people quickly. Her boss, a political appointee who did not understand the system, also blamed the federal agency office.[9]

7. Publicly blowing the whistle within the organization. John W. Young, the chief of NASA's astronaut office, wrote a 12-page internal memorandum to 97 people after the Challenger explosion that killed seven crew members. The memo listed a large number of safety-related problems that Young said had endangered crews since October 1984. According to Young, "If the management system is not big enough to stop the space shuttle program whenever necessary to make flight safety corrections, it will not survive and neither will our three space shuttles or their flight crews." The memo was instrumental in the decision to broaden safety investigations throughout the total NASA system.[10]

8. Quietly refraining from implementing an unethical order/policy. Frank Ladwig was a top salesman and branch manager with a large computer company for more than 40 years. At times, he had trouble balancing his responsibilities. For instance, he was trained to sell solutions to customer problems, yet he had order and revenue quotas that sometimes made it difficult for him to concentrate on solving problems. He was responsible for signing and keeping important customers with annual revenues of between $250,000 and $500,000 and for aggressively and conscientiously representing new products that had required large R&D investments. He was required to sell the full line of products and services, and sometimes he had sales quotas for products that he believed were not a good match for the customer or appeared to perform marginally. Ladwig would quietly not sell those products, concentrating on selling the products he believed in. He would quietly explain the characteristics of the questionable products to his knowledgeable customers and get their reactions, rather than making an all-out sales effort. When he was asked by his sales manager why a certain product was not moving, he explained what the customers objected to and why. However, Ladwig thought that a salesman or manager with an average or poor performance record would have a difficult time getting away with this type of solution to an ethical dilemma.[11]

9. Conscientiously objecting to an unethical policy or refusing to implement it. Francis O'Brien was a research director for the pharmaceutical company Searle & Co. O'Brien conscientiously objected to what he believed were exaggerated claims for the Searle Copper 7 intrauterine contraceptive. When reasoning with upper-level management failed, O'Brien wrote them the following:

> Their continued use, in my opinion, is both misleading and a thinly disguised attempt to make claims which are not FDA approved. . . . Because of personal reasons I do not consent to have my name used in any press release or in connection with any press release. In addition, I will not participate in any press conferences.

O'Brien left the company ten years later. Currently, several lawsuits are pending against Searle, charging that its IUD caused infection and sterility.[12]

10. Indicating uncertainty about or refusing to support a cover-up in the event that the individual and/or organization gets caught. In the Boston office of Bear Stearns, four brokers informally work together as a group. One of the brokers had been successfully trading on insider information, and he invited the other three to do the same. One of the three told the others that such trading was not worth the risk of getting caught, and if an investigation ever occurred, he was not sure he would be able to participate in a cover-up. The other two brokers decided not to trade on the insider information, and the first broker stopped at least that type of insider trading.[13]

11. Secretly blowing the whistle outside the corporation. William Schwartzkopf of the Commonwealth Electric Company secretly and anonymously wrote a letter to the Justice Department alleging large-scale, long-time bid rigging among many of the largest U.S. electrical contractors. The secret letter accused the contractors of raising bids and conspiring to divide billions of dollars of contracts. Companies in the industry have already paid more than $20 million in fines to the government in part as a result of this letter, and they face millions of dollars more in losses when the victims sue.[14]

12. Publicly blowing the whistle outside the organization. A. Earnest Fitzgerald, a former high-level manager in the U.S. Air Force and Lockheed CEO, revealed to Congress and the press that the Air Force and Lockheed systematically practiced a strategy of underbidding in order to gain Air Force contracts for Lockheed, which then billed the Air Force and received payments for cost overruns on the contracts. Fitzgerald was fired for his trouble, but eventually received his job back. The underbidding/cost overruns, on at least the C-5/A cargo plane, were stopped.[15]

Limitations of Intervention

The intervention strategies described above can be very effective, but they also have some important limitations.

1. The individual can be wrong about the organization's actions. Lower-level employees commonly do not have as much or as good information about ethical situations and issues as higher-level managers. Similarly, they may not be as experienced as higher-level managers in dealing with specific ethical issues. The quality of experience and information an individual has can influence the quality of his or her ethical judgments. To the extent that this is true in any given situation, the use of intervention may or may not be warranted. In Case 9, for example, if Frank Ladwig had limited computer experience, he could have been wrong about some of the products he thought would not produce the promised results.

2. Relationships can be damaged. Suppose that instead of identifying with the individuals who want an organization to change its ethical behavior, we look at these situations from another perspective. How do we feel when we are forced to change our behavior? Further, how would we feel if we were forced by a subordinate to change, even though we thought that we had the position, quality of information, and/or quality of experience to make the correct decisions? Relationships would probably be, at the least, strained, particularly if we made an ethical decision and were nevertheless forced to change. If we are wrong, it may be that we do not recognize it at the time. If we know we are wrong, we still may not like being forced to change. However, it is possible that the individual forcing us to change may justify his or her behavior to us, and our relationship may actually be strengthened.

3. The organization can be hurt unnecessarily.   If an individual is wrong in believing that the organization is unethical, the organization can be hurt unnecessarily by his or her actions. Even if the individual is right, the organization can still be unnecessarily hurt by intervention strategies.

4. Intervention strategies can encourage "might makes right" climates. If we want "wrong" people, who might be more powerful now or in the future than we are, to exercise self-restraint, then we may need to exercise self-restraint even when we are "right." A problem with using force is that the other side may use more powerful or effective force now or later. Many people have been punished for trying to act ethically both when they were right and when they were wrong. By using force, one may also contribute to the belief that the only way to get things done in a particular organization is through force. People who are wrong can and do use force, and win. Do we want to build an organization culture in which force plays an important role? Gandhi's response to "an eye for an eye" was that if we all followed that principle, eventually everyone would be blind.

Being as a Part

While the intervention strategies discussed above can be very effective, they can also be destructive. Therefore, it may be appropriate to consider the advantages of leading an ethical change effort (being as a part) as well as intervening against unethical behaviors (being as an individual).

Tillich maintains that the courage to be as a part is the courage to affirm one's own being through participation with others. He writes,

> The self affirms itself as participant in the power of a group, of a movement. . . . Self-affirmation within a group includes the courage to accept guilt and its consequences as public guilt, whether one is oneself responsible or whether somebody else is. It is a problem of the group which has to be expiated for the sake of the group, and the methods of punishment and satisfaction . . . are accepted by the individual. . . . In every human community, there are out-standing members, the bearers of the traditions and leaders of the future. They must have sufficient distance in order to judge and to change. They must take

responsibility and ask questions. This unavoidably produces individual doubt and personal guilt. Nevertheless, the predominant pattern is the courage to be a part in all members of the . . . group. . . . The difference between the genuine Stoic and the neocollectivist is that the latter is bound in the first place to the collective and in the second place to the universe, while the Stoic was first of all related to the universal Logos and secondly to possible human groups. . . . The democratic-conformist type of the courage to be as a part was in an outspoken way tied up with the idea of progress. The courage to be as a part in the progress of the group to which one belongs . . .[16]

Leading Ethical Change

A good cross-cultural conceptualization of leadership is offered by Yoshino and Lifson: "The essence of leadership is the influential increment over and above mechanical compliance with routine directives of the organization."[17] This definition permits comparisons between and facilitates an understanding of different leadership styles through its use of a single variable: created incremental performance. Of course, different types of leadership may be more or less effective in different types of situations; yet, it is helpful to understand the "essence" of leadership in its many different cultural forms as the creation of incremental change beyond the routine.

For example, Yoshino and Lifson compare generalizations (actually over-generalizations) about Japanese and American leadership styles:

> In the United States, a leader is often thought of as one who blazes new trails, a virtuoso whose example inspires awe, respect, and emulation. If any individual characterizes this pattern, it is surely John Wayne, whose image reached epic proportions in his own lifetime as an embodiment of something uniquely American. A Japanese leader, rather than being an authority, is more of a communications channel, a mediator, a facilitator, and most of all, a symbol and embodiment of group unity. Consensus building is necessary in decision making, and this requires patience and an ability to use carefully cultivated relationships to get all to agree for the good of the unit. A John Wayne in this situation might succeed temporarily by virtue of charisma, but eventually the inability to build strong emotion-laden relationships and use these as a tool of motivation and consensus building would prove fatal.[18]

A charismatic, "John Wayne type" leader can inspire and/or frighten people into diverting from the routine. A consensus-building, Japanese-style leader can get people to agree to divert from the routine. In both cases, the leader creates incremental behavior change beyond the routine. How does leadership (being as a part) in its various cultural forms differ from the various intervention (being as an individual) strategies and cases discussed above? Some case data may be revealing.

Cases

1. Roger Boisjoly and the Challenger launch.[19]

In January 1985, after the post-flight hardware inspection of Flight 52C, Roger Boisjoly strongly suspected that unusually low temperatures had compromised the performance effectiveness of the O-ring seals on two field joints. Such a performance compromise could cause an explosion. In March 1985, laboratory tests confirmed that low temperatures did negatively affect the ability of the O-rings to perform this sealing function. In June 1985, the post-flight inspection of Flight 51B revealed serious erosion of both primary and backup seals that, had it continued, could have caused an explosion.

These events convinced Boisjoly that a serious and very dangerous problem existed with the O-rings. Instead of acting as an individual against his supervisors and the organization, for example, by blowing the whistle to the press, he tried to lead a change to stop the launching of flights with unsafe O-rings. He worked with his immediate supervisor, the director of engineering, and the organization in leading this change. He wrote a draft of a memo to Bob Lund, vice-president of engineering, which he first showed and discussed with his immediate supervisor to "maintain good relationships." Boisjoly and others developed potential win-win solutions, such as investigating remedies to fix the O-rings and refraining from launching flights at too-low temperatures. He effectively established a team to study the matter, and participated in a teleconference with 130 technical experts.

On the day before the Challenger launch, Boisjoly and other team members were successful in leading company executives to reverse their tentative recommendation to launch because the overnight temperatures were predicted to be too low. The company recommendation was to launch only when temperatures were above 53 degrees. To this point, Boisjoly was very effective in leading a change toward what he and other engineering and management people believed was a safe and ethical decision.

However, according to testimony from Boisjoly and others to Congress, the top managers of Morton Thiokol, under pressure from NASA, reversed their earlier recommendation not to launch. The next day, Challenger was launched and exploded, causing the deaths of all the crew members. While Boisjoly was very effective in leading a change within his own organization, he was not able to counteract subsequent pressure from the customer, NASA.

2. Dan Phillips and Genco, Inc.[20]

Dan Phillips was a paper products group division manager for Genco, whose upper-level management adopted a strategy whereby several mills, including the Elkhorn Mill, would either have to reduce costs or close down. Phillips was concerned that cost cutting at Elkhorn would prevent the mill from meeting government pollution-control requirements, and that closing the mill could seriously hurt the local community. If he reduced costs, he would not meet pollution-control requirements; if he did not reduce costs, the mill would close and the community would suffer.

Phillips did not secretly or publicly blow the whistle, nor did he sabotage, conscientiously object, quietly refrain from implementing the plan, or quit; however, he did lead a change in the organization's ethical behavior. He asked research and development people in his division to investigate how the plant could both become more cost efficient and create less pollution. He then asked operations people in his division to estimate how long it would take to put such a new plant design on line, and how much it would cost. He asked cost accounting and financial people within his division to estimate when such a new operation would achieve a break-even payback. Once he found a plan that would work, he negotiated a win-win solution with upper-level management: in exchange for not closing the plant and increasing its investment in his division, the organization would over time benefit from lower costs and higher profitability. Phillips thus worked with others and the organization to lead an inquiry and adopt an alternative ethical and cost-effective plan.

3. Lotus and Brazilian Software Importing.[21]

Lotus, a software manufacturer, found that in spite of restrictions on the importing of much of its software to Brazil, many people there were buying and using Lotus software. On further investigation, the company discovered that Brazilian businessmen, in alliance with a Brazilian general, were violating the law by buying Lotus software in Cambridge, Massachusetts and bringing it into Brazil.

Instead of blowing the whistle on the illegal behavior, sabotaging it, or leaving Brazil, Lotus negotiated a solution: In exchange for the Brazilians' agreement to stop illegal importing, Lotus helped set them up as legitimate licensed manufacturers and distributors of Lotus products in Brazil. Instead of working against them and the Lotus salespeople supplying them, the Lotus managers worked with these people to develop an ethical, legal, and economically sound solution to the importing problem.

And in at least a limited sense, the importers may have been transformed into ethical managers and business people. This case may remind you of the legendary "Old West," where government officials sometimes negotiated win-win solutions with "outlaw gunfighters," who agreed to become somewhat more ethical as appointed sheriffs. The gunfighters needed to make a living, and many were not interested in or qualified for such other professions as farming or shopkeeping. In some cases, ethical behavior may take place before ethical beliefs are assumed.

4. Insurance company office/sales manager and discrimination.[22]   The sales-office manager of a very large Boston-area insurance company tried to hire female salespeople several times, but his boss refused to permit the hires. The manager could have acted against his boss and the organization by secretly threatening to blow the whistle or actually blowing the whistle, publicly or secretly. Instead, he decided to try to lead a change in the implicit hiring policy of the organization.

The manager asked his boss why he was not permitted to hire a woman. He learned that his boss did not believe women made good salespeople and had never worked with a female salesperson. He found that reasoning with his boss about the capabilities of women and the ethics and legality of refusing to hire women was ineffective.

He inquired within the company about whether being a woman could be an advantage in any insurance sales areas. He negotiated with his boss a six-month experiment whereby he hired on a trial basis one woman to sell life insurance to married women who contributed large portions of their salaries to their home mortgages. The woman he hired was not only very successful in selling this type of life insurance, but became one of the office's top salespeople. After this experience, the boss reversed his policy of not hiring female salespeople.

Limitations to Leading Ethical Organizational Change

In the four cases described above, the individuals did not attack the organization or people within the organization, nor did they intervene against individuals and/or the organization to stop an unethical practice. Instead, they worked with people in the organization to build a more ethical organization. As a result of their leadership, the organizations used more ethical behaviors. The strategy of leading an organization toward more ethical behavior, however, does have some limitations. These are described below.

1. In some organizational situations, ethical win–win solutions or compromises may not be possible. For example, in 1975 a pharmaceutical company in Raritan, New Jersey decided to enter a new market with a new product.[23] Grace Pierce, who was then in charge of medical testing of new products, refused to test a new diarrhea drug product on infants and elderly consumers because it contained high levels of saccharin, which

was feared by many at the time to be a carcinogen. When Pierce was transferred, she resigned. The drug was tested on infant and elderly consumers. In this case, Pierce may have been faced with an either–or situation that left her little room to lead a change in organizational behavior.

Similarly, Errol Marshall, with Hydraulic Parts and Components, Inc.,[24] helped negotiate the sale of a subcontract to sell heavy equipment to the U.S. Navy while giving $70,000 in kickbacks to two materials managers of Brown & Root, Inc., the project's prime contractor. According to Marshall, the prime contractor "demanded the kickbacks. . . . It was cut and dried. We would not get the business otherwise." While Marshall was not charged with any crime, one of the upper-level Brown & Root managers, William Callan, was convicted in 1985 of extorting kickbacks, and another manager, Frank DiDomenico, pleaded guilty to extorting kickbacks from Hydraulic Parts & Components, Inc. Marshall has left the company. In this case, it seems that Marshall had no win–win alternative to paying the bribe. In some situations it may not be possible to lead a win–win ethical change.

2. Some people do not understand how leadership can be applied to situations that involve organizational ethics issues. Also, some people—particularly those in analytical or technical professions, which may not offer much opportunity for gaining leadership experience—may not know how to lead very well in any situation. Some people may be good leaders in the course of their normal work lives, but do not try to lead or do not lead very well when ethical issues are involved. Some people avoid discussing ethical, religious, and political issues at work.

For example, John Geary was a salesman for U.S. Steel when the company decided to enter a new market with what he and others considered an unsafe new product.[25] As a leading salesman for U.S. Steel, Geary normally was very good at leading the way toward changes that satisfied customer and organizational needs. A good salesman frequently needs to coordinate and spearhead modifications in operations, engineering, logistics, product design, financing, and billing/payment that are necessary for a company to maintain good customer relationships and salary. Apparently, however, he did not try to lead the organization in developing a win-win solution, such as soliciting current orders for a later delivery of a corrected product. He tried only reasoning against selling the unsafe product and protested its sale to several groups of upper-level engineers and managers. He noted that he believed the product had a failure rate of 3.6% and was therefore both unsafe and potentially damaging to U.S. Steel's longer-term strategy of entering higher technology/profit margin businesses. According to Geary, even though many upper-level managers, engineers, and salesmen understood and believed him, "the only desire of everyone associated with the project was to satisfy the instructions of Henry Wallace (the sales vice-president). No one was about to buck this man for fear of his job."[26] The sales vice-president fired Geary, apparently because he continued to protest against sale of the product.

Similarly, William Schwartzkopf of Commonwealth Electric Co.[27] did not think he could either ethically reason against or lead an end to the large-scale, long-time bid rigging between his own company and many of the largest U.S. electrical contractors. Even though he was an attorney and had extensive experience in leading organizational changes, he did not try to lead his company toward an ethical solution. He waited until he retired from the company, then wrote a secret letter to the Justice Department accusing the contractors of raising bids and conspiring to divide billions of dollars of contracts among themselves.

Many people—both experienced and inexperienced in leadership— do not try to lead their companies toward developing solutions to ethical problems. Often, they do not understand that it is possible to lead such a change; therefore, they do not try to do so—even though, as the cases here show, many succeed when they do try.

3. Some organizational environments—in both consensus-building and authoritarian types of cultures—discourage leadership that is non-conforming. For example, as Robert E. Wood, former CEO of the giant international retailer Sears, Roebuck, has observed, "We stress the advantages of the free enterprise system, we complain about the totalitarian state, but in our individual organizations we have created more or less a totalitarian system in industry, particularly in large industry."[28] Similarly, Charles W. Summers, in a *Harvard Business Review* article, observes, "Corporate executives may argue that . . . they recognize and protect . . . against arbitrary termination through their own internal procedures. The simple fact is that most companies have not recognized and protected that right."[29]

David Ewing concludes that "It [the pressure to obey unethical and illegal orders] is probably most dangerous, however, as a low-level infection. When it slowly bleeds the individual conscience dry and metastasizes insidiously, it is most difficult to defend against. There are no spectacular firings or purges in the ranks. There are no epic blunders. Under constant and insistent pressure, employees simply give in and conform. They become good 'organization people.' "[30]

Similar pressures can exist in participate, consensus-building types of cultures. For example, as mentioned above, Yoshino and Lifson write,

"A Japanese leader, rather than being an authority, is more of a communications channel, a mediator, a facilitator, and most of all, a symbol and embodiment of group unity. Consensus building is necessary to decision making, and this requires patience and an ability to use carefully cultivated relationships to get all to agree for the good of the unit."[31]

The importance of the group and the position of the group leaders as a symbol of the group are revealed in the very popular true story, "Tale of the Forty-Seven Ronin." The tale is about 47 warriors whose lord is unjustly killed. The Ronin spend years sacrificing everything, including their families, in order to kill the person responsible for their leader's death. Then all those who survive the assault kill themselves.

Just as authoritarian top-down organizational cultures can produce unethical behaviors, so can participative, consensus-building cultures. The Japanese novelist Shusaku Endo, in his *The Sea and Poison*, describes the true story of such a problem.[32] It concerns an experiment cooperatively performed by the Japanese Army, a medical hospital, and a consensus-building team of doctors on American prisoners of war. The purpose of the experiment was to determine scientifically how much blood people can lose before they die.

Endo describes the reasoning and feelings of one of the doctors as he looked back at this behavior:

> "At the time nothing could be done. . . . If I were caught in the same way, I might, I might just do the same thing again. . . . We feel that getting on good terms ourselves with the Western Command medical people, with whom Second [section] is so cozy, wouldn't be a bad idea at all. Therefore we feel there's no need to ill temperedly refuse their friendly proposal and hurt their feelings. . . . Five doctors from Kando's section most likely will be glad to get the chance. . . . For me the pangs of conscience . . . were from childhood equivalent to the fear of disapproval in the eyes of others—fear of the punishment which society would bring to bear. . . . To put it quite bluntly, I am able to remain quite undisturbed in the face of someone else's terrible suffering and death. . . . I am not writing about the experiences as one driven to do so by his conscience . . . all these memories are distasteful to me. But looking upon them as distasteful and suffering because of them are two different matters. Then why do I bother writing? Because I'm strangely ill at ease. I, who fear only the eyes of others and the punishment of society, and whose fears disappear when I am secure from these, am now disturbed. . . . I have no conscience, I suppose. Not just me, though. None of them feel anything at all about what they did here." The only emotion in his heart was a sense of having fallen as low as one can fall.[33]

What to Do and How to Be

In light of the discussion of the two approaches to addressing organizational ethics issues and their limitations, what should we do as individuals and members of organizations? To some extent that depends on the circumstances and our own abilities. If we know how to lead, if there's time for it, if the key people in authority are reasonable, and if a win-win solution is possible, one should probably try leading an organizational change.

If, on the other hand, one does not know how to lead, time is limited, the authority figures are unreasonable, a culture of strong conformity exists, and the situation is not likely to produce a win–win outcome, then the chances of success with a leadership approach are much lower. This may leave one with only the choice of using one of the intervention strategies discussed above. If an individual wishes to remain an effective member of the organization, then one of the more secretive strategies may be safer.

But what about the more common, middle range of problems? Here there is no easy prescription. The more win–win potential the situation has, the more time there is, the more leadership skills one has, and the more reasonable the authority figures and organizational cultures are, the more likely a leadership approach is to succeed. If the opposite conditions exist, then forcing change in the organization is the likely alternative.

To a large extent, the choice depends on an individual's courage. In my opinion, in all but the most extreme and unusual circumstances, one should first try to lead a change toward ethical behavior. If that does not succeed, the mustering the courage to act against others and the organization may be necessary. For example, the course of action that might [have saved] the Challenger crew was for Boisjoly or someone else to act against Morton Thiokol, its top managers, and NASA by blowing the whistle to the press.

If there is an implicitly characteristic American ontology, perhaps it is some version of William James' 1907 *Pragmatism*, which, for better or worse, sees through a lens of interactions the ontologies of being as an individual and being as a part. James explains our situation as follows:

> What we were discussing was the idea of a world growing not integrally but piecemeal by the contributions of its several parts. Take the hypothesis seriously and as a live one. Suppose that the world's author put the case to you before creation, saying: "If I am going to make a world not certain to be saved, a world the perfection of which shall be conditional merely, the condition being that each several agent does its own 'level best.' I offer you the chance of taking part in such a world. Its safety, you see, is unwarranted. It is a real adventure, with real danger, yet it may win through. It is a social scheme of co-operative work genuinely to be done. Will you join the procession? Will you trust yourself and trust the other agents enough to face the risk?" . . . Then it is perfectly possible to accept sincerely a drastic kind of a universe from which the element

of "seriousness" is not to be excelled. Who so does so is, it seems to me, a genuine pragmatist. He is willing to live on a scheme of uncertified possibilities which he trusts; willing to pay with his own person, if need be, for the realization of the ideals which he frames. What now actually are the other forces which he trusts to co-operate with him, in a universe of such a type? They are at least his fellow men, in the stage of being which our actual universe has reached.[34]

In conclusion, there are realistic ethics leadership and intervention action strategies. We can act effectively concerning organizational ethics issues. Depending upon the circumstances including our own courage, we can choose to act and be ethical both as individuals and as leaders. Being as a part and leading ethical change is the more constructive approach generally. However, being as an individual intervening against others and organizations can sometimes be the only short or medium term effective approach.

Notes

1. Paul Tillich, *The Courage To Be*. New Haven: Yale University Press, 1950.
2. See Endnote 1, p. 159.
3. David Ewing, *Freedom Inside the Organization*. New York: McGraw-Hill, 1977.
4. The person blowing the whistle in this case wishes to remain anonymous. See also Elizabeth Neuffer, "GE Managers Sentenced For Bribery." *The Boston Globe*, 26 July 1988, p. 67.
5. Barbara Ley Toffler, *Tough Choices: Managers Talk Ethics*. New York: John Wiley, 1986, pp. 153–169.
6. Richard P. Nielsen, "What Can Managers Do About Unethical Management?" *Journal of Business Ethics* (April 1987), 153–161. See also Nielson's "Limitations of Ethical Reasoning As An Action Strategy", *Journal of Business Ethics* 7 (November 1988), 725–733, and "Arendt's Action Philosophy and the Manager as Eichmann, Richard III, Faust or Institution Citizen." *California Management Review* 26, 3 (Spring 1984), 191–201.
7. The person involved wishes to remain anonymous.
8. The person involved wishes to remain anonymous.
9. See Endnote 6.
10. R. Reinhold, "Astronauts Chief Says NASA Risked Life For Schedule", *The New York Times* 36, 22 August 1986, p. 1.
11. Personal conversation and letter with Frank Ladwig, 1986. See also Frank Ladwig and Associates, *Advanced Consultative Selling For Professionals*. Stonington, CT, 1988.
12. W. G. Glaberson, "Did Searle Lose Its Eyes to a Health Hazard?" *Business Week*, 14 October 1985, pp. 120–122.
13. The person involved wishes to remain anonymous.
14. Andy Pasztor, "Electrical Contractors Reel Under Charges The They Rigged Bids," *The Wall Street Journal*, 29 November 1985, pp. 1, 14.
15. A. Ernest Fitzgerald, *The High Priests of Waste*. New York: McGraw-Hill, 1977.

16. See Endnote 1, pp. 89, 93.

17. M. Y. Yoshino and T. B. Lifson, *The Invisible Link: Japan's Saga Shosha and the Organization of Trade*. Cambridge: MIT Press, 1986.

18. See Endnote 17, p. 178.

19. Roger Boisjoly, address given at Massachusetts Institute of Technology on January 7, 1987. Reprinted in *Books and Religion*, March/April 1987, 3–4, 12–13. See also Carolyn Whitbeck, "Moral Responsibility and the Working Engineer," *Books and Religion*, March/April 1987, 3, 22–23.

20. Personal conversation with Ray Bauer, Harvard Business School, 1975. See also R. Ackerman and Ray Bauer, *Corporate Social Responsiveness*. Reston, VA: Reston Publishing, 1976.

21. The person involved wishes to remain anonymous.

22. The person involved wishes to remain anonymous.

23. David Ewing, *Do It My Way Or You're Fired*. New York: John Wiley, 1983.

24. E. T. Pound, "Investigators Detect Pattern of Kickbacks For Defense Business," *The Wall Street Journal*, 14 November 1985, pp. 1, 25.

25. See Endnote 23. See also *Geary vs. U.S. Steel Corporation*, 319 A. 2nd 174, Supreme Court of Pa.

26. See Endnote 23, p. 86.

27. See Endnote 14.

28. See Endnote 3, p. 21.

29. C. W. Summers, "Protecting All Employees Against Unjust Dismissal," *Harvard Business Review* 58, 1980, 132–139.

30. See Endnote 3, pp. 216–217.

31. See Endnote 17, p. 187.

32. Shusaku Endo, *The Sea and Poison*. New York: Taplinger Publishing Co., 1972. See also Y. Yasuda, *Old Tales of Japan*, Tokyo: Charles Tuttle Co., 1947.

33. See Endnote 32.

34. William James, *Pragmatism: A New Name for Some Old Ways of Thinking*. New York: Longmans, Green and Co., 1907, pp. 290, 297–298.

CASE I

PERSONALITIES OR PEEVES?

This case concerns the management of a 35-bed special care nursery in a moderate-sized teaching hospital. The unit is a regional referral and transport center for sick and premature newborns. It has grown rapidly with a tripling of census in five years accompanied by the mushrooming of sophisticated technology. Much of this growth has occurred in the past two years. Expansion of equipment and personnel resources have often lagged behind need and demand. As might be expected, with rapid growth in size and complexity, it has been a time of stress and change for the unit.

There are approximately 90 personnel in the unit, including 4 assistant head nurses under the direction of Gertrude the head nurse. Gertrude reports both to Charlotte the clinical specialist, and to Adam the administrative supervisor. Approximately three years ago, several major changes occurred in nursing service administration:

1. The obstetric-gynecological (Ob-Gyn) nursing supervisor was promoted to assistant director of hospital nursing with responsibility for specialty units. She has been at the institution for 20 years and has risen through the ranks from staff nurse.
2. The head nurse of the special care nursery was promoted to Ob-Gyn nursing supervisor. She has been at the hospital for 13 years, receiving her basic education there and working there since graduation.
3. The assistant head nurse in the special care nursery was promoted to head nurse. In the ten years since her graduation, she has

worked exclusively at the hospital. She has been with the special care nursery for five years.

About two years ago Charlotte, the clinical specialist, arrived at the special care nursery having worked peripherally with the nursery under a grant for outreach education. She received her basic education from a university in New York City; worked in several different clinical settings with various clinical, administrative, and supervisory responsibilities; and received advanced clinical preparation in her area of specialization. Although she occupies a supervisory line position, her role is primarily clinical, ensuring excellence of care provided to the patient. The Ob-Gyn supervisor, Adam, also responsible for the special care nursery, assumes the administrative duties. This fine line between clinical and administrative tasks regularly creates confusion, as responsibilities often overlap.

In the role of clinical specialist, responsible for patient care and staff education, Charlotte interacts daily with the staff. It appears that the staff sees her more as a resource person and colleague than as a supervisor. Approximately a year-and-a-half ago, she began to receive a series of informal complaints from staff and attending physicians regarding the "attitude" and "personality" of the head nurse, Gertrude. These concerns expressed a general lack of respect and loss of confidence in Gertrude's leadership abilities. She was labeled lazy, unresponsive, hostile, and tactless. There were also reports of her being judgmental toward patients. She rarely participated in patient care. Staff were unwilling to confront her directly as they felt she was "punitive" and would retaliate through assignment of undesirable duties, manipulation of time, and rendering of poor evaluations. Her style was demolishing staff morale, diminishing staff involvement and productivity, and, according to some, contributing to an increased turnover of experienced personnel. She received little or no support from staff, and the physicians pushed for her replacement.

When Charlotte discussed these concerns with Gertrude the head nurse denied problems with the staff and was generally uncommunicative. Most of the allegations were difficult to confirm. Most involved what might be viewed as "personality" problems, and Gertrude always had explanations or "reasons" for the observed behaviors. In addition, she was administratively competent and had never demonstrated difficulties in dealing with her superiors. She had no previous poor evaluations.

Charlotte brought her concerns to the administrative supervisor and assistant director. They were concerned about overreacting and bending to the power of the physicians. After all, every leader meets with some criticism. One can not hope to please everyone all the time. Gertrude deserved due process and verification and confirmation of the problems. The managers met with the director of personnel and developed a plan to monitor the problem over a period of time. They clarified expectations of Gertrude and defined parameters for evaluation. They made a commitment to offer their support in order to promote her growth. Counseling sessions were to be fairly and carefully documented. Gertrude attributed some of the identified problems to her overload of administrative duties. As it is true that she was responsible for an unusually large number of personnel and patients, the managers developed the position of administrative assistant head nurse and made plans to delegate duties. Gertrude agreed to the plan.

Things appeared to be improving but, after awhile, individual staff began to express concern. They again refused to speak with Gertrude. She became less and less communicative; her sick time increased. One day, Gertrude had a major disagreement with one of the attendings. He threatened to "go to the top" if something wasn't done.

The administrative supervisor, assistant director, and clinical supervisor met and decided that although Gertrude was extremely capable in her administrative duties, she indeed appeared to have difficulties in interpersonal relations with staff, physicians, and patients. They had spent a great deal of effort during the past two years attempting to encourage staff participation and decision making to improve morale and job satisfaction. They had hopes, supported by experience and current literature, that this would increase retention and recruitment of qualified personnel and would promote optimal performance. They felt that many of these efforts were negated, undermined, or at least not vigorously supported by Gertrude. While Gertrude's experience and administrative competence were valuable, there were other competent, caring, and capable persons who could assume these tasks and bring with them the creative energy and sensitivity needed in the head nurse position.

The issues were complicated by personal concerns for Gertrude. She still lived at home, with a strict, high-achieving family. There was apparently little warmth, sharing, or communication. In addition, Gertrude was in the process of repaying a significant sum of money to the hospital for tuition reimbursement. Moreover, she was obese. Despite support and encouragement, she had failed to participate in counseling to assist her with her personal situation.

Despite all of these considerations, delays in talking with Gertrude continued. After a period of time, she abruptly resigned from her position as head nurse. The assistant director then offered Gertrude a day position on the postpartum unit, a position for which two other qualified staff nurses had been waiting. Neither the supervisor nor the assistant director

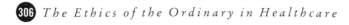

have to date spoken to Gertrude to clarify the problem, and neither has offered assistance.

Questions for Discussion

1. Have all ethical obligations been met?
2. Is Gertrude being treated ethically?
3. Should Gertrude be treated as "sick" and in need of professional help? Should she be disciplined for incompetence? Should she be kept from interpersonal roles?
4. Is it ethical to place Gertrude ahead of the two qualified nurses awaiting the position in the postpartum unit?
5. Did the clinical supervisor behave ethically in not communicating directly with Gertrude?
6. Has a win–win alternative been sought? Does such an alternative exist?

CASE J

MORAL MANIPULATION?

What is the ethical thing to do when a healthcare manager's professional judgment conflicts with the judgment of higher authority? This case traces the evolution of such a dilemma as encountered by a midlevel supervisor working at a state facility for the mentally disabled. The case probes fiscal, intergovernmental, organizational, and personal realities that complicated the situation. A major focus is the tension between funding constraints and professional wisdom, a tension commonly experienced by healthcare managers.

Amber Good, a unit supervisor at a state developmental center, has been directed to prepare written plans for the transfer of her unit's 66 clients to a level of care that she and her staff firmly view as inappropriate. The directive came through her immediate boss from the facility director in an effort to comply with a new regulation of the federal Health Care Financing Administration (HCFA). Since 80 percent of the unit's funding comes from the Medicaid program administered by HCFA, failure to meet the federal requirements will have a devastating impact on the facility.

In order to continue to qualify for the federal funds, the facility is required to certify, in a written plan, that each of the unit's 66 severely retarded clients is projected to be moved to a lower level of care within three to five years. The problem is that the unit staff—clinical as well as administrative—are convinced that, with a few exceptions, the clients will continue to require the same level of care as that currently provided.

Fred Cower, Amber's boss, has told her that plans "must be in the charts of every client within two weeks," when the federal utilization review (UR) team is due to inspect the facility. While aware of the ramifications—for her clients, her staff, her facility, and her own career—of failing to comply, Amber Good has serious ethical concerns about carrying out the directive. As she has told her boss: "I'm very disturbed over the ethics of putting something in writing which neither I nor my team can truly support." She has been chided for being argumentative about a task that, in Fred's words, "simply must be done." Amber is in the grip of an ethical dilemma.

The Organizational Setting

Treatment team leaders (TTLs) like Amber are individuals with professional credentials in a clinical field and may also have a professional management degree. Generally, as in Amber's case, they have advanced through the system to positions of increasing clinical responsibility until they are recognized for their experience and demonstrated skills and are promoted to the more managerial position of TTL. A TTL has supervisory power over all professional clinicians and therapy aides, including other supervisory-level staff on the treatment team.

The facility, which is charged with the care and treatment of the mentally retarded and developmentally disabled, receives most of its funding through the federal government's Medicaid program for intermediate care facilities (ICFs). It is, thus, subject to regulation and regular inspection by HCFA. Federal guidelines, which include significant restrictions, then set the tone for state regulation and policy.

Because a large sum of federal money does go to support the Medicaid ICF program, many regulations and inspection criteria focus on utilization review for all of the clients supported. Specifically, the federal government looks, first, for verification of those diagnoses that are deemed appropriate for treatment at an ICF. Second, HCFA requires documented and obtainable client benefit from each individually prescribed treatment program. Third, HCFA mandates specific formalized plans developed by the treatment team for the client's movement to another—lower—level of care. In meeting these requirements, and formally stating so in its annual case review report for each client, the treatment team is expected to actually verify the appropriateness of using federal monies to maintain the client at the current care level. Taking this one step further, team leaders at Amber's facility have been advised both formally and informally of their superiors' expectation that, without preapproved exceptions, all clients are to meet federal UR criteria.

The rationale given by Amber's superiors for this approach has been that, without federal funding to support continued care, these clients would have to be placed elsewhere where they might not receive care and services that they need; or, failing to gain their admission to these alternative care facilities, the facility might have to maintain them and provide for their care and treatment at a rate of reimbursement that would be $20,000 per client less per year. That is, noncompliance with the new regulations will likely result in a major reduction of federal funding, and loss of such funding will result in major job cutbacks and loss of ICF status for the facility.

It is specifically the third federal UR requirement that is the source of Amber Good's ethical dilemma. The formal organizational expectation is that her treatment team identify and document for each of its clients a clearly articulated post-institutional plan that includes specification of services required when, within three to five years, the client will move to a facility providing a lower level of care. But Amber's treatment team has concluded that, with few exceptions, the clients will not be able to be moved to a lower level of care within that time frame.

Further complicating the situation for Amber is the concern, previously expressed by some of her team members, about routinely verifying the appropriateness of the expensive care provided at the facility. These team members have suggested that, given fiscal constraints and the remote likelihood that many of the clients will noticeably benefit from the ICF level of care, perhaps a lower level of care is, indeed, more appropriate immediately. In Amber's unit (ITT 007), the client population consists entirely of severely or profoundly retarded clients. All of them have significant physical limitations that, combined with their mental limitations, preclude any active assistance in their own personal care. Most of them are also severely limited in communications skills.

Initial Responses

Prior to introduction of the organizational expectation of compliance with the post-institutional plans requirement, ITT 007 had, as a team, determined that it would handle the problem as follows:

1. Whittle down to the smallest number possible the estimate of clients who could benefit as much from a lower level of care as from the current level; then, document in the record that they are receiving active treatment and apparently benefiting. The chart will state that these clients would be suited for a lower level of care within three to five years.
2. Monitor the status of those currently "on the border," while similarly verifying in the record their need for active treatment with the intent of modifying the plan downward should that become appropriate.

Amber's team is concerned about what "they" are really trying to accomplish with the new directive. Amber has used her influence to suggest that the new instructions might be intended only as a means of improving team planning on behalf of the clients. But suspicions have been raised by the governor's recent announcement that the facility will be closed within four years, with all residents moved to community placements. Clinical professionals on the team are convinced that development of appropriate community sites and services must precede formulation of any placement plans for their clients. A fear of being a party to the "dumping" of clients is widespread as is concern about job loss.

As noted previously, Amber's team has worked through its reservations about even routinely validating that client needs are being met by the current level of care. Now, the new directive is forcing the team to step well beyond what it previously agreed was acceptable.

Reality Sets In

Amber Good receives notification on April 14 from the utilization review coordinator of the change in federal requirements for the post-institutional plans. The new requirement, which went into effect on April 1, stipulates that all post-institutional plans must specify a projected level of care other than that provided at the facility. The UR inspection team is due at the facility during the first week of May to verify compliance with this new regulation.

Amber is aware that failure to act on the compliance directive will have serious ramifications, but she has some grave reservations as to whether it is ethical to follow through as expected. Her professional perspective leads her to believe that her clients should have the opportunity for treatment and program services that can be provided only in an ICF unit. In addition, however, her clinical judgment is that the clients served by her team are more likely to regress than to progress because of the severity of their disabilities. Yet the new directive requires her to project so much progress that the supports and services provided in her unit will no longer be required.

Amber previously engaged in discussions of related matters with her treatment team and suspects that they will resist the new requirement. Thus, not only is she unsure whether she can support the directive, but she anticipates that the team might flatly refuse to cooperate. Before this she has enjoyed an open, honest, and mutually respectful relationship with her team members, and has never asked them to participate in something with which she does not agree. She fears that if she supports the new directive, her own integrity might be questioned.

In the past, Amber has felt that Fred Cower, her boss, both liked her and respected her competence. Their relationship has been honest and friendly. Of late, however, Fred has become rather abrupt with all of the team leaders and argumentative over small matters. They have begun to regard him as someone quick to comply with whatever senior administration wants. Amber does not know whether this apparent shift in Fred's managerial style has resulted from job pressure, personal problems, or some other causes. She has been trying to avoid him but, given the current situation, she feels that some guidance and direction from him is needed.

After waiting a week for him to return from a conference, Amber meets with Fred and is informed that Bob Barsky himself—the facility director—has ordered Fred and all unit chiefs to have client charts in full compliance with the new UR criteria before the UR team visitation. Fred tells Amber that he knew she "would be mad" about this. He then produces the draft of a form which, he has assured Barsky, will be used to bring all charts into compliance.

Amber begins to outline her concerns, but Fred says flatly that the new post-institutional plans must be in the charts of every client on time, and that the new form will help "take care of it." The other treatment team leaders, Fred stresses to Amber, have already begun the task. Amber then expresses her concern over the basic ethical question of putting something in writing that neither she nor her team can truly support. She reminds Fred that the clinical judgment of the team is that the current ICF program is the only level of care suitable for most of the clients. She also tells him that she is uncomfortable with some of the wording on the form and asks if it can be changed. Fred chides her for being argumentative and says the meeting is over.

Between a Rock and a Hard Place

At this point, Amber Good feels that she has two choices. One, she can set aside personal reservations and call a team meeting (or write a memo) advising ITT 007 of the need to comply with the directive, and specifying assignments and time frames for completing the task. If she does not allow for discussion to ventilate feelings, she thinks, this option is likely to result in hostility and anger from team members and possible refusal to comply. Whether the refusal might come in a confrontational manner or through a more passive-aggressive act of noncompliance within the required time, Amber will be forced to deal with the matter through disciplinary action and that, in turn, is likely to damage her relationship with the team. The only virtue in this is that the expectations of Barsky and Cower might be satisfied, and they would probably view Amber as having done a good job. If she presents the directive to the team with a face-to-face discussion and explanation, team members might be more generally expected to follow through, she reasons. However, a loss of respect for Amber might still result from feelings that she has compromised her integrity by "selling out" to the administration. Still, the expectations of the director and the unit chief will have been met.

Alternatively, Amber can adhere strictly to her professional judgment and not comply with the directive. While this, likewise, could be done in several ways, the end result would be similar, she thinks. She could confront Fred, up front, and refuse to comply. Such a response could be viewed as insubordinate. This would probably force him to deal with her in a disciplinary manner and could jeopardize her career. Or, rather than refusing compliance, Amber reasons, she could simply fail to inform the team of the directive, thus assuring that the distasteful task will not be accomplished. This less open, but perhaps more expedient, approach might still result in a reprimand for her, but any sanctions might be less severe than in the more confrontational and deliberate approach. In any case, she feels that this would at least temporarily maintain the professional judgment of the treatment team and undermine the administrative judgment of her bosses.

Toward Creative Resolution

Amber Good concludes that neither course of action is responsible, and she gropes for an escape from the dilemma. Drawing from her experience, she surmises that, of all the alternatives open to the federal government UR team when a facility fails a compliance inspection, the least likely course of action is formal sanction. Rather, historically, UR teams more often advise the facility of its deficiencies and propose a time frame within which compliance would be expected. No formal check would likely be initiated prior to the next regularly scheduled UR visitation six months hence.

In this case, however, there is an additional factor to consider: the most recent HCFA site visit resulted in an initially favorable report that was later changed to one noting noncompliance with active treatment mandates. Fallout from that report included an increased sense of concern at administrative levels, as well as substantial efforts to demonstrate sufficient intent to comply with regulations prior to the follow-up visit. Thus, anxiety and pressure are now ongoing realities among her facility's administrative staff. Clearly, administrators are not interested in a repeat performance of the HCFA experience, a factor that is contributing to their current attitudes and actions regarding the pending UR inspection. The trickle-down effect of this anxiety is aggravating everyone's sense of job insecurity brought on by the planned closure of the facility.

Further reflection leads Amber to believe that she might still be able to influence the situation positively. Her history of competence and loyalty, she believes, gives her some leverage with Fred, who she senses is personally feeling the weight of a dilemma beneath his hard-nosed administrative behavior. Perhaps a "creative" proposal can be developed.

She decides to call a team meeting to discuss the problem face-to-face within the context of a clear understanding that the team members, like herself, have some ethical problems with the directive as well as with the regulatory guideline that prompted it—but with the similarly clear expectation that some course of action has to be identified that will allow the team both to preserve its ethical standards and values, and still honor the directive and the UR guideline.

At the meeting Amber does exert her authority and influence in bringing the team to consensus that compliance, in some form, is necessary. She also tries to work through the team's feelings regarding the matter and to clarify what the UR guideline *minimally* requires. This necessitates two tense hours of discussion at a time when there are only four working days left before the UR team arrives.

In concert with her team members Amber then develops a plan that includes modifying the form provided by Cower. The modification accommodates the requirement of projected placement at a different level of care, while also allowing the team to maintain its own position by not specifying any *currently* known and approved alternative levels of care. The modified form specifically includes the following:

- More individualization of information on supports and services required by each client in any projected alternative placement;
- A clear statement that the client currently does require ICF level of care and will be receiving that level in the next planned community placement when the facility closes.
- A statement of the precise requirements of alternative placement beyond the facility, followed by a description of an alternative living program setting that is not currently assigned to any known level of care at all. Specifically, the phraseology selected is "a small community-based facility with capacity to provide treatment programs on-site and in a day program setting that offers special supports and services."

The team then agrees to follow through on this approach in a timely manner, with Amber checking on compliance. She advises Fred only that problems have arisen with her team, as expected, but that a workable solution has been developed that will be implemented within the desig-nated time frame. "So long as it meets the UR team requirements," he responds. Amber assures him that it will.

Fred Cower thus has been sufficiently apprised to keep him from being "blind-sided" in the event that anyone questions the approach being taken by ITT 007; but he is not being confronted in a way that might force him to deal directly with the specifics. Amber assumes that his confidence in the clinical as well as administrative judgment she has demonstrated in the past will preclude any necessity to inform him more specifically.

The course of action agreed to is followed to the letter. The entire ITT 007 team works cooperatively to ensure completion of the newly defined task within the short time frame. The team adopts the attitude that doing so is the best way to protect all interests, especially the clients' interests.

The utilization review group does, indeed, arrive at the anticipated time. After only brief questioning of Amber regarding what level of care is actually being specified (to which she responds "no specific level of care is being specified since we do not know what to label the specific alternative that would best meet our peoples' needs") the UR group determines that ITT 007 has met the criteria. They require only that some level of care other than ICF be projected. All the ITT 007 clients are subsequently certified as meeting UR criteria.

Since no deficiency is identified, no further check is made on the ITT 007 course of action either by Fred Cower or other facility administra-tors. While Fred never specifically says so, he appears pleased with the outcome, as are Amber Good and her team members.

Interestingly, three other ITTs at the facility fail the inspection. Although they had no ethical problem with the directive, they were unable to complete the required documentation within the UR time limit.

Questions for Discussion

1. Did Amber Good behave ethically? Did she treat her boss fairly? Was her approach dishonest? Did she use her moral imagination to uphold the dignity of her patients? Did she unethically manipulate the situation? What, specifically, distinguishes ethical from unethical behavior in cases like this?

2. Distinguish the macroethics issues of the case—those involving HCFA and the facility's top echelon—from the microethics issues that confronted Amber Good.

3. Identify the values that were important in this case. Clarify the power that Amber had for dealing with the situation. Specify

the external and internal controls that were present. Discuss the dynamics that unfolded amidst these realities.

4. Was legitimate organizational authority undermined?
5. When managerial judgment differs, as in this case, from clinical/professional judgment, whose judgment should prevail? Which is the "ethical" judgment?
6. What, if anything, does this case suggest regarding the contention that "good ethics is good business"?

Annotated Bibliography

Donaldson, T., and T. Dunfee. "Toward a Unified Conception of Business Ethics." *Academy of Management Review* 19, no. 2 (April 1994): 252–84. A first-rate analysis of moral risk and limitations of ethical maturity together with presentation of an approach to ethical development.

Frank, R. *Passions Within Reason*. New York: Norton, 1988. A compelling discourse on the link between good ethics and good business.

Glaser, J. *Three Realms of Ethics*. Kansas City, MO: Sheed and Ward, 1994. A splendidly presented perspective on the nature of healthcare ethics and the human limitations endemic.

Gustafson, J. "Moral Discourse About Medicine," *Journal of Medicine and Philosophy* 15, no. 2 (April 1990): 125–42. An enlightening commentary on the boundedness of our healthcare enterprise.

Harrington, S. "What Corporate America Is Teaching About Ethics." *Academy of Management Executive* 5, no. 1 (February 1991): 21–30. A candid and surprising report on the perceived relationship of ethics to good business.

APPENDIX A

American College of Healthcare Executives Code of Ethics[*][1]

Preamble

The purpose of the *Code of Ethics* of the American College of Healthcare Executives is to serve as a guide to conduct for members. It contains standards of ethical behavior for healthcare executives in their professional relationships. These relationships include members of the healthcare executive's organization and other organizations. Also included are patients or others served, colleagues, the community, and society as a whole. The *Code of Ethics* also incorporates standards of ethical behavior governing personal behavior, particularly when that conduct directly relates to the role and identity of the healthcare executive.

The fundamental objectives of the healthcare management profession are to enhance overall quality of life, dignity, and well-being of every individual needing healthcare services; and to create a more equitable, accessible, effective, and efficient healthcare system.

Healthcare executives have an obligation to act in ways that will merit the trust, confidence, and respect of healthcare professionals and the general public. Therefore, healthcare executives should lead lives that embody an exemplary system of values and ethics.

In fulfilling their commitments and obligations to patients or others served, healthcare executives function as moral advocates. Since every management decision affects the health and well-being of both individuals and communities, healthcare executives must carefully evaluate the possible outcomes of their decisions. In organizations that

[*]As amended by the Council of Regents at its annual meeting on August 22, 1995.
[1]Appendices I and II, entitled "American College of Healthcare Executives Grievance Procedure" and "Ethics Committee Action," respectively, are a material part of this *Code of Ethics* and are incorporated herein by reference.

deliver healthcare services, they must work to safeguard and foster the rights, interests, and prerogatives of patients or others served. The role of moral advocate requires that healthcare executives speak out and take actions necessary to promote such rights, interests, and prerogatives if they are threatened.

I. The Healthcare Executive's Responsibilities to the Profession of Healthcare Management

The healthcare executive shall:

A. Uphold the values, ethics and mission of the healthcare management profession;

B. Conduct all personal and professional activities with honesty, integrity, respect, fairness, and good faith in a manner that will reflect well upon the profession;

C. Comply with all laws pertaining to healthcare management in the jurisdictions in which the healthcare executive is located, or conducts professional activities;

D. Maintain competence and proficiency in healthcare management by implementing a personal program of assessment and continuing professional education;

E. Avoid the exploitation of professional relationships for personal gain;

F. Use this *Code* to further the interests of the profession and not for selfish reasons;

G. Respect professional confidences;

H. Enhance the dignity and image of the healthcare management profession through positive public information programs; and

I. Refrain from participating in any activity that demeans the credibility and dignity of the healthcare management profession.

II. The Healthcare Executive's Responsibilities to Patients or Others Served, to the Organization and to Employees

A. RESPONSIBILITIES TO PATIENTS OR OTHERS SERVED
   The healthcare executive shall, within the scope of his or her authority:
   1. Work to ensure the existence of a process to evaluate the quality of care or service rendered;
   2. Avoid practicing or facilitating discrimination and institute safeguards to prevent discriminatory organizational practices;
   3. Work to ensure the existence of a process that will advise patients or others served of the rights, opportunities, responsibilities, and risks regarding available healthcare services;
   4. Work to provide a process that ensures the autonomy and self-determination of patients or others served; and
   5. Work to ensure the existence of procedures that will safeguard the confidentiality and privacy of patients or others served.

B. RESPONSIBILITIES TO THE ORGANIZATION
   The healthcare executive shall, within the scope of his or her authority:

1. Provide healthcare services consistent with available resources and work to ensure the existence of a resource allocation process that considers ethical ramifications;
2. Conduct both competitive and cooperative activities in ways that improve community healthcare services;
3. Lead the organization in the use and improvement of standards of management and sound business practices;
4. Respect the customs and practices of patients or others served, consistent with the organization's philosophy; and
5. Be truthful in all forms of professional and organizational communication, and avoid disseminating information that is false, misleading, or deceptive.

C. RESPONSIBILITIES TO EMPLOYEES

Healthcare executives have an ethical and professional obligation to employees of the organizations they manage that encompass but are not limited to:

1. Working to create a working environment conducive for underscoring employee ethical conduct and behavior;
2. Working to ensure that individuals may freely express ethical concerns and providing mechanisms for discussing and addressing such concerns;
3. Working to ensure a working environment that is free from harassment, sexual and other; coercion of any kind, especially to perform illegal or unethical acts; and discrimination on the basis of race, creed, color, sex, ethnic origin, age or disability;
4. Working to ensure a working environment that is conducive to proper utilization of employees' skills and abilities;
5. Paying particular attention to the employee's work environment and job safety; and
6. Working to establish appropriate grievance and appeals mechanisms.

III. Conflicts of Interest

A conflict of interest may be only a matter of degree, but exists when the healthcare executive:

A. Acts to benefit directly or indirectly by using authority or inside information, or allows a friend, relative, or associate to benefit from such authority or information.
B. Uses authority or information to make a decision to intentionally affect the organization in an adverse manner.

The healthcare executive shall:

A. Conduct all personal and professional relationships in such a way that all those affected are assured that management decisions are made in the best interests of the organization and the individuals served by it;
B. Disclose to the appropriate authority any direct or indirect financial or personal interests that pose potential or actual conflicts of interest;
C. Accept no gifts or benefits offered with the express or implied expectation of influencing a management decision; and
D. Inform the appropriate authority and other involved parties of potential or actual conflicts of interest related to appointments or elections to boards or committees inside or outside the healthcare executive's organization.

IV. The Healthcare Executive's Responsibilities to Community and Society

The healthcare executive shall:

A. Work to identify and meet the healthcare needs of the community;

B. Work to ensure that all people have reasonable access to healthcare services;

C. Participate in public dialogue on healthcare policy issues and advocate solutions that will improve health status and promote quality healthcare;

D. Consider the short-term and long-term impact of management decisions on both the community and on society; and

E. Provide prospective consumers with adequate and accurate information, enabling them to make enlightened judgments and decisions regarding services.

V. The Healthcare Executive's Responsibility to Report Violations of the *Code*

A member of the College who has reasonable grounds to believe that another member has violated this *Code* has a duty to communicate such facts to the Ethics Committee.

Appendix I

American College of Healthcare Executives Grievance Procedure

1. In order to be processed by the College, a complaint must be filed in writing to the Ethics Committee of the College within three years of the date of discovery of the alleged violation, and the Committee has the responsibility to look into incidents brought to its attention regardless of the informality of the information, provided the information can be documented or supported or may be a matter of public record. The three-year period within which a complaint must be filed shall temporarily cease to run during intervals when the accused member is in inactive status, or when the accused member resigns from the College.

2. The Committee chairman initially will determine whether the complaint falls within the purview of the Ethics Committee and whether immediate investigation is necessary. However, all letters of complaint that are filed with the Ethics Committee will appear on the agenda of the next committee meeting. The Ethics Committee shall have the final discretion to determine whether a complaint falls within the purview of the Ethics Committee.

3. If a grievance proceeding is initiated by the Ethics Committee:

   a. Specifics of the complaint will be sent to the respondent by certified mail. In such mailing, committee staff will inform the respondent that the grievance proceeding has been initiated, and that the respondent may respond directly to the Ethics Committee; the respondent also will be asked to cooperate with the Regent investigating the complaint.

   b. The Ethics Committee shall refer the matter to the appropriate Regent who is deemed best able to investigate the alleged infraction. The Regent shall make inquiry into the matter, and in the process the respondent shall be given an opportunity to be heard.

   c. Upon completion of the inquiry, the Regent shall present a complete report and recommended disposition of the matter in writing to the Ethics Committee. Absent unusual circumstances, the Regent is expected to complete his or her report and recommended disposition, and provide them to the Committee, within 60 days.

4. Upon the Committee's receipt of the Regent's report and recommended disposition, the Committee shall review them and make its written recommendation to the Board of Governors as to what action shall be taken and the reason or reasons therefor. A copy of the Committee's recommended decision along with the Regent's report and recommended disposition to the Board will be mailed to the respondent by certified mail. In such mailing, the respondent will be notified that within 30 days after his or her receipt of the Ethics Committee's recommended decision, the respondent may file a written appeal of the recommended decision with the Board of Governors.

5. Any written appeal submitted by the respondent must be received by the Board of Governors within 30 days after the recommended decision of the Ethics Committee is received by the respondent. The Board of Governors shall not take action on the Ethics Committee's recommended decision until the 30-day appeal period has elapsed. If no appeal to the Board of Governors is filed in a timely fashion, the Board shall review the recommended decision and determine action to be taken.

6. If an appeal to the Board of Governors is timely filed, the College Chairman shall appoint an ad hoc committee consisting of three Fellows to hear the matter. At least 30 days' notice of the formation of this committee, and of the hearing date, time and place, with an opportunity for representation, shall be mailed to the respondent. Reasonable requests for postponement shall be given consideration.

7. This ad hoc committee shall give the respondent adequate opportunity to present his or her case at the hearing, including the opportunity to submit a written statement and other documents deemed relevant by the respondent, and to be represented if so desired. Within a reasonable period of time following the hearing, the ad hoc committee shall write a detailed report with recommendations to the Board of Governors.

8. The Board of Governors shall decide what action to take after reviewing the report of the ad hoc committee. The Board shall provide the respondent with a copy of its decision. The decision of the Board of Governors shall be final. The Board of Governors shall have the authority to accept or reject any of the findings or recommended decisions of the Regent, the Ethics Committee, or the ad hoc committee, and to order whatever level of discipline it feels is justified.

9. At each level of the grievance proceeding, the Board of Governors shall have the sole discretion to notify or contact the complainant relating to the grievance proceeding; provided, however, that the complainant shall be notified as to whether the complaint was reviewed by the Ethics Committee and whether the Ethics Committee or the Board of Governors has taken final action with respect to the complaint.

10. No individual shall serve on the ad hoc committee described above, or otherwise participate in these grievance proceedings on behalf of the College, if he or she is in direct economic competition with the respondent or otherwise has a financial conflict of interest in the matter, unless such conflict is disclosed to and waived in writing by the respondent.

11. All information obtained, reviewed, discussed, and otherwise used or developed in a grievance proceeding that is not otherwise publicly known, publicly available, or part of the public domain is considered to be privileged and strictly confidential information of the College, and is not to be disclosed to anyone outside of the grievance proceeding except as determined by the Board of Governors or as required by law; provided, however, that an individual's membership status is not confidential and may be made available to the public upon request.

Appendix II

Ethics Committee Action

Once the grievance proceeding has been initiated, the Ethics Committee may take any of the following actions based upon its findings:

1. Determine the grievance complaint to be invalid.
2. Dismiss the grievance complaint.
3. Recommend censure.
4. Recommend transfer to inactive status for a specified minimum period of time.
5. Recommend expulsion.

APPENDIX B

American Hospital Association
Ethical Conduct for Health Care Institutions

Introduction

Health care institutions, by virtue of their roles as health care providers, employers, and community health resources, have special responsibilities for ethical conduct and practices. Their broad range of patient care, education, public health, social service, and business functions is essential to the health and well-being of their communities. In general, the public expects that they will conduct themselves in an ethical manner that emphasizes a basic community service orientation.

This management advisory is intended to assist members of the American Hospital Association to better define the ethical aspects and implications of institutional policies and practices. It is offered with the understanding that individual decisions seldom reflect an absolute ethical right or wrong, and that each institution's leadership in making policy and decisions must take into account the needs and values of the institution, its medical community, and employees and those of individual patients, their families, and the community as a whole.

The governing board of the institution is responsible for establishing and periodically evaluating the ethical standards that guide institutional practices. The chief executive officer is responsible for assuring that hospital medical staff, employees, and volunteers and auxilians understand and adhere to these standards and for promoting an environment sensitive to differing values and conducive to ethical behavior.

This management advisory examines the hospital's ethical responsibilities to its community and patients as well as those deriving from its organizational roles as employer and a business entity. Although some responsibilities also may be included in legal and accreditation requirements, it should be remembered that legal, accreditation, and ethical obligations often overlap and that ethical obligations often extend beyond legal and accreditation requirements.

Community Role

- Health care institutions should be concerned with the overall health status of their communities while continuing to provide direct patient services. This principle requires them to communicate and work with other health care and social agencies to improve the availability and provision of health promotion and education and services as well as patient care and to take a leadership role in enhancing public health and continuity of care in the community.

- Health care institutions are responsible for fair and effective use of available health care delivery resources to promote access to comprehensive and affordable health care services of high quality. This responsibility extends beyond the resources of the given institution to include efforts to coordinate with other health care providers and to share in community solutions for providing care for the medically indigent and others.

- All health care institutions have community service responsibilities which may include care for the poor and the uninsured, provision of needed services, and education and various programs designed to meet the specific needs of their communities. Not-for-profit institutions, in consideration of their community service origins, Hill-Burton obligations, and tax status, should be particularly sensitive to the importance of providing and designing services for their communities.

- Health care institutions, being dependent upon community confidence and support, are accountable to the public, and therefore their communications and disclosure of information and data related to the institution should be clear, accurate, and sufficiently complete to assure that it is not misleading. Such disclosure should be aimed primarily at better public understanding of health issues, the services available to prevent and treat illness, and patients' rights and responsibilities relating to health care decisions.

- As health care institutions operate in an increasingly competitive environment, they should consider the overall welfare of their communities and their own missions in determining their activities, service mixes, and business ventures and conduct their business activities in an ethical manner.

Patient Care

- Health care institutions are responsible for assuring that the care provided to each patient is appropriate and of the highest quality they are able to provide. Health care institutions should establish and follow procedures to verify the credentials of physicians and other health professionals, assess and improve quality of care, and review appropriateness of utilization.

- Health care institutions should have policies and practices that support the process of informed consent for diagnostic and therapeutic procedures and that respect and promote the patient's responsibility for decision making.

- Health care institutions are responsible for assuring confidentiality of patient-specific information. They are responsible for providing safeguards to prevent unauthorized release of information and establishing procedures for authorizing release of data.

- Health care institutions should assure that the psychological, social, spiritual, and physical needs and cultural beliefs and practices of patients and families are recognized and should promote employee and medical staff sensitivity to the full range of such needs and practices.
- Health care institutions should assure respect for and reasonable accommodation of individual religious and social beliefs and customs of patients whenever possible.
- Health care institutions should have specific mechanisms or procedures to resolve conflicting values and ethical dilemmas among patients, their families, medical staff, employees, the institution, and the community.

Organizational Conduct

- The policies and practices of health care institutions should respect the professional ethical codes and responsibilities of their employees and medical staff members and be sensitive to institutional decisions that employees might interpret as compromising their ability to provide high-quality health care.
- Health care institutions should have policies and practices that provide for equitably administered employee policies and practices.
- To the extent possible and consistent with the ethical commitments of the institution, health care institutions should accommodate the desires of employees and medical staff to embody religious and moral values in their professional activities.
- Health care institutions should have written policies on conflict of interest that apply to officers, governing board members, physicians, and others who make or influence decisions for or on behalf of the institution. These policies should recognize that individuals in decision-making or administrative positions often have duality of interests that may not ordinarily present conflicts. But they should provide mechanisms for identifying and addressing conflicts when they do exist.
- Health care institutions should communicate their mission, values, and priorities to the employees and volunteers, whose patient care and service activities are the most visible embodiment of the institution's ethical commitments and values.

AHA Resources

This management advisory identifies the major areas affecting the ethical conduct of health care institutions. It would be impossible for one advisory document to detail all of the factors and issues relating to each area. Additional information and guidance is available in the following AHA management advisories:

A Patient's Bill of Rights
Advertising
Discharge Planning
Disclosure of Financial and Operating Information
Disclosure of Medical Record Information
Establishment of an Employee Grievance Procedure
Ethics Committees
Imperatives of Hospital Leadership

Quality Management
Resolution of Conflicts of Interest
The Patient's Choice of Treatment Options
Verifying Physician Credentials
Verifying Credentials of Medical Students and Residents

The following AHA publications may also be useful:

Values in Conflict: Resolving Ethical Issues in Hospital Care (AHA #025002)
Effective DNR Policies: Development, Revision, and Implementation (AHA #058750)

INDEX

ABOUT THE AUTHOR

The University Professor of Public Administration at Seton Hall University, John Abbott Worthley is an educator and public service professional with extensive experience in healthcare, higher education, government, and ministry. His career in the academy includes faculty and administrative positions at both public and private universities. He was dean of the Center for Public Affairs at Briarcliff College, and program director at an international research unit of the State University of New York. In 1980 John Worthley went to Seton Hall as director of the graduate public management program, which he led to accreditation and developed into a university center. He became a deputy chancellor and headed task forces that designed new administrative structures.

Author of six books and a host of articles, cases, and essays on various aspects of public service management and policy, Worthley is internationally active in the field of professional ethics. He has served as principal ethics consultant to New York state government, and has lectured on the subject in settings that range from Mother Teresa's headquarters in Calcutta to the United Nations European center in Geneva. Known in healthcare circles as the author of *Managing Computers in Healthcare*, he recently co-developed a special learning series for the American College of Healthcare Executives. His considerable healthcare consulting includes work with hospitals, with state and local government health departments, with hospice and home care agencies, and with health-related corporations.

In addition to higher education and healthcare, Worthley has been engaged in military service, politics, and pastoral work. A naval aviator, he served as commanding officer of a reserve unit and retired with the rank of commander. Twice nominated for the New York state senate, he has held state and local appointive positions. He has been a trustee for several organizations and holds editorial board memberships. Since entering ordained ministry in 1990, he has served at large suburban parishes, at homeless shelters, in hospital chaplaincies, and in overseas missions.

A graduate of the College of the Holy Cross, John Worthley holds Master's degrees in foreign affairs from the University of Virginia and in theology from the Seton Hall Seminary as well as a doctorate from the State University of New York at Albany. At this writing, he is 52 years of age and recently completed his third and last New York City marathon.